The Dutch Response to HIV

Social Aspects of AIDS
Series Editor: Peter Aggleton
(Institute of Education, University of London)

AIDS is not simply a concern for scientists, doctors and medical researchers, it has important social dimensions as well. These include individual, cultural and media responses to the epidemic, stigmatization and discrimination, counselling, care and health promotion. This series of books brings together work from many disciplines including psychology, sociology, cultural and media studies, anthropology, education and history. The titles will be of interest to the general reader, those involved in education and social research, and scientific researchers who want to examine the social aspects of AIDS.

Recent titles include:

Power and Community: Organizational and Cultural Responses to AIDS
Dennis Altman

Moral Threats and Dangerous Desires: AIDS in the News Media
Deborah Lupton

Last Served? Gendering the HIV Pandemic
Cindy Patton

Crossing Borders: Migration, Ethnicity and AIDS
Edited by Mary Haour-Knipe

Bisexualities and AIDS: International Perspectives
Edited by Peter Aggleton

Sexual Interactions and HIV Risk: New Conceptual Perspectives in European Research
Edited by Luc Van Campenhoudt, Mitchell Cohen, Gustavo Guizzardi and Dominique Hausser

AIDS: Activism and Alliances
Edited by Peter Aggleton, Peter Davies and Graham Hart

AIDS as a Gender Issue
Edited by Lorraine Sherr, Catherine Hankins and Lydia Bennett

Drug Injecting and HIV Infection: Global Dimensions and Local Responses
Edited by Gerry Stimson, Don C. Des Jarlais and Andrew Ball

Sexual Behaviour and HIV/AIDS in Europe: Comparisons of National Surveys
Edited by Michel Hubert, Nathalie Bajos and Theo Sandfort

Men Who Sell Sex: International Perspectives on Male Prostitution and AIDS
Edited by Peter Aggleton

The Dutch Response to HIV
Pragmatism and Consensus

Edited by

Theo Sandfort

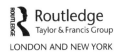

Routledge
Taylor & Francis Group

LONDON AND NEW YORK

First published in 1998 by UCL Press
Reprinted 2003
By Routledge
11 New Fetter Lane, London EC4P 4EE

Transferred to Digital Printing 2003

The name of University College London (UCL) is a registered trade mark
used by UCL Press with the consent of the owner.

British Library Cataloguing-in-Publication Data
A CIP catalogue record for this book is available from the British Library.

Library of Congress Cataloging-in-Publication Data are available

ISBN: 1-85728-816-5 HB
     1-85728-817-3 PB

Typeset by Best-set Typesetter Ltd., Hong Kong

Contents

Contents

Figures

Figures

Tables

Abbreviations

NCAB   Nationale Commissie AIDS Bestrijding (National Committee on AIDS Control)

NcGv   Nationaal Centrum Geestelijke Volksgezondheid (National Institute on Mental Health)

NIAD   Nederlands Instituut voor Alcohol en Drugs (Netherlands Institute on Alcohol and Drugs)

NISSO   Nederlands Instituut voor Sociaal-Seksuologisch Onderzoek (Netherlands Institute of Social Sexological Research)

NIGZ   Nationaal Instituut voor Gezondheidsbevordering en Ziektepreventie (Netherlands Institute for Health Promotion and Disease Prevention)

NVIH COC   Nederlandse Vereniging tot Integratie van Homoseksualiteit COC (Dutch Society for the Integration of Homosexuality COC)

PccAo   Programma en coördinatie commissie AIDS onderzoek (Programme Coordination Committee for AIDS Research)

RIVM   Rijksinstituut voor Volksgezondheid en Milieu (National Institute of Public Health and the Environment)

Series Editor's Preface

It goes without saying that some countries have responded more effectively to HIV and AIDS than others. While many governments procrastinated pretending that AIDS would not become a major public health issue, a few reacted more positively acting quickly to control the epidemic and to provide care and support to people who were directly affected. Without doubt, the Netherlands' response was of the latter kind. In contrast to some other European countries and the United States, little attempt was made to pretend either that AIDS did not exist or that swift action would not be needed to arrest the growth of the epidemic. A combination of factors ensured that this was the case. These included the far sighted actions of courageous individuals, a government willing to heed scientific advice and to provide clear messages about how HIV could be prevented through safer sex and safer drug use, and a sense of pragmatism which ensured that a wide range of measures were rapidly put in place to prevent new infections and to provide care to people living with HIV and AIDS. In many ways the Netherlands' response was exemplary and it is a privilege to publish a book describing the nature of that response, the factors which gave rise to it, and the lessons that can be learned. An enormous range of issues are discussed in the chapters that comprise this volume, the majority published for the first time in English. If others can learn from the experiences described here, our goals will have been more than achieved.

Peter Aggleton

Preface

The most important aims of Dutch HIV/AIDS policy have always been, and continue to be; promoting primary prevention, optimizing the system for care and support for people with HIV/AIDS, and ensuring an equal position for people with HIV/AIDS in society. Although AIDS is increasingly viewed as an 'ordinary' chronic disease, epidemiological, medical-technological and societal developments continue to demand extraordinary vigilance from government, researchers, treating physicians and prevention workers. This is especially true in relation to developments in combination therapies and early treatment, and the (up to now largely unknown) consequences these have for the need for and provision of care.

The major achievement in the fight against AIDS, which in the Netherlands has been quite successful, lie in prevention. The most important challenge is to establish lasting behaviour change to prevent new infections. The goal is, naturally, to encourage as many people as possible to practise safe sex. This endeavour is particularly difficult since our behaviours are determined by habits, traditions and emotions. Important questions relating to this are:

- Are there limits to the impact of education and how can education be carried out most effectively for the various target groups?
- Might contact tracing contribute to the prevention of HIV transmission?
- Should people be encouraged to get tested?
- Who, in fact, is supposed to take responsibility for what?

In answering these questions, we may have to differentiate between people with HIV and people who are not infected; and between people with symptoms and those without. We should at all times, however, guard against social exclusion and stigmatization.

However difficult it may be to answer the above questions, I am strongly convinced that by mobilizing the knowledge and experience which has been acquired, we will make major progress in the Netherlands, as well as in other parts of the world.

Preface

It is with great pleasure that I recommend to you this book about Dutch AIDS policy and prevention.

E. Borst-Eilers, MD, PhD
Minister of Health, Welfare and Sports

Introduction

Chapter 1

Pragmatism and Consensus:
The Dutch Response to HIV

Theo Sandfort

The way in which the Netherlands has responded to AIDS is widely regarded as well organized and effective. To a certain extent this response was possible because of some unique features of the Netherlands. At the time AIDS was first detected, a number of organizations already existed with sufficient knowledge and experience to meet the needs of groups most at risk for HIV infection. Before AIDS, there had already been several campaigns to promote health behaviour within the general population and even one on the secondary prevention of STDs. Furthermore, although the epidemic had a major impact on the lives of many people, AIDS did not develop into a major societal disaster and, relative to the small size of the epidemic, the resources available for a response were extensive. Virtually the entire Dutch population is insured for the cost of medical care. Finally, Dutch society is characterized by a liberal climate with a long tradition of tolerance and acceptance of different religious, ideological and political positions. Although the Dutch response to AIDS might to some extent be a consequence of this unique situation, the Netherlands also provides an instructive example for other countries. This book describes various aspects of the Dutch response to AIDS.[1] This introductory chapter presents a general overview of the major principles underpinning the Dutch policy response, epidemiology, the organizations involved in AIDS prevention and societal responses to AIDS.[2]

Pragmatism and Consensus

Pragmatism and consensus are the keys to understanding the way in which public problems are dealt with in the Netherlands. An awareness that decisions made by only a few are likely to be ineffective was an important guiding principle in public decision making back in the seventeenth century (Van der Horst, 1996). The regents at the time knew that as many parties as possible had to be involved in decision making if decisions were to be endorsed by the majority, and therefore likely to solve a problem.

Closely related to consensus is pragmatism. Except for values such as individual rights and tolerance, public decisions are not primarily directed by moral considerations. Policy solutions to public problems are primarily arrived at on the basis of whether they are likely to be effective. A cornerstone of this pragmatism is the awareness that social ills are not always completely controllable and the best one can sometimes do is to try to contain them and to prevent them from getting worse. This principle of pragmatism is clearly present in Dutch policy responses to drug use. Although drug use – injecting as well as other forms – is illegal in the Netherlands, extensive needle exchange programmes had been developed before the onset of AIDS to prevent transmission of other infectious diseases. Furthermore, the use of hard drugs is combatted by accepting the use of so-called soft drugs like marijuana and hashish, and by targeting major dealers instead of the individual user.

Consensus and pragmatism also characterize the way in which the problem of AIDS has been understood in the Netherlands and the way in which it has been responded to (Van Wijngaarden, 1992). Ever since the first cases of AIDS were diagnosed, there has been a general awareness that AIDS is not just a biomedical problem, but also has major social and political dimensions, more so than other diseases. AIDS is not just a serious medical condition; it carries the potential for stigmatization and discrimination and it predominantly affects groups of people who already have a marginal position in society. The major aims of Dutch prevention policy were not simply the prevention of further infections and the development of adequate care, but included the prevention and counteracting of potential negative societal consequences of HIV/AIDS. In order for a policy to be effective, a multidisciplinary approach was required, involving the various groups affected by HIV/AIDS.

Neither the government nor the medical authorities dictated how transmission of HIV was to be prevented (Moerkerk, 1990). Instead, AIDS policy in the Netherlands resulted from private initiative in which various interested parties of different backgrounds and sometimes conflicting interests collaborated (Schnabel, 1989). This consensus approach was possible since, with the exception of the 'general population', all the groups involved were well-organized: the gay movement (which was fairly influential in Dutch society), the society for people with haemophilia, and even injecting drug users (through the National Federation of Junkie Unions). AIDS, in turn, resulted in the formation of new groups and societies such as the Dutch HIV Society.

In preventing HIV infection, the starting principle was that people are responsible for both their own and other people's health and that moralizing doesn't help: the government should refrain from interfering in people's private lives. People's basic human rights also had to be protected. Characteristic of the pragmatic approach was the rejection of legal regulations to control AIDS. Although the Netherlands has a Communicable Diseases Act dating from 1928, which makes the compulsory notification of certain diseases possible as well as the temporary quarantine of persons infected, this law was not applied to HIV. Measures based on freedom of choice were expected to be more effective than regulatory ones. Compulsory notification was thought likely to result in stigmatization and discrimination, and might possibly have counterproductive effects. It could discourage members of high risk groups from seeking medical advice or treatment, or voluntarily choosing to have a test. The few legislative measures introduced as a consequence of AIDS were not of a restrictive nature, but of a promotional, supportive character, such as directives for planning of health care facilities and for subsidizing the provision of drugs (Roscam Abbing, 1988).

Pragmatism also underpinned the decision not to close the saunas and other public places where gay men meet and have sex. Although it was occasionally suggested that such venues should be closed, it was never clear to what extent sexual activities in these public places contributed to HIV transmission. Data suggest that most unprotected anal sex with casual partners occurred in private homes (De Wit *et al.*, 1997). A further compelling reason not to close these venues was that closing them would result in the same amount of sexual activity in places where gay men would not be accessible for prevention efforts. Additionally, it was suggested that closing saunas might break the relationship of trust between gay men and the health care system, with potential detrimental consequences for public health.

One of the consequences of the consensus approach was that general population prevention campaigns came to focus not so much on condom use as on safer sex in general. Simply promoting condom use might have antagonized some groups in society, so safer sex included postponing sexual intercourse, restricting sexual contact to a mutually monogamous relationship, and practising other forms than penetrative sex. Although the promotion of safer sex is still the common denominator of most campaigns, over the years safer sex has become more closely associated with condom use, a phenomenon reflected in public perceptions of safer sex (De Vroome *et al.*, 1994).

The promotion of condoms to the general public was initially also objected to by gay groups. It was suggested that such an approach might be confusing to gay men who were strongly advised to abstain from penetrative sex all together. For pragmatic reasons, gay men were included in general population campaigns at a later stage, by featuring gay couples in posters displayed in public places. The assumption was that this was the only way to reach gay men who could not be reached by more targeted kinds of prevention. In addition, the inclusion of images of homosexuality in general campaigns was felt likely to contribute to the reduction of stigmatization and discrimination.

Human Rights and HIV-Testing

Although legal regulations have not been a part of prevention policy, some idiosyncrasies in Dutch AIDS policy can only be understood by taking into account questions of human rights and the fundamental freedoms embedded in the Dutch Constitution. Central to the Dutch Constitution are principles of non-discrimination, the right to bodily integrity, and the right to privacy. In the context of health care, these rights translate into the principle of informed consent prior to any medical action, the right to confidentiality in the doctor–patient relationship, and the protection of professional confidentiality.

Infringements to these human rights are only possible under specific circumstances. Measures which might place restrictions on individual freedom can only be imposed after the social benefits of these measures have been demonstrated. Subsequently, the least restrictive alternative that could achieve the desired social benefit has to be given priority. Furthermore, restrictions have to be based on the law and should be exceptional (Roscam Abbing, 1988). The importance of the human rights perspective is reflected in the fact that of the three sections in the (former) National Committee on AIDS Control (NCAB), one was entirely devoted to ethical and legal issues (the other two were prevention and public education, and care and treatment).

The importance of the human rights perspective in relation to HIV/AIDS can best be illustrated in relation to HIV testing in the Netherlands. Following from the right to bodily integrity and the right to privacy, the basic principle is that serological testing can only be conducted on a voluntary basis and is subject to strict requirements of confidentiality. Informed consent is necessary before testing occurs, in whatever setting. These rights imply the right 'not to know' or not be informed involuntarily about one's HIV status. Disclosing someone's HIV status to third parties against the person's will is only allowed if imminent and grave harm to others can be prevented by doing so.

This perspective on testing implied that testing without informing the people is not considered ethical and legal since blood samples can only be used for the reasons for which they were originally intended and for which donors have given their consent. This also applied to specific risk groups, such as sex workers, prison inmates and injecting drug users. Scientific research using bodily materials such as blood, which were gathered for other purposes, is allowed only if the people, from whom these materials came, do not object to this use.

This perspective has had important consequences for large-scale anonymous seroprevalence studies, preoperative testing, testing as part of assessment procedures in job applications, and testing for health care workers. When epidemiologists stressed the importance of reliable data on HIV prevalence, the official response was that since there was no evidence that a substantial spread of HIV was likely, such surveillance was not warranted. Some concluded that in this case the right to privacy had triumphed over the need for appropiate epidemiological data. Others questioned the relevance of these studies for health promotion. In consequence, epidemiological studies have only been carried out on a small scale and in selected groups, and subjects involved had to give their informed consent.

When in the late 1980s some surgeons demanded routine HIV tests prior to operations, the official response was that if the right precautions were taken, routine testing was unnecessary, given the small risks involved. HIV testing was not considered to be an adequate means of reducing the risk of infection through needle stick accidents. Testing here was allowed only if the patient had given his consent.

Testing is not allowed as part of assessment procedures by job applications, since being HIV infected does not imply an inability to work and since transmission of HIV does not usually occur at the work place. The government has also rejected the testing of health care workers for HIV. Introducing HIV testing into the health care sector might lead to a false sense of security when the outcome of a test is negative, and possible over-reaction after a positive test result. Special measures for HIV infected health careworkers, such as not allowing them to continue to work, have been officially rejected as well. It was reasoned that the risk of patients being infected with HIV through invasive procedures carried out by infected health care workers was negligible compared with other risks involved in such procedures. The potential effect of these measures would not justify transgressing the rights of an individual health care worker.

Central to the Dutch perspective on testing are the potentially negative consequences of finding out that one is HIV positive. When in 1985 preparations were made to initiate screening in blood banks, a campaign was in fact undertaken to urge gay men to think twice before undergoing testing. Implementing HIV testing on a large scale as a means in HIV prevention was, and still is, rejected for various reasons (Reinking, 1993). First of all, there is no cure for people who turn out to be HIV positive and an HIV test only reflects the situation at a given moment. A negative test result, moreover, might induce a false sense of security. Furthermore, since HIV cannot be transmitted in ordinary interactions in society, large-scale testing could result in unwarranted social unrest and divert people's attention from education and prevention. In relation to prevention, one's serostatus is assumed to be irrelevant: everybody has to practise safe sex. Avoiding infection is not only the responsibility of the person infected, but both people involved in a sexual interaction.

The advent of early medical intervention has only mildly affected general attitudes towards testing. Whereas before, testing was initially discouraged, there is a more neutral attitude now, in which balancing the various costs and benefits of knowing one's HIV serostatus is recommended.

Epidemiological Situation

The first official cases of AIDS in the Netherlands were diagnosed in 1982 in gay men and in people who had received contaminated blood products. It is likely, however, that there were earlier unreported deaths caused by HIV (Goudsmit, 1997). As of January 1997, there were 4350 cumulative reported cases of people with AIDS. About 10 per cent of these cases consisted of women. Since the reporting of AIDS cases is voluntary, the actual number of people who have died should be assumed to be somewhat higher. Geographically, most Dutch cases of AIDS have been reported in the western, urbanized part of the Netherlands.

From a European perspective, the Netherlands, together with Austria, Belgium and the United Kingdom, are not as strongly affected by AIDS as France, Italy, Spain and Switzerland. However, the cumulative number of AIDS cases per million inhabitants in the Netherlands is substantially higher than in Germany, Greece, Ireland and Sweden. It should be realized, however, that comparing relative prevalences has its limitations since countries differ regarding the stage of the epidemic they have reached.

When the total number of new cases of AIDS per million people total population in 1996 is computed for all European countries, the Netherlands, with an incidence of 25 cases, is in the middle range of countries. The rate is clearly higher than in countries such as Finland, Austria, and Germany (with an incidence of 4, 16 and 18 per million people respectively), but lower than in countries such as France, Portugal and Spain, with an incidence of 72, 81 and 162 per million people respectively (European Centre for the Epidemiological Monitoring of AIDS, 1996).

In 1992, the highest number of new cases of AIDS in one year, 509, was recorded. In 1996, when 342 new cases were reported, a significant decline was observed for the first time. This decrease in annual AIDS incidence, which is partly a consequence of the increasing use of new anti-retroviral therapies, has been observed in most European countries. In some countries such as Portugal and Spain, with a different epidemiological pattern, and in Poland and Romania, where the spread of HIV started later, the incidence is still increasing (Coates *et al.*, 1996; European Centre for the Epidemiological Monitoring of AIDS, 1996).

In the Netherlands, as in some other countries, the relative contribution of the various transmission routes is changing (Houweling *et al.*, 1994). At the start of the epidemic, 89 per cent of all new cases per year came in the category men who have sex with men. By 1996, this percentage had decreased to 64 per cent. This decrease masks the fact, however, that in younger cohorts of gay men the incidence of AIDS is increasing. Injecting drug users used to be the second most vulnerable group in the Netherlands, and 11 per cent of all AIDS cases belong to this category. Now, however, the cumulative number of reported cases of AIDS among heterosexual people is higher than among injecting drug users. The proportion of people who acquired AIDS through heterosexual transmission of HIV is slowly increasing, from 3 per cent of new cases in 1986 to 23 per cent in 1996. Of all people who acquired AIDS through heterosexual means, 337 were men and 225 were women. In about two-thirds of these cases, the person had a HIV-infected partner who belonged to an-other risk group, or came from a country where AIDS is more prevalent among heterosexual people. In about one-third of the cases, no clear transmission route, other than having had multiple sex partners, could be identified. Among people with haemophilia and people who have received blood products, the incidence of AIDS has become very small; cumulatively they constitute 3 per cent of all cases. Cases of AIDS as a consequence of mother–child transmission constitute less than 1 per cent of the total number of cases. In an absolute, as well as a relative sense, gay men are still the most affected group in the Netherlands. This is the same in the United Kingdom where 59 per cent of all AIDS cases have been diagnosed among gay men (compared to 64 per cent in the Netherlands). In other countries, the cumulative proportion of AIDS cases among gay men is smaller. In France, gay men constitute 38 per cent of all AIDS cases, and in Spain this is 11 per cent.

The number of people with HIV infection in the Netherlands is estimated to be between 8000 and 12000 (525 to 790 per million people). Actual figures are not known since seroprevalence studies have not been carried out in the Netherlands. Initially, when it was unclear on what scale HIV might spread, much higher numbers were predicted. Around 1987, it was generally expected that HIV might not be contained to the so-called risk groups but would slowly permeate into the population more generally. At that time it was expected that up to 2000 new cases of AIDS might be expected every year in the late 1990s. As more information became available these predictions were adjusted.

Participating Institutions and Organizational Structure

Chronologically, the first activities in the field of AIDS prevention, safeguarding the blood supply and informing gay men, resulted from the initiative of a small group of gay men, people with haemophilia and medical doctors working under the auspices of the Amsterdam Municipal Health Service (Van Wijngaarden, 1992). It was largely a private initiative, not one instigated by the government. Out of this group an informal National AIDS Policy Coordination Team developed, which was empowered and funded by the Ministry of Health; the Ministry did not actively participate in this committee, but had an observer on it. While this coordinating team focused on practical matters, such as distributing information and providing psychosocial care, there was also a Standing Committee on AIDS, established by the National Health Council, whose task it was to provide scientific advice on medical matters to the government.

Initially, the Ministry of Health, which is ultimately responsible for the AIDS policy in the Netherlands, kept at a distance. This is a typical government response when several social partners are seen to be working together effectively. This changed, however, when the devastating effect of AIDS in other parts of the world, especially in sub-Saharan Africa and in the Carribean, became clear. It henceforth seemed unlikely that AIDS would be confined to gay men and injecting drug users, and it was anticipated that AIDS would spread among the population more generally as well.

This new situation required a national response and a new structure for formal decision making. This structure became the NCAB, a temporary committee created by the government, which existed between 1987 and 1995. The task of the NCAB was to provide advice, both solicited and unsolicited, to the government on policy measures regarding AIDS and to monitor the implementation of policy decisions. The NCAB coordinated the work of various NGOs involved, taking advantage of the knowledge and skills already available in these organizations, and coordinating their activities with one another. The major parties involved in AIDS care and prevention, as well as affected groups, were represented on the committee. In 1992, experts on women's health care and health care for ethnic minorities were included as well. The creation of the NCAB did not imply a disruption to the policy developed by the former Coordinating Team. In fact, the NCAB continued to work with many of the same principles developed by this team and also pursued a policy of consensus. It facilitated consistency among AIDS messages and the pursuit of a coherent set of public policy goals.

By creating a national committee, the government remained at a distance; its involvement consisted primarily of establishing major directions, approving the policy developed by the NCAB, creating the conditions for policy implementation and providing the necessary resources. The advantage of this position was that AIDS remained largely unpoliticized. This does not, however, imply that the role of politics can be completely disregarded.

Several national NGOs were involved in AIDS work. The most important were the Dutch Foundation for STD Control; gay organizations involved in prevention and counselling: the Schorerstichting and the SAD (Ancillary Services Department), which merged into one organization; the Rutgers Stichting predominantly involved in sex education and contraception; the Netherlands Institute for Alcohol and Drugs; and the National Centre for Health Education.

Parallel to the National Committee, local AIDS Platforms were established to provide an infrastructure for implementing national policy. In these local platforms, people from the Municipal Health Services and members of specific interest groups (like the gay movement) collaborated. In 1990, there were about 40 of these platforms throughout the Netherlands. Their role became more crucial in the early 1990s when the Law on Collective Prevention in Public Health came into effect. This law was part of a decentralization policy by national government and implied that responsibility for funding health promotion and disease prevention should be transferred from the central government to local governments. Henceforth, it was up to local government to decide what they wanted to spend their money on.

In the following years, the AIDS policy structure further evolved. The intention of the Ministry was that the tasks which were carried out by the NCAB would gradually be transferred to social and health care organizations involved with AIDS. At the time of writing, the major coordinating tasks are undertaken by the AIDS Fund, initially an institution which raised private funds to support research and to provide affected individuals with financial support. The AIDS Fund, a private institution, is now responsible for advising the government on AIDS policy and distributing government funds to other NGOs.

Soon, the AIDS Fund will also have a responsibility for programming and coordinating research on AIDS. Earlier, from 1988 until 1997, this task was carried out by the Programme Coordination Committee on AIDS Research. Research is considered to be one of the key elements in Dutch policy against AIDS. One of the criteria by which social science research proposals have been judged has been their potential to contribute to the control of AIDS-related problems.

Societal Response

Unlike in other countries, AIDS did not create high levels of anxiety among the Dutch population. Moral panic and outrage did not occur. The way people feel about AIDS in relation to other social issues has been regularly monitored since 1986 (NSS Research & Consultancy, 1997). Several dimensions are evaluated including level of interest, perceived importance of the issue to other people, level of emotional involvement, willingness to do something about the issue, and a general index of involvement.

Given the relatively small size of the problem, AIDS is not an issue most people in the Netherlands are overly concerned about. More important issues include health care, criminal behaviour, and the environment. On the other hand, people are more concerned about AIDS than issues such as emancipation, development aid, the European Union, and inflation. Men and women do not differ concerning their involvement in AIDS. Younger people, people living in the three major urbanized areas in the Netherlands, and people with higher levels of education are, however, relatively more concerned about AIDS.

Over time, a rapid rise in concern about AIDS can be traced to the moment when the first campaign aimed at the general population was launched. Levels of involvement have remained relatively stable over time, although they have slowly decreased in the last few years. The number of people who assume that others think that AIDS is not an important issue has, in particular, increased.

The calm response of the Dutch to AIDS is partly due to the way in which the media has portrayed AIDS. In the beginning some inaccuracies were difficult to avoid since early news came from far away, was hard to check, and little was actually known. Most media, however, reported on AIDS in a matter of fact style. As Wellings and Field (1996) observed, the supportive approach of the media made it possible for AIDS educators to make good use of it. As a consequence, accurate knowledge about HIV/AIDS in the general population was already relatively high before the Netherlands had a general population information campaign. This situation is in contrast with, for example, the United Kingdom where, according to Wellings and Field, the tone of media reporting was initially highly retributive, suggesting that AIDS was a disease which was visited upon deserving minorities.

While the threat of STDs has in earlier times been used to combat sex work and promiscuity, and to promote sexual abstinence in defence of traditional marriage, AIDS was not used to moralize about sexuality. Although some gay activists feared that AIDS might negatively affect the position of homosexuality in society, undoing the major successes which the gay and lesbian movement had accomplished, this clearly did not happen. Opinion polls have not shown any decline in the societal acceptance of homosexuality. Since AIDS was not used to threaten sex work, drug use or homosexuality, it may even have contributed to the acceptance or even legitimacy of these lifestyles. Regarding attitudes towards sexuality and sexual behaviour in general, AIDS and HIV/AIDS prevention have, if anything, led to greater openness rather than repression (STG, 1992).

The few attempts of small right-wing groups and Christian fundamentalists to present AIDS as a punishment of God never gained much ground in the Netherlands. On a small scale, incidents of discrimination against people with HIV/AIDS have been reported; these cases, however, have been relatively less severe than those which have happened in other countries.

The absence of a strong moralizing response can be understood as a consequence of the Dutch AIDS policy as well as other factors. Mooij (1993) has suggested that various factors played a role, each one reinforcing the other. Unlike in earlier societal debates about STDs, AIDS rapidly became seen as a medical not a moral problem. Whether people got infected was therefore less a consequence of the social category to which they belonged, as a consequence of what they did sexually and their place in a network of relationships. The dominance of the medical perspective also implied that, in contrast to earlier debates about sexually transmitted diseases, affected people were no longer guilty of their condition. If there was anybody or anything to blame, it was the virus.

Mooij furthermore showed that the distance between the people who controlled debates about STDs (the narrators) and affected people has become smaller. Affected people have organized themselves and, in so doing, have become some of the narrators in the debate. The diminishing power difference between the positions made it more difficult to be judgemental about specific behaviours, other than those which affect people's health status, since the debate is now being led by all the parties involved.

It is unclear what would have happened if the AIDS epidemic had followed a different course in the Netherlands, affecting heterosexual society more than it did. For most people, AIDS remains a rather distant disease. It is quite likely that a more severe epidemic might have induced higher levels of anxiety and that the need for scapegoats would have been stronger. Furthermore, the absence of a moralizing approach does not imply that AIDS did not have consequences for the societal regulation of sexuality. Much more than ever before there is a strong appeal to people to take responsibility for living a healthy sexual life.

This Book

The contributions in this book about the Dutch response to AIDS explore a variety of issues. The first section covers prevention as it has been focused so as to meet the needs of various groups. General population campaigns and the reasoning behind the approaches taken, are discussed by Kok *et al.* Hospers and Blom present an overview of prevention activities developed at a national level and directed at gay men. Van Ameijden and Van den Hoek demonstrate how various preventive measures have effectively slowed down the development of the HIV epidemic among injecting drug users. Vanwesenbeeck and De Graaf describe prevention aimed at sex workers and their clients, including findings from their own studies; while Singels discusses the organization of prevention aimed at migrants and ethnic minorities in the Netherlands.

The second section deals with broader policy issues. First, Veenker demonstrates that although the issue of AIDS was never politicized, formal politics played a major role in bringing about an adequate response to AIDS. In the subsequent chapter, one of the few major controversies in Dutch AIDS prevention is analyzed. During the first decade of AIDS, gay men in the Netherlands, unlike gay men in other Westernized countries, were instructed to abstain from anal sex. De Zwart *et al.* explore the origins of this message and how it finally changed. Van den Boom and Schnabel then describe the rationale behind dominant patterns of health care response, as well as the way in which AIDS has affected the health care system. Acknowledging the emergency of the problem of AIDS in developing countries, the Dutch government has attributed much importance to prevention activities abroad. The Dutch international response is described in detail by Moerkerk.

In the final section, findings from a number of major Dutch research studies are presented. Special attention is given to those studies which, due to the language barrier and despite their relevance, have minimally found their way abroad. Van Zessen and Sandfort report on the Dutch general population survey on sexuality and AIDS, which was one of the first of its kind to be carried out in Western Europe. Bakker *et al.* present an in-depth overview of Dutch research examining the social psychological determinants of safe sex among adult heterosexuals. Vogels *et al.* present data from a large national sex survey among young people. Since data was collected in both 1990 and 1995, it was possible to examine changes in sexual behaviour among young people over this time. Based on a longitudinal, national study, De Vroome *et al.* finally describe the diffusion of safer sex in the gay population.

Future Developments

Over its 15 years' existence, the AIDS epidemic has changed significantly. The progress made regarding the medical treatment of HIV has considerably altered the face of the disease, but it also presents us with various new challenges. One of them is transmission of new drug-resistant strains of HIV. Experiences with other STDs have taught us that even when effective treatment and vaccines are available, the fight against a disease such as AIDS will not be over (Brandt, 1987). As Coates *et al.* (1996, p. 1143) put it: 'HIV disease is here to stay. Even if HIV preventive vaccines pass the rigours of clinical trials and become available for general use, they are unlikely to be effective, to provide sterilising immunity, or to reach critical proportions of the population, especially in the parts of the world that need them most.' Furthermore, it is still unclear what the consequences of medical accomplishments will be for people's preventive behaviours.

From a political perspective the challenge will be one of maintaining sufficient support for the necessary prevention, care and research. In the Netherlands there are clear signs that political commitment is weakening. This is partly a result of the fact that AIDS is now seen as less serious than when it first appeared. Among the general population, AIDS seems to be losing some of its importance. The continuing need for prevention aimed at the general population is openly called into question by the media. Major cuts in the budget for biomedical and social science research have been announced.

If support for a comprehensive AIDS policy disappears, we run the risk of losing what has been accomplished. More attention may need to be given to the serious impact of AIDS in other parts of the world. At the same time, there is a continued need in the Netherlands to understand how AIDS affects people and their behaviours; to help people maintain acquired preventive behaviours; and to reach young people before they become sexually active.

Notes

1 I would like to thank everyone who assisted in putting this book together, especially Maarten van Doorninck, Jan Visser, Jan van Wijngaarden and Jeffrey Weiss, and most particularly Peter Aggleton, Editor of the Social Aspects of AIDS Series, for his critical support and enduring patience.
2 For a more detailed description of the first ten years of Dutch AIDS policy see Van Wijngaarden (1992).

References

BRANDT, A.M. (1987) *No Magic Bullet. A Social History of Venereal Disease in the United States since 1880*, New York: Oxford University Press.

COATES, T.J., AGGLETON, P., GUTZWILLER, F., DES JARLAIS, D., KIHARA, M., KIPPAX, S., SCHECHTER, M. and VAN DEN HOEK, J.A.R. (1996) 'HIV prevention in developed countries', *Lancet*, **348**, pp. 1143–8.

EUROPEAN CENTRE FOR THE EPIDEMIOLOGICAL MONITORING OF AIDS (1996) 'AIDS cases reported by 31 December 1996', *HIV/AIDS Surveillance in Europe, Fourth Quarterly Report no. 52.*

GOUDSMIT, J. (1997) *Viral Sex. The Nature of AIDS*, New York: Oxford University Press.

VAN DER HORST, H. (1996) *The Low Sky. Understanding the Dutch*, Schiedam: Scriptum.

HOUWELING, H., HEISTERKAMP, S.H., VAN WIJNGAARDEN, J.K., WIESSING, L.G., COUTINHO, R.A. and JAGER, J.C. (1994) 'Analyse van de AIDS-epidemie in Nederland, 1982–1993', *Nederlands Tijdschrift voor Geneeskunde*, **138**, 1954–9.

MOERKERK, H. (1990) 'AIDS prevention strategies in European countries', in M.E.M. PAALMAN (Ed.) *Promoting Safer Sex. Proceedings of an International Workshop, May 1989, the Netherlands*, Amsterdam: Swets & Zeitlinger.

MOOIJ, A. (1993) *Geslachtsziekten en Besmettingsangst. Een Historisch-sociologische Studie 1850–1990*, Amsterdam: Boom.

NSS RESEARCH & CONSULTANCY (1997) *Multi dimensionele Indicatoren voor Betrokkenheid bij Maatschappelijke Problemen*, Den Haag.

REINKING, D. (1993) *Aids-beleid in Nederland*, Utrecht: NcGv.

ROSCAM ABBING, H.D.C. (1988) 'AIDS, human rights and legislation in the Netherlands', in M. BREUM and A. HENDRIKS (Eds) *AIDS and Human Rights. An International Perspective*, Copenhangen: Akademisk Forlag.

SCHNABEL, P. (1989) 'De diepten van een epidemie; over de maatschappelijke gevolgen van AIDS', in A. NOORDHOF-DE VRIES (Ed.) *AIDS; een Nieuwe Verantwoordelijkheid voor Gezondheidszorg en Onderwijs*, Amsterdam: Swets & Zeitlinger.

STG; STEERING COMMITTEE ON FUTURE HEALTH SCENARIOS (1992) *AIDS up to the Year 2000; Epidemiological, Sociocultural and Economic Scenario Analysis for the Netherlands*, Dordrecht: Kluwer Academic Publishers.

DE VROOME, E.M.M., PAALMAN, M.E.M., DINGELSTAD, A.A.M., KOLKER, L. and SANDFORT, TH.G.M. (1994) 'Increase in safe sex among the young and nonmonogamous: knowledge, attitudes and behavior regarding safe sex and condom use in the Netherlands from 1987 to 1993', *Patient Education and Counselling*, **24**, pp. 279–88.

WELLINGS, K. and FIELD, B. (1996) *Stopping AIDS. AIDS/HIV Public Education and the Mass Media in Europe*, London: Longman.

VAN WIJNGAARDEN, J.K. (1992) 'The Netherlands: AIDS in a consensual society', in D.L. KIRP and R. BAYER (Eds) *AIDS in the Industrialized Democracies. Passions, Politics, and Policies*, New Brunswick, NJ:

Rutgers University Press.

DE WIT, J.B.F., DE VROOME, E.M.M., SANDFORT, TH.G.M., VAN GRIENSVEN, G.J.P. (1997) 'Homosexual encounters in different venues', *International Journal of STD & AIDS*, **8**, pp. 130–4.

Part 1

HIV Prevention Strategies and Outcomes

Chapter 2

'Safe Sex' and 'Compassion': Public Campaigns on AIDS in the Netherlands

*Gerjo Kok, Lilian Kolker, Ernest de Vroome
and Anton Dijker*

In two separate series of public information campaigns, people in the Netherlands are being encouraged to have safe sex in order to prevent STDs/AIDS and to react with compassion towards HIV-infected people and people with AIDS. These public information campaigns are part of a broader AIDS education programme, including specific preventive activities developed for risk groups. We will describe the theoretical and empirical background of the two public information campaigns, the difficulties in evaluating their effects, the development and implementation of both campaigns, and the available process and effect evaluations. In reality however, the campaigns did not explicitly follow theory and research in the way it is presented here, as research results often become available only after they are desperately needed and theoretical principles are often difficult to apply in practice.

Planned AIDS Education

AIDS prevention through public information campaigns is a form of health education. Health education is a planned activity stimulating learning through communication to promote healthy behaviour (Green and Kreuter, 1991). The concept of health education needs to be distinguished from the concept of health promotion. Health promotion refers to 'any planned combination of educational, political, regulatory, and organizational supports for actions and conditions of living conducive to the health of individuals, groups, or communities' (Green and Kreuter, 1991, p. 432). The goals of health promotion include three types of prevention: 1) primary prevention; 2) early detection and treatment (which used to be questionable for AIDS); and 3) patient care and support. Health education on the other hand refers to 'any planned combination of learning experiences designed to predispose, enable, and reinforce voluntary behaviour conducive to health in individuals, groups, or communities' (Green and Kreuter, 1991, p. 432). As such, health education is one means of achieving the goals of health promotion. Other health promotion means are resource provision (for AIDS prevention for instance: availability of testing facilities), pricing (cheap or free condoms) and regulation (mandatory AIDS education in schools). Whereas health education relies on voluntary behaviour change to bring about its effects, regulation is based on forced compliance. This implies that regulation may only be effective in combination with control and sanctions. Health promotion is the combination of the above mentioned goals and means. Generally, health promotion programmes using various means will be most effective (De Leeuw, 1989; Milio, 1988; Simons-Morton *et al.*, 1988). In this chapter we will focus on health education for primary prevention of AIDS.

Health education should be a planned activity. One of the best known and most frequently used planning models in health education and health promotion is Green's PRECEDE/PROCEED model (Green and Kreuter, 1991). This model states that health promotion should start with a *social diagnosis*, also called social needs assessment or social reconnaissance. Social diagnosis is defined as the process of determining people's perceptions of their own needs or quality of life, and their aspirations for the common good (Green and Kreuter, 1991, p. 45). The second phase in the model is the *epidemiological diagnosis* which is conducted to determine two things: 1) which health problems are important 'objectively' and 2) which behavioural and environmental factors contribute to the occurrence of those health problems (Green and Kreuter, 1991, p. 90). The third phase of the model, the *behavioural and environmental diagnosis*, includes the systematic analysis of the behavioural, social and environmental factors that are linked to the goals or problems that were identified in the epidemiological or social diagnosis. In this phase the determinants of health are analyzed in terms of behaviour, lifestyle, and environment. The fourth phase, the *educational and organizational diagnosis*, examines the determinants of the behavioural and environmental conditions that are linked to health status or quality-of-life concerns. It also identifies the factors that must be changed to initiate and sustain the process of behavioural and environmental change. Three categories of factors can be distinguished: 1) predisposing factors, referring to behavioural antecedents that provide a rationale or motivation for behaviour; 2) enabling factors, referring to behavioural antecedents that enable the realization of a motivation; and 3) reinforcing factors, referring to factors subsequent to a behaviour that enhance its persistence or repetition. The model's fifth phase, the *administrative and policy diagnosis*, addresses the analysis of the possible usefulness of health education and other potential interventions (resources, regulations). This phase also refers to the political, regulatory, and organizational factors that may facilitate or hinder the development and widespread implementation of a health promotion programme. Subsequent phases of the model refer to the actual implementation of the intervention, and the evaluation of the process, impact, and outcome of the intervention, resulting in feedback and improvement of the programmes.

The development of public information campaigns on AIDS in the Netherlands did not follow this planning model exactly. An epidemiological analysis and a behavioural analysis had been executed, but the educational analysis on determinants of behaviour only became available during the course of the campaigns. Nevertheless, the campaign developers tried to follow the planning model as well as possible.

Planned AIDS Education Campaigns

Epidemiological Analysis of the Problem

The best indicator of the size of the HIV epidemic would in theory be large-scale testing for HIV antibodies. National policy in the Netherlands has been to advise against testing: first, because of the lack of effective treatment (from the perspective of testing as early detection); second, because of unclear preventive effects (from the perspective of primary prevention). Testing was therefore seen as having mostly negative effects, such as discrimination. Large-scale anonymous testing was judged to be against the Dutch Constitution. Instead, a monitoring system reliant on voluntary HIV testing in samples of different populations and risk groups was established to offer an overall impression of the prevalence of HIV infection in different groups. There is formal registration of diagnosed cases of AIDS. However, because of the long delay between infection and diagnosis, the latter data are not appropriate for adequate policy development.

Behavioural Analysis of Risk Groups and Risk Behaviours

The data on AIDS diagnoses show roughly that homosexual or bisexual men constitute the major risk group (comprising cumulatively about 70 per cent of AIDS cases, currently 60 per cent), followed by injecting drug users (about 15 per cent). In the last few years, the percentage of gay and bisexual men has decreased, while the other percentages have increased. The percentage of (young) heterosexual adults is low, but slowly rising. Many prevention activities have been directed at specific groups, such as gay men, injecting drug users, adolescents and young adults, migrants and sex workers. Alongside these specific campaigns, mass media campaigns have taken place on a regular basis.

The Campaigns

From 1987 until 1995, AIDS prevention activities were coordinated by the National Committee on AIDS Control (NCAB) financed by the Ministry of Health. After 1995 they were coordinated by the Dutch AIDS Fund. Most of the mass media campaigns were designed and executed by the Dutch Foundation for STD Control. The NCAB formulated some basic principles in 1987 which AIDS education, including the mass campaigns, had to fulfil (De Vroome et al., 1994). These include the beliefs that:

1. a moralistic approach is not very useful; so AIDS prevention was not to be restricted to promoting abstinence or monogamy but also adressed other risk reduction behaviours, especially condom use;
2. sexuality should be approached positively and as a healthy and pleasant activity; the battle should be against AIDS, not sex;
3. safe sex campaigns should not inadvertently stigmatize or discriminate against certain social groups: people who are seropositive, people with AIDS, gay and bisexual men or injecting drug users;
4. behaviour change should be stimulated by persuasion, not by compulsory measures, mainly because the last would be impossible to enforce;
5. safe sex campaigns should not create undue anxiety; and
6. the tone and language of the campaigns should be such that people from all layers of society could understand and relate to the message.

In practice, the focus of safe sex mass media campaigns was on the promotion of condom use. A complicating factor was that the public campaign was also directed at gay men, while the specific prevention activities developed for gay men started with an abstinence message for anal sex, emphasizing no anal sex, based on data about relatively high percentages of condom failure in anal sex. Over time, that message shifted to a 'double' message, emphasizing no anal sex or using a special condom (see Kok, Hospers and De Wit, 1997). In the general public safe sex mass media campaigns, both messages were combined: condom use for heterosexual contacts, the double message for homosexual contacts. Both messages were presented in a common framework of *Safe Sex or No Sex*.

One of the pitfalls in health education planning, causing non-effective campaigns, is a 'jump' from problem analysis to campaigns without sufficient analysis of determinants of behaviour and with insufficient attention to theoretical principles of behaviour change (Kok, 1993). In reality, however, campaigns often have to start without sufficient information, and the best strategy is to gather the necessary data as early as possible in order to adapt the campaign as it develops. Before describing the campaigns further, we will briefly describe the theoretical and empirical bases of public information campaigns in general.

Theories of Behaviour and Behaviour Change through Communication

Having analyzed the epidemiological and behavioural aspects of the problem, we need more knowledge on the determinants of behaviour and on adequate intervention strategies. On the one hand, we have theories on behaviour and on behaviour change through communication (Kok *et al.*, 1996), and on the other hand we have data to operationalize concepts derived from those theories (Meibach and Parrot, 1995).

Theories of Behaviour

Various general social-psychological models predicting goal-oriented behaviour can be applied to health-related behaviours. Although these models include a broad range of variables, three basic general categories of behavioural determinants can be distinguished (Ajzen, 1988; Bandura, 1986):

- *Attitudes*: beliefs and evaluations about advantages and disadvantages (for example health risks) of behaviour, resulting in an attitude about the behaviour, also referred to as outcome expectations.
- *Social influences*: subjective beliefs about social norms and expectations (Cialdini, Reno and Kallgren, 1990); observed behaviour of others, also referred to as modelling (Bandura, 1986); and direct social pressures (De Vries *et al.*, 1995; Evans *et al.*, 1978).
- *Self-efficacy*: beliefs about perceived behavioural control, or self-efficacy expectations (Strecher *et al.*, 1986).

These three categories of behavioural determinants can be seen as social cognitive perceptions or predisposing factors. These should be distinguished from reinforcing factors (for example actual social support) and enabling factors (for example actual skills or facilities) (Green and Kreuter, 1991). Ajzen (1988) and Bandura (1986) call attention to the potential discrepancy between perceptions of social norms and actual norms, and between perceptions of self-efficacy and actual skills or barriers. Improving people's self-efficacy for healthy behaviour through health education should be combined with lowering barriers that hinder healthy behaviour, through health promotion.

Models of behavioural determinants do not imply a unidirectional influence; attitudes, social influences and self-efficacy can be consequences as well as antecedents of behaviour (Zimbardo and Leippe, 1991). Educational programmes try to change behavioural determinants in order to change behaviour, but when possible, techniques are also used to influence behaviour directly, such as commitment procedures and practice of behaviour followed by feedback and reinforcement. Positive experiences when a desired behaviour is exhibited may in turn change psychosocial determinants of behaviour, thus creating reciprocal determinism (Bandura, 1986).

Theories of Behaviour Change through Communication

Current social psychological models of behaviour change distinguish steps, phases or stages of change. Within those steps, various specific theories can be applied. One general framework for theories of behaviour change is provided by McGuire's (1985) persuasion-communication model. This model describes the various steps that people take, from the initial response to an educational message to, hopefully, a more enduring change of behaviour in the desired direction. This framework has been simplified and extended into seven steps: 1) attention, 2) comprehension, 3) attitude change, 4) changes in social influences, 5) improved self-efficacy, 6) behaviour change, and 7) maintenance of behaviour change (Kok *et al.*, 1996). Interventions may be different for each step, and the decisions that have to be made about categories of communication variables (message, target group, channel, and source) may be different too, and may even conflict. This is one of the reasons why we should always pilot-test an intervention with a sample from the target population to find out if there are any 'unwanted' effects (Romano, 1984).

Another general theory, or theoretical framework, covering both determinants of behaviour and the process of behaviour change is Bandura's (1986) social cognitive theory (SCT). In SCT, the relationships between cognitive, environmental and behavioural variables are seen as interactive and bi-directional. The reinforcement of behaviour is a key environmental factor studied by social cognitive theorists. Other people in the environment can also affect behaviour because a person learns through observing others and receiving reinforcement. In SCT cognitive variables include outcome expectations and self-efficacy expectations. Modelling and incentives are SCT's major intervention methods for influencing behaviour.

Mass Media and Behaviour Change

The mass media are certainly not the best media to use if we want to change people's behaviour (Rice and Atkin, 1989; Atkin and Wallack, 1990). Going through the persuasion-communication steps, the impact of mass media relative to interpersonal channels decreases. Mass media may be effective in getting initial attention or awareness for an issue, but as a result of the one-directional nature of the communication, there is a risk of miscomprehension, which cannot easily be corrected. Mass media may have some impact on attitudes, social influence and self-efficacy or skills, but that influence is limited. Examples of mass media health education programmes that have affected behaviour are scarce. However, the mass media can be supportive of other forms of health education. Moreover, mass media campaigns are sometimes the only feasible way to reach groups that are very difficult to locate, such as non-monogamous young adults.

Health educational interventions should be adapted in accordance with evaluation findings. However, in the case of mass media campaigns, evaluation is especially difficult, if not impossible.

Evaluation of Public Information Campaigns

Evaluation research, especially effect or impact evaluation, is usually grounded in experimental research design. Here, an experimental group that is exposed to an intervention is compared to a control group that is not exposed, while people are divided at random into experimental and control groups. Where complete randomization is not possible, there are many kinds of acceptable quasi-experimental designs (Cook and Campbell, 1979), but for public or mass campaigns it is basically impossible to randomize exposure to the campaign. As a result, it is nearly always impossible to claim direct effects (or lack of effects) for large-scale mass media campaigns.

A common practice in campaign evaluation research is the comparison of exposed people with non-exposed people based on a post-test. This procedure, however, lacks the rigour of a randomized design because we may expect major differences between exposed and non-exposed groups even before the intervention. Obviously there may be hidden variables, such as involvement in the issue, that determine why some people will be exposed to the campaign and others will not. It is also possible that behaviour change may be the cause of exposure instead of the effect.

We do not mean to suggest that evaluation research for mass media campaigns is useless – quite the contrary. But we have to be aware of design difficulties and possible threats to validity inherent in the evaluation of public campaigns. Sometimes we can find alternative control groups; longitudinal analyses can be very convincing, while process evaluation may show changes following a predicted route. The most convincing outcome is a change in behaviour which is relatively new, in the sense that the behaviour has not been demonstrated before, and which is measured shortly after the campaign (Cook and Campbell, 1979, p. 103).

'Safe Sex' Campaigns

Research Data and the Development of the Safe Sex Campaign

In 1987, the Foundation for STD Control developed a long-term strategy to promote safe sex among heterosexual people who are potentially at risk of becoming infected with HIV or other STDs (De Vroome *et al.*, 1994), in accordance with the available data at the time. The objective of the first safe sex campaign was to make condom use socially acceptable. Since the first general population survey (April 1987) indicated that most people already knew that condoms protected against STDs and AIDS, and general acceptance of condoms in the Netherlands was nearly 100 per cent, the first campaign primarily emphasized personal acceptance of condom use. This was tried by using several well-known Dutch men and women who announced that they 'used them' (that is that they used condoms).

Subsequent safe sex campaigns were specifically targeted at young people. With a tinge of the romantic, the 1988 *Safe Sex on Holidays* campaign emphasized the importance of safe sex while on holidays. Attention was paid not only to condom use, but also to postponing the first sexual encounter, monogamy, and sexual activities not including intercourse. Holidays were chosen because it was believed that young people are particularly likely to start their sexual relationships in this context. In the accompanying brochure, attention was also given to the skills needed to communicate about safe sex. Part of the campaign was a television programme in which a young couple offer a very explicit real life demonstration of adequate condom use. Anticipating resistance, the programme was broadcast late in the evening and was preceded by warnings. In practice, however, most complaints concerned the late broadcasting hour and the programme was subsequently repeated at an earlier time!

Research data showed that by 1988 young people knew they should practise safe sex, and also had the intention to do so (De Vroome *et al.*, 1994). However, the well-known gap between intention and behaviour was also found to be present. Focus-group discussions showed that young people used many excuses or self-justifications for not practising safe sex. Thus, the *Excuses* campaign was started in 1989 (Figure 2.1). Its goal was to blunt some of the self-justifications used, and to make young people conscious of the fact that

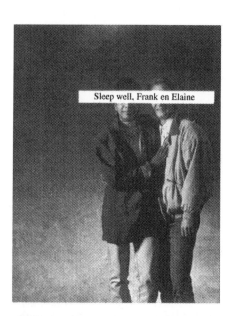 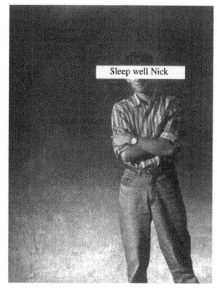

Figure 2.1 *A low risk perception seemed to be a major barrier for not using condoms amongst youngsters. A message that it is important to use condoms as a protection against HIV infection was not enough. The campaign tried to confront young people in a very straightforward way in order to convince them that the possible consequences of unsafe sex had a relation with their own behaviour. In 1989 and 1990 a total of 12 different excuses for not having safe sex or not using condoms were given with a photo of either a young man, a woman, or a couple. Reprinted with kind permission from the Dutch Foundation for STD Control.*

they are at risk. From the survey conducted after this campaign, however, it appeared that those with a lower educational level were less comprehending of the ironic undertone of the campaign (De Vroome *et al.*, 1991). Thus, adjustments were made to some of the excuses when the campaign was continued in 1990. However, evaluation showed that lower educated young people still did not interpret the message correctly.

Moreover, research revealed that overall knowledge about AIDS was less among those with lower educational levels (De Vroome *et al.*, 1994). Since it was also found that those with lower educational levels have sex at a somewhat earlier age, AIDS education specifically targeted at this group was warranted. The 1992 safe sex campaign, the *Cupid* campaign, was directed primarily at young people with lower educational levels. Part of the campaign was the provision of information and distribution of free condoms during disco shows. Moreover, the disc jockeys emphasized the importance of practising safe sex. The *Cupid* campaign shifted from a mass media campaign to a risk-group approach.

In 1993 the Foundation for STD Control started the campaign *Safe Sex or No Sex*. The target group of this campaign was the general population and specifically the young and those having occasional as well as perhaps regular partners (including gay men). New research data were available (De Vroome *et al.*, 1994), indicating a need for education on practical and social skills. As well as the original principles, new objectives for this new campaign included:

1. reinforcing the social norm of safe sex;
2. improving practical and social skills for safe sex;
3. integrating HIV prevention and the prevention of other STDs;
4. integrating health promotion work on homosexuality and heterosexuality;
5. explicit promotion of condom use; and
6. serving as an 'umbrella' for various risk-group oriented and local interventions.

The visual part of the campaign presented five couples, three heterosexual and two gay (men), in intimate poses suggesting that sex was going to own. Using a condom was presented as the major HIV and STD preventive behaviour. The emphasis in the accompanying text was not on knowledge or attitudes, but on strengthening the social norm of condom use and improving self-efficacy in negotiating and decision-making about condom use (Figure 2.2). Based on research data, the campaign was continued in 1994, 1995 and 1996 with improved materials (for example better visibility of the condoms) and clearer messages. Within this general framework, the focus of the 1995 campaign was on 'how' to start talking with the partner about condoms, while in 1996 the focus was on 'the right moment' to start talking about condoms with the partner.

To communicate the messages in the various campaigns, outdoor advertising, magazine advertisements, leaflets, brochures, and commercials in movie

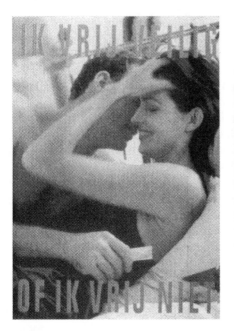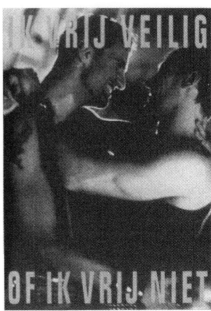

Figure 2.2 *In 1993 the campaign 'I'll have safe sex or no sex' (Ik vrij veilig of ik vrij niet) was launched. The campaign was based on 'lifestyle', and aimed to support the social norm to practise safe sex. To stress this message only the slogan next to a sensual picture appeared on the posters. After the campaign 59 per cent of the Dutch people were able to recall this slogan and 88 per cent said that they endorsed the message. Reprinted with kind permission from the Dutch Foundation for STD Control.*

theatres and on radio and TV, were the principal means used. All campaigns were pilot-tested with communication experts and a sample of the target population. In addition, many free condoms with instructions have been handed out. Finally, newspapers, magazines, television, and radio have all provided extensive free publicity in support of the safe sex message.

Effects: Exposed Compared to Non-exposed People

The *Excuses* campaign was evaluated with a quasi-experimental design, comparing exposed and non-exposed people with each other, and with a pre-test (De Vroome *et al.*, 1991). A representative sample of the target population for this campaign, 18–24-year-olds, was interviewed by telephone: 481 at pre-test (response 47 per cent), and 495 at post-test after six months (response 56 per cent). Both samples were similar with respect to demographic characteristics. The mean age was 21.0 and women were slightly overrepresented (53 per cent).

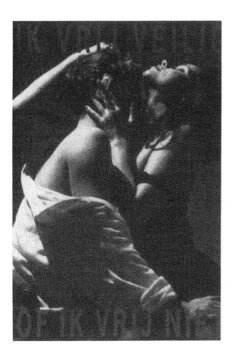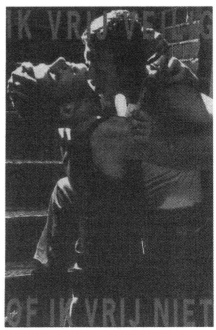

Figure 2.3 *In 1994 a follow-up of the 1993 campaign was introduced. New photos were made but the headings stayed the same. The couples on the these pictures showed more passion to give the situations a more realistic look. On the back of the postcards and in the advertisements reminders were given how people could let their partners know that they wanted to practise safer sex. After the campaign 91 per cent of the Dutch could remember having seen something of the campaign. Sixty five per cent of the people felt that this campaign was also targeted at themselves. Reprinted with kind permission from the Dutch Foundation for STD Control.*

At post-test, 70 per cent of the respondents remembered the *Excuses* campaign (the 'exposed'), against 30 per cent who did not remember the campaign (the 'non-exposed'). The highly educated were more often exposed: 75 per cent against 65 per cent of the less educated ones. Treating the exposed and non-exposed as quasi-experimental and quasi-control groups respectively, comparison with the pre-test scores showed some significant differences between the two groups. Respondents who were exposed to the campaign were more aware of their personal risk of HIV infection. Also, they showed a reduction in the endorsement of the excuses that were the focus of the campaign. As mentioned earlier, it is not certain that the campaign is the cause of these changes, especially when we notice that the groups differ with respect to education. There were no significant differences between the non-exposed group and the pre-test group, which at least supports the idea that the improvement in the exposed group may partly be an effect of the campaign.

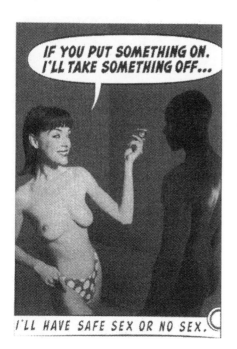

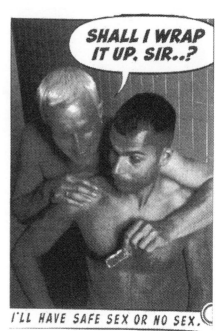

Figure 2.4 *Many people remembered the slogan after two years of campaigning. So the heading 'I'll have safe sex or no sex' became a pay-off in future campaigns. To focus on the self-efficacy regarding talking about condom use several examples were given for how to bring up the subject of condom use and negotiate on using them with a partner. When the picture 'If you'll put something on . . .' appeared on the bus stops all over the country, questions were asked in Parliament. However, the Minister of Health supported the campaign. And as a result of the public discussion on this poster many people saw the message.*

Effects: Changes in Longitudinal Data

Twice a year, from 1987 to 1994, a telephone survey regarding safe sex and condom use has been conducted (see De Vroome *et al.*, 1991; 1994; Dingelstad *et al.*, 1994). Approximately 1000 residents of the Netherlands, ranging from 15 to 45 years of age, participated in each of the 14 surveys. In each survey a new sample was recruited through random selection from telephone subscriber lists. The response rate has varied from 37 to 56 per cent. All surveys combined, the studied group consists of 13,200 respondents of whom 16 per cent are young (15–20 years of age) and 8 per cent are non-monogamous. The mean age is 29.9 years and women are overrepresented (52–63 per cent).

In the first eight surveys (April 1987–October 1990), respondents were asked what they understood to be safe sex. The percentage mentioning condom use increased significantly from 43 to 72 per cent. That 'properly used

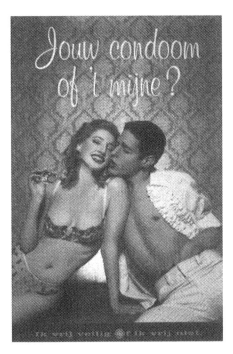 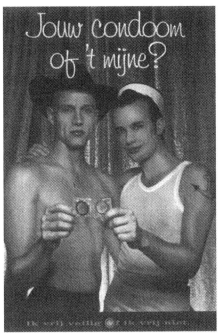

Figure 2.5 *'Your condom or mine'. 'I'll have safe sex or no sex.' On a series of posters put out in 1996 the theme again was to negotiate with your partner about condom use. An important difference was that in the earlier pictures you just saw a couple in an erotic situation, in the new pictures one of them was holding a condom; also the negotiations were depicted as being less combative. In this same year an STD Top 10 was presented to raise awareness of the most common but less known STD in the Netherlands: Chlamydia. After the campaign, the recognition of the name Chlamydia as an STD had increased by 15 per cent.*

condoms protect against AIDS', was confirmed by 74 per cent in 1987, rising to 98 per cent in 1988 and following years. There was no change over the years in attitudes and risk awareness. Attitudes towards condoms were relatively positive (76 per cent), especially among young people (86 per cent). Of the entire group, 15 per cent acknowledged their personal risk awareness for AIDS. Young people were more aware than the older respondents (32 versus 12 per cent). Non-monogamous individuals were more aware than monogamous (58 versus 11 per cent).

There was a significant increase over the years among the young who during the previous six months had done something to prevent HIV infection, from 10 per cent to 55 per cent. In the non-monogamous group, the increase was from 29 per cent to 82 per cent. Most people mention condom use as their main prevention strategy. Among young people, occasional or consistent condom use increased from 11 per cent to 62 per cent; among the non-monogamous any condom use has increased from 30 per cent to 85 per cent, while consistent condom use has increased from 9 per cent to 51 per cent. The intention to use condoms in the future has also increased over the years, especially among young respondents (from 43 to 80 per cent), and the non-monogamous (from 65 to 83 per cent).

In summary (see De Vroome *et al.*, 1994), there has been an increase in condom intention and reported behaviour over the years, probably as a result of many kinds of educational activities, of which the public information campaigns were a part. There have been no major changes in attitudes and risk awareness, possibly because the increase in these variables occurred in the Netherlands before the onset of these studies. Moreover, behaviour change may not be determined by attitudes or risk awareness, but by social influence or self-efficacy. Based on these research data, attention in the later campaigns shifted to increasing social support and self-efficacy. As for any validation of the self-reported behavioural data, condom sales by London Rubber Company Netherlands, which covers 90 to 95 per cent of the Dutch market, increased by a factor 1.50 between 1986 to 1995. The use of the contraceptive pill has also increased in that period, which previously would have been associated with a decrease in condom use.

'Compassion' Campaigns

The first compassion campaign, *A Little Understanding Never Gave Anyone AIDS*, began in 1990. The general target of these campaigns was to increase and support awareness and involvement in AIDS. Prior to the advent of the campaign, there had been repeated incidents of stigmatization and discrimination, which the campaigns were intended to prevent. The theoretical underpinning for the campaign was social cognitive theory or modelling; the visual part of the campaign showed a 'healthy' person throwing his arm around the shoulder of a 'seropositive' person. The idea was that people who are seropositive and people with AIDS need social support in interpersonal contact. However, most people have never had any contact with people who were seropositive or people with AIDS. Also, appropriate research data were not available. As a result, the specific objectives of the compassion campaigns were quite vague at the time.

Preventing stigmatization and discrimination is an area where much research data are lacking (Stephan, 1985). Most available data concern discrimination towards minority ethnic groups. In relation to the stigmatization of diseases or disability, uncertainty about how to behave has been shown to be an important determinant (Jones *et al.*, 1984). In the area of AIDS, studies in the USA and in the Netherlands have shown that people who are seropositive and people with AIDS are 'blamed', and that the perceived chance of infection through social contact and a negative attitude towards homosexuals are positively related to stigmatization (Peters *et al.*, 1994).

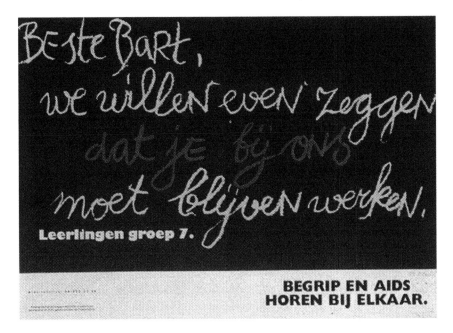

Figure 2.6 *'Dear Bart, we just want you to know that you have to stay working with us.'*
Pupils group 7. 'AIDS and understanding make a good team.'

In 1993–94, a new campaign *AIDS and Understanding Make a Good Team* started. The campaign was directed at the general public and intended to stimulate and support positive attitudes and behaviours. The central theme was how to handle uncertainties in contact with people with HIV and AIDS. Three real-life situations were chosen to illustrate potential uncertainties: work, sport and school. The accompanying texts follow the same possible reactions: the first is *shock and fear*, followed by a period of *searching for a solution* (for instance talking about it), and finally *acceptance*. The texts used were literal citations derived from focus group interviews conducted with people that had been involved in situations like those in the campaign (Figure 2.6). Along with the campaign, studies started to analyze people's reactions to persons with AIDS.

Theory and Research

On the basis of their research during the last three years, Dijker and colleagues have formulated a theoretical model of emotional reactions to ill and handicapped people that proved especially useful in understanding the nature of responses to persons with AIDS (PWAs). Briefly, the model specifies different illness dimensions that in various combinations are associated with different diseases. In the case of AIDS, reactions to ill persons are influenced by the seriousness and perceived contagiousness of the disease, and the extent to which the ill person is thought to be responsible for getting ill. Which of these dimensions will be most salient depends on the type of contact with the ill person. Once activated, a particular dimension will arouse characteristic emotions. For example, perceived contagiousness will arouse fear, seriousness will arouse feelings of pity, sadness, and helplessness, and personal responsibility will arouse feelings of anger. Situational factors will further moderate the arousal of emotions. Thus fear of contact with an infectious disease like AIDS may be moderated by increase in personal control and predictability, whereas feelings of helplessness may be reduced by an ill person showing successful coping behaviour. In addition, anger may be inhibited by making salient the suffering of the ill person, thereby inducing feelings of pity. This model has received some support in several empirical studies.

The Relation between Contagiousness of Disease and Fear

Dijker, Kok and Koomen (1996) have demonstrated that, in addition to anger and pity, fear may be an important determinant of readiness to engage in everyday contact with PWAs. Dijker, Stam and Kok (1996) examined whether stigmatizing responses to PWAs could be influenced by reducing fear responses to PWAs through education about the low risks involved in everyday contact with PWAs. It was found that an educative brochure was effective in reducing risk perception and (self-reported) fear responses to PWAs among individuals who expressed low involvement in the issue of 'AIDS'. No effects were found, however, for persons who were strongly involved and who were motivated to seek contact with persons with AIDS. One of the authors' conclusions was that important aspects of the experience of fear may not be easily influenced by information about risks alone, but should be complemented by attempts to influence aspects of the interaction situation. Indeed, when Dijker, Koomen and Kok (1997) examined the influence of predictability information on fear responses to PWAs, they found that, although subjects who anticipated working with a colleague with or without AIDS show more anxiety and avoidance of physical contact for the former than the latter, differential avoidance responses disappeared when the target was presented as a predictable and controllable person.

The Relation between Seriousness of Disease and Helplessness

Dijker and Raeijmaekers (in print) studied nursing students' reactions to the prospects of caring for patients with various serious and lethal diseases. They found that when subjects imagined personal contact with the patient in which thoughts and feelings about the nature of the disease would be exchanged, subjects' anxiety reactions were influenced by the seriousness of the disease. That is, the lethal diseases cancer and AIDS evoked equal anxiety but more anxiety than the non-lethal diseases appendicitis and hepatitis. In contrast, when anticipating close physical contact with the target (for example while giving an injection to the patient), subjects' anxiety responses were primarily determined by the contagiousness of the disease. Specifically, AIDS and hepatitis caused equal anxiety, but more anxiety than cancer and appendicitis.

Dijker and colleagues hypothesize that information about the target's efforts and ability to cope successfully with his or her lethal condition – information that may, for example, be provided by the target during disclosure of HIV infection – will moderate the influence of seriousness on feelings of helplessness. Findings from two studies, although not specifying the kinds of emotions involved, are consistent with this argument. Schwarzer and Weiner (1991) found that stigmatizing responses to different chronic illnesses could be reduced when the chronically ill person was described as highly motivated to cope effectively with, and improve, his or her condition. Silver *et al.* (1990) demonstrated that a cancer patient who communicated successful efforts to cope with her health condition, aroused less feelings of discomfort in prospective interaction partners than a patient who reported that she had lost hope.

The Relation between Responsibility for Getting a Disease and Anger

Consistent with earlier findings of Weiner, Perry and Magnusson (1988), Schaalma, Peters and Kok (1993) and Peters *et al.* (1994) found that angry reactions to PWAs are influenced by attributions that are based on knowledge of the causal origin of the medical condition.

That pity arousal can moderate the influence of responsibility on anger is suggested by the negative relationship between pity and anger. Dijker and colleagues hypothesize that information about the ill person's responsibility for acquiring the disease will exert relatively less influence on anger towards the person when this person also arouses pity. For pity to be aroused, the affected person should show signs of physical or psychological suffering (Batson, Fultz and Schoenrade, 1987; Silver, Wortman and Crofton, 1990). As Silver, Wortman and Crofton (1990) note, however, seriously ill persons are faced with a 'self-presentational dilemma'. These authors argue that a minimum amount of observable distress and suffering is necessary to motivate social support from others. At the same time, feelings of depression and helplessness at the side of potential support providers have to be reduced (for example by the affected person showing good coping efforts). This is a complicated issue that demands further reflection before practical recommendations can be formulated. Future research needs to be directed at finding fruitful combinations of both factors that may prove effective in everyday interactions between ill persons and their environment.

In sum, reactions to persons with AIDS are influenced not only by beliefs about the nature and background of the disease (how serious and infectious it is, and what behaviour might be responsible for it), but also by concerns and uncertainties about future interactions with these same individuals (how should I help, if necessary?; how much can I personally control these encounters and reduce feelings of unsafety?). The latter worries especially may have been ignored by ongoing campaigns in the Netherlands as these do not acknowledge people's concern for safety during interactions with a person with AIDS (indeed they try to demonstrate that these concerns are largely unfounded!). Neither do they focus sufficient attention on the role of the persons with AIDS themselves in reducing fear responses and inviting helpful social reactions.

How can such campaigns be improved? The interaction between the healthy person and the person with AIDS should be characterized as an interaction between people who have different needs (the need to be safe and the need to be accepted), and who are willing to take the needs of the other into account. People who are afraid should be convinced that people with HIV or AIDS know about their fear, and are willing to help them feel safe. On the other hand, in order to motivate helpful responses, the campaign could provide information about the extent to which persons with AIDS suffer and about the successful ways in which they can cope with their condition. At present, however, a public campaign following these principles has yet to be realized. It may be that these principles can only be applied in settings in which interpersonal interactions with persons with AIDS can be actually practised.

Conclusions

What is the use of mass media campaigns for AIDS prevention? In 1987, such a question was not really relevant. The main goal of the campaign then was to give as many people as possible correct information about a new infectious disease and the ways to protect oneself against it. Moreover, the 1987 campaign was not underpinned by research data of the kind that should have been available for adequate planning. Later, as research data became available, other, local and risk-group oriented types of health promotion interventions were developed. So the question now is: what is the use of mass media campaigns for AIDS prevention in the coming years?

In themselves, mass media campaigns are not the most effective method of influencing people's behaviour. Mass media are important, however, for getting people's attention and involvement, and for reinforcing social norms. Moreover, mass media campaigns may serve as an 'umbrella' for other, local and risk-group oriented interventions. Such campaigns will be more effective with optimal planning and evaluation, based on relevant theories and research data. The evaluation of mass media campaigns is difficult if not impossible, yet a careful process and effect evaluation will serve as feedback for improvement of the campaigns. Mass media campaigns for AIDS prevention, including the prevention of stigmatization, should always be accompanied by various specific, more interpersonal, communication campaigns, targeted at specific risk groups and executed at local and community levels. For these specific interventions, a careful planning and evaluation is again necessary.

Since the first campaigns in 1987, the focus of public information campaigns in the Netherlands has shifted from AIDS to STDs *and* AIDS. The assumption is that for most people, especially women, these two issues are related. Health educators assumed that people could be better motivated to use condoms by linking AIDS prevention to STD prevention, STDs having short-term consequences and a much higher prevalence. At present, there is no specific research supporting this assumption. It will be important to see if and how AIDS prevention improves as a result of the integration with STDs, or even with sexual health in general.

References

AJZEN, I. (1988) *Attitudes, Personality, and Behaviour*, Milton Keynes: Open University Press.

ATKIN, C. and WALLACK, L. (Eds) (1990) *Mass Communication and Public Health*, London: Sage.

BANDURA, A. (1986) *Social Foundations of Thought and Action*, Englewood Cliffs, NJ: Prentice-Hall.

BATSON, C.D., FULTZ, J. and SCHOENRADE, P.A. (1987) 'Adults' emotional reactions to the distress of others', in N. EISENBERG and J. STRAYER (Eds) *Empathy and its Development*, New York: Cambridge University Press.

CIALDINI, R.B., RENO, R.R. and KALLGREN, C.A. (1990) 'A focus theory of normative conduct: recycling the concept of norms to reduce littering in public places', *Journal of Personality and Social Psychology*, **58**, pp. 1015–26.

COOK, T.D. and CAMPBELL, D.T. (1979) *Quasi-experimentation, Design and Analysis Issues for Field Settings*, Boston: Houghton Mifflin.

DIJKER, A.J. and RAEIJMAEKERS, F. (in print) 'Emotional reactions to ill persons: the influence of seriousness and contagiousness of disease, and kind of interpersonal contact', Psychology & Health.

DIJKER, A.J., KOK, G. and KOOMEN, W. (1996) 'Emotional reactions to people with AIDS', *Journal of Applied Social Psychology*, **26**, pp. 731–48.

DIJKER, A.J., KOOMEN, W. and KOK, G. (1997) 'Interpersonal determinants of fear of people with AIDS: the moderating role of predictable behaviour', *Basic and Applied Social Psychology*, **19**, pp. 61–79.

DIJKER, A.J., STAM, H. and KOK, G. (1996) 'Beinvloeding van stigmatisering van mensen met AIDS door middel van voorlichting: de rol van betrokkenheid en voorlichtingsbron' (Reduction of stigmatization of PWAs by education: the role of involvement and source), in E. VAN SCHIE, D. DAAMEN, A. PRUYN, and W. OTTEN (Eds), *Sociale Psychologie en haar Toepassingen (Applied Social Psychology)*, Delft: Eburon.

DINGELSTAD, A., DE VROOME, E., PAALMAN, M. and SANDFORT, TH. (1994) 'Trends in condom use among non-monogamous heterosexual men in the Netherlands', *American Journal of Public Health*, **84**, p. 1184.

EVANS, R.I., ROZELLE, R.M., MITTELMARK, M.B., HANSEN, W.B., BANE, A.L. and HAVIS, J. (1978) 'Deterring the onset of smoking in children: knowledge of immediate physiological effects and coping with peer pressure, media pressure and parental modeling', *Journal of Applied Social Psychology*, **8**, pp. 126–35.

GREEN, L.W. and KREUTER, M.W. (1991) *Health Promotion Planning; An Educational and Environmental Approach*, Mountain View, CA: Mayfield.

JONES, E.E., FARINA, A., HASTORF, A.H., MARKUS, H., MILLET, D.T. and SCOTT, R.A. (1984) *Social Stigma: The Psychology of Marked Relationships*, New York: Freeman.

KOK, G.J. (1993) 'Why are so many health promotion programs ineffective?', *Health Promotion Journal of Australia*, **3**, pp. 12–17.

KOK, G., HOSPERS, H. and DE WIT, J. (1997) 'Applying social psychology to HIV prevention', in D.C. UMEH (Ed.), *Cross-cultural Perspectives on HIV/AIDS Education*, Lawrenceville, NJ: Africa World Press.

KOK, G., SCHAALMA, H., DE VRIES, H., PARCEL, G. and PAULUSSEN, TH. (1996) 'Social psychology and health education', in W. STROEBE and M. HEWSTONE (Eds), *European Review of Social Psychology*, **7**, Chichester: Wiley.

DE LEEUW, E. (1989) *The Sane Revolution. Health Promotion: Backgrounds, Scope, Prospects*, Maastricht: Van Gorkum.

McGUIRE, W.J. (1985) 'Attitudes and attitude change', in M. LINDSAY and E. ARONSON (Eds), *The Handbook of Social Psychology, vol. 2*, New York: Random House.

MEIBACH, E. and PARROT, R.L. (1995) *Designing Health Messages: Approaches from Communication Theory and Public Health Practice*, Thousand Oaks: Sage.

MILIO, N. (1988) 'Strategies for health promoting policy: a study of four national case studies', *Health Promotion International*, **3**, pp. 307–11.

PETERS, L., DEN BOER, D.J., KOK, G. and SCHAALMA, H.P. (1994) 'Public reactions towards people with AIDS: an attributional analysis', *Patient Education and Counseling*, **24**, pp. 323–35.

RICE, E. and ATKIN, C. (1989) *Public Communication Campaigns*, London: Sage.

ROMANO, R. (1984) *Pretesting in Health Communications*, Bethesda, MI: NCI.

SCHAALMA, H.P., PETERS, L. and KOK, G. (1993) 'Reactions among Dutch youth toward people with AIDS', *Journal of School Health*, **63**, pp. 182–7.

SCHWARZER, R. and WEINER, B. (1991) 'Stigma controllability and coping as predictors of emotions and social support', *Journal of Social and Personal Relationships*, **8**, pp. 133–40.

SILVER, R.C., WORTMAN, C.B. and CROFTON, C. (1990) 'The role of coping in support provision: the self-presentational dilemma of victims of life crises', in I.G. SARASON, B.R. SARASON and P.R. PIERCE (Eds), *Social Support: An Interactional View*, New York: Wiley.

SIMONS-MORTON, D.G., BUNKER, J.F., PARCEL, G.S. and SIMONS-MORTON, B.G. (1988) 'Influencing personal and environmental conditions for community health: a multilevel intervention model', *Family and Community Health*, **11**, pp. 25–35.

STEPHAN, W.G. (1985) 'Intergroup relations', in G. LINDSEY and E. ARONSON (Eds), *Handbook of Social Psychology, vol. 2*, New York: Random House.

STRECHER, V.J., DEVELLIS, B.M., BECKER, M.H. and ROSENSTOCK, I.M. (1986) 'The role of self efficacy in achieving health behavior change', *Health Education Quarterly*, **13**, pp. 73–91.

DE VRIES, H., BACKBIER, E., KOK, G. and DIJKSTRA, M. (1995) 'The impact of social influences in the context of attitude, self-efficacy, intention and previous behaviour as predictors of smoking onset', *Journal of Applied Social Psychology*, **25**, pp. 237–57.

DE VROOME, E.M.M., PAALMAN, M.E.M., DINGELSTAD, A.A.M., KOLKER, L. and SANDFORT, TH. G.M. (1994) 'Increase in safe sex among the young and non-monogamous: knowledge, attitudes and behaviour regarding safe sex and condom use in the Netherlands from 1987 till 1993', *Patient Education and Counseling*, **24**, pp. 279–88.

DE VROOME, E.M.M., DE VRIES, K.J.M., PAALMAN, M.E.M., SANDFORT, TH.G.M. and TIELMAN, R.A.P. (1991) 'Evaluation of a safe sex campaign regarding AIDS and other STDs among young people in the Netherlands', *Health Education Research*, **6**, pp. 317–25.

WEINER, B., PERRY, R.P. and MAGNUSSON, J. (1988) 'An attributional analysis of reactions to stigmas', *Journal of Personality and Social Psychology*, **55**, pp. 738–48.

ZIMBARDO, PH.G. and LEIPPE, M.R. (1991) *The Psychology of Attitude Change and Social Influence*, Philadelphia: McGraw-Hill.

Chapter 3

HIV Prevention Activities for Gay Men in the Netherlands 1983–93

Harm Hospers and Cor Blom

This chapter offers an overview of HIV prevention activities for gay men that were developed and implemented in the Netherlands between 1983 and 1993. We begin with a concise history of the development of HIV prevention interventions. The core of this chapter summarizes the wide range of interventions that have been developed and implemented, including each intervention's characteristics and goals and, if available, evaluation results. Then we describe future directions of HIV prevention for gay men. The chapter concludes with a brief discussion of the issues raised earlier.

We have limited ourselves to the period up to 1993 because the majority of HIV prevention funds – and thus activities – were decentralized in that year. Small group projects as well as outreach activities for gay men are now carried out at a local level where once they were developed at a national level. The interventions that were developed at the national level during the first ten years of the epidemic are still influential in HIV prevention today: many current activities are derivatives of the national projects described in this chapter.

The First Campaign

In 1983, the Dutch Blood Bank intended to exclude gay men from donating blood in order to safeguard the Dutch blood supply. This led to upheaval among gay advocacy organizations. Concurrent deliberations between the Blood Bank and representatives from gay organizations led to the agreement that the Blood Bank would start a campaign, together with the Health Education Division of the Amsterdam Public Health Service, the SAD (initially an Amsterdam based STD clinic for gay men run by gay physicians), and the Dutch Gay and Lesbian Association (NVIH COC). The goal was to inform blood donors and gay men about AIDS. The campaign was funded by the Ministry of Health, the City of Amsterdam, and the Central Committee for Medical Blood Transfusion. The campaign for gay men consisted of several elements: a brochure, information meetings at 10 local chapters of the Dutch Gay and Lesbian Association, activities in two gay bars and a gay sauna, and articles in the gay press (Van der Linden, 1984).

The brochure for gay men (circulation 400000 copies) was published in June 1983 concurrent with the brochure for blood donors. The latter brochure asked members of so-called risk groups (that is gay men) to voluntarily withdraw themselves from blood donation programmes. The brochure for gay men reminded readers that there was considerable uncertainty about the aetiology of the disease at that time. It stated that the exact cause of the

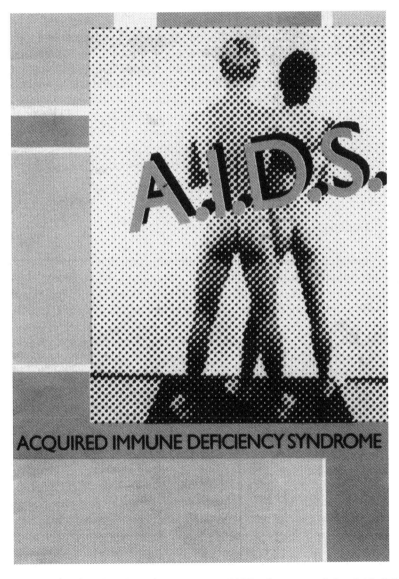

Figure 3.1 *The first brochure for gay men (1983). Courtesy of the SAD-Schorer Foundation.*

disease was as yet unknown, and that the latest theories suggested a viral origin. It further asserted that anal sex could be involved in transmission and 'that there are strong indications that the disease is passed on via blood'. Clear behavioural advice was not given. The brochure told gay men that receptive anal sex was probably associated with an elevated risk, if it occurs with multiple partners. It also stated that 'No one will be advised to have less sex. Maybe one could consider to have sex with less men, especially if one does not know them.'

The first information campaign was considered successful (Van der Linden, 1984). The information brochure was widely disseminated, the information meetings proved popular among gay men, and almost without exception, owners of gay bars agreed to cooperate. This first campaign was followed up by many small-scale initiatives conducted at a local level for which representatives from the gay community were primarily responsible. For example, a local Amsterdam radio station aired a special programme on HIV and AIDS once a year between 1984 and 1987, a number of gay health care workers published a magazine that contained narratives on sexual encounters with a safer sex twist, and the Amsterdam Jacks started to organize safer sex parties in 1986 (Algra, 1988).

The Organizations Involved

The cooperation between the three organizations that organized the first campaign was institutionalized in a task force (Van Wijngaarden, 1984). As a consequence, gay men contributed at an early stage in the AIDS epidemic to the development and execution of prevention activities. The task force focused initially on HIV prevention for gay men. The task force later developed into an official advisory organ to the Dutch government, the National Committee on AIDS Control (NCAB) which became responsible for the formulation of the general HIV/AIDS policy in the Netherlands.

From 1984 until 1993 there were a large number of mass media campaigns, small group interventions, and outreach activities involving gay men. These activities were organized by a small number of providers. The SAD became responsible for all small group and outreach activities that were organized nationally in the first decade, while the Health Education Division of the Amsterdam Public Health Service became responsible for the development and publication of HIV prevention brochures and posters. The Dutch Gay and Lesbian Association has always played an important role in the distribution of written materials and at a later stage in the distribution of condoms. Since 1992 they have operated an organization called Safe Service which distributes condoms to their local chapters, to gay bars and discos and, in the larger cities, to drugstores (chemists).

Almost without exception, funding for HIV prevention activities has come directly or indirectly from government agencies. Of the total national budget for HIV prevention campaigns and activities, approximately 20 per cent has been earmarked specifically for work with gay men.

Prevention Messages

The content of prevention messages for gay men is an aspect of Dutch HIV prevention that is worth mentioning, since it has long been markedly different from prevention messages in other European countries. Until 1992, the Netherlands adopted a so-called 'double message'. The primary focus in the message was on abstinence from anal sex, with condom use in anal sex being seen as an inferior behavioural option. Thus, the initial message said: 'Avoid anal sex. If you can't avoid anal sex, use special condoms.' In most other European countries, the focus of HIV prevention for gay men was almost exclusively on condom use.

Although the motives behind the decision to adopt a 'double message' are not well documented (see also Chapter 8 in this book), it seems that the following factors contributed to a greater or lesser extent. Key persons at that time were convinced that extreme efforts had to be made to prevent an epidemic similar to that then unfolding in the United States. Decisions had to be made quickly since evidence on the sexual behaviour of Dutch gay men, let alone information on their attitudes towards anal sex, was scarce. In addition, at that time there was considerable doubt about the reliability of condoms. These doubts were based on a report that showed high failure rates for six condom brands that were developed for anal sex (Oud, 1986). From the moment the 'double message' was adopted, there were reservations, especially among HIV educators, about the feasibility of advocating abstinence. In the years that followed, research showed that a considerable number of gay men continued to have anal sex, and studies demonstrated the important role that anal sex played in the lives of many gay men (De Wit, 1994). Based partly on these results, prevention workers began to develop activities around condom promotion for men who could not or would not refrain from anal sex. In 1992 the NCAB advised that both abstinence and condom use were to be considered equivalent risk-reducing behavioural options, and that both behavioural options should be addressed in HIV prevention (De Zwart and Sandfort, 1993). From that moment condom promotion became a standard component of HIV prevention for gay men in the Netherlands. The change instigated the development of new brochures and small group activities that focused on promoting condom use with anal sex.

Prevention of Discrimination

Besides information materials and activities that specifically targeted gay men, the Dutch policy also explicitly attempted to prevent discrimination and stigmatization of people with HIV and AIDS (and hence gay men, since they were and are the largest subgroup within the population with HIV or AIDS). In order to achieve this goal, mass media campaigns were launched, in which risk *behaviours* were emphasized as opposed to risk *groups*, an attempt to weaken the almost unavoidable association people made between homosexuality and HIV. Also, mass media campaigns for the general public – especially the more recent ones – have focused within the same campaign on both heterosexual and homosexual contact, using the same format and the same message. The goal was to disseminate the notion that preventing AIDS is relevant to everyone regardless of sexual orientation. Finally, concurrent to primary prevention campaigns for the general public there have been mass media campaigns – with the slogan 'No one has acquired AIDS by showing compassion' – that seek to promote greater understanding for people living with HIV or AIDS.

In sum, characteristic of HIV prevention activities among gay men in the Netherlands in the first decade of the AIDS epidemic has been the notable influence and substantial participation of gay men in shaping and executing the Dutch policy. During that decade a substantial number of prevention activities were developed and implemented, while the prevention message for gay men changed from an emphasis on refraining from anal intercourse to addressing condom use. Finally, activities for gay men were reinforced by campaigns for the general public that promoted safer sex and attempted to prevent stigmatization and discrimination towards people with HIV and AIDS.

Overview of HIV Prevention Interventions

Activities with respect to HIV prevention among gay men in the Netherlands can be placed in the following categories: written HIV prevention materials, posters, other AIDS information materials, small group HIV prevention activities, and outreach activities.

Written Materials

Between 1983 and 1993, 11 brochures with background information for gay men on HIV and AIDS were published in the Netherlands. Almost from the beginning the development of brochures included an extensive pre-testing phase using a standard protocol (Van Kalmthout, 1993). Communication experts, medical specialists and gay men themselves evaluated the first drafts of brochures. Consequently, these drafts were adjusted according to their comments. Table 3.1 shows the year of publication for each brochure as well as a summary of the information and safe sex guidelines provided in these brochures. Several of the brochures in Table 3.1 were also available in foreign

Table 3.1 HIV prevention brochures for gay men

Brochure title	Year	Background information	Safe sex guidelines
A.I.D.S. Important announcement for blood donors	1983	AIDS infection probably via blood Three risk groups: gay men, IVDUs and haemophiliacs Symptoms of AIDS	See a physician if you belong to a risk group Stop donating blood if you belong to a risk group
A.I.D.S. Acquired Immune Deficiency Syndrome	1983	Probably a virus Anal sex probably involved Symptoms of AIDS No test	Anal sex, especially receptive, is risky Multiple anonymous partners risky
A.I.D.S. The situation at this moment	1984	Cause unknown No cure No test Infection via blood and sex, mechanism unknown Anal sex, oral sex, and probably rimming risky Number of AIDS cases	Limit the number of sex partners Avoid anal sex Using condoms for anal sex strongly reduces the risk

Table 3.1 *Continued*

Brochure title	Year	Background information	Safe sex guidelines
AIDS Information 1985	1985	AIDS caused by virus (LAV/HTLV-III) Infection does not have to result in AIDS No cure Mechanism unknown Bloodtests soon available Number of AIDS cases	Do not donate blood Limit the number of sex partners Avoid anal and oral sex Avoid rimming If you want to have anal sex use a condom Testing discouraged, instead behaviour change encouraged
STOP AIDS. Have Safe Sex.	1986	AIDS caused by virus (LAV/HTLV-III) Mechanism: blood–blood and blood–semen contact	Avoid anal sex, especially receptive Condom use limits but not eliminates risk Rimming possibly risky Avoid 'dirty sex' Oral sex with ejaculation is risky Stop use of amyl nitrites Kissing and masturbation no risk
AIDS Information 1987	1987	Caused by HIV Difference between HIV infection and AIDS Some people who are infected do not get sick, others do. Chances of developing AIDS probably higher than 30% No cure Symptoms of AIDS Number of AIDS cases	Do not donate blood Avoid anal sex Avoid oral sex with ejaculation No need to limit the number of sex partners Use a special condom for anal sex if you want to have anal sex Condoms are not 100% safe Do not get tested but have safe sex

		Knowledge	Behaviour
Information 1988	1988	Infection mechanism of HIV (blood–blood/blood–semen) Difference between HIV infection and AIDS Symptoms of infection Syndromes: AIDS, ARC, ADC 30% will develop AIDS 30% will develop other syndromes AZT Number of AIDS cases	Avoid anal sex Use a special condom for anal sex if you want to have anal sex Condoms are not 100% safe Avoid oral sex with ejaculation Carefully consider the advantages and disadvantages of testing Get anonymous testing Report discrimination
The State of Affairs	spring 1990	Infection mechanism of HIV (blood–blood/blood–semen) Difference between HIV infection and AIDS Symptoms of infection Symptoms of AIDS (opportunistic infections, Kaposi's sarcoma) AZT, DDI Early treatment Advantages and disadvantages of testing Number of AIDS cases	Avoid anal sex Use a special condom for anal sex if you want to have anal sex Condoms are not 100% safe Avoid oral sex with ejaculation Discuss safe sex with steady partner Carefully consider the advantages and disadvantages of testing Get anonymous testing Report discrimination

Table 3.1 *Continued*

Brochure title	Year	Background information	Safe sex guidelines
The State of Affairs	autumn 1990	Infection mechanism of HIV (blood–blood/blood–semen) Difference between HIV infection and AIDS Symptoms of infection Symptoms of AIDS (opportunistic infections, Kaposi's sarcoma) AZT, DDI, Kemron Early treatment Referral to AIDS Info for latest news Advantages and disadvantages of testing Number of AIDS cases	Refraining from anal sex is the safest option Use a special condom for anal sex if you want to have anal sex Avoid oral sex with ejaculation Discuss safe sex with steady partner Carefully consider the advantages and disadvantages of testing Get anonymous testing Report discrimination Extensive and explicit instruction how to use condoms properly
Info for Men who Have Sex with Men	1991	History, epidemiology, HIV, AIDS, infections mechanism, unsafe and safe techniques, other STDs, condom use, coping with being HIV+, solidarity testing, AIDS medication.	No behavioural advice Unprotected anal sex unsafe Oral sex with ejaculation unsafe List of safe techniques (e.g. kissing, masturbation)
Do it with	1991		There is nothing wrong with wanting to have anal sex Use special condoms made for anal sex Extensive and explicit instruction how to use condoms properly

languages (English, German, French, Italian, Spanish, Arabic, Turkish, and Papiemento), and targeted both migrants and tourists.

These brochures usually targeted all gay men, and provided safe sex guidelines as well as background information on HIV and AIDS. In the early years of the epidemic, new brochures were published every year, containing the latest medical and epidemiological facts. As more became known, the text in the brochures got lengthier. While the first brochure contains four pages, the 1990 brochure contains 32 pages of information.

The earlier brochures clearly discouraged men from taking HIV tests, while the later brochures gave extensive information on the advantages and disadvantages of testing, and urged men to consider these carefully before getting tested. As of 1988, brochures provided information about the treatment of AIDS. Furthermore, the brochures became more realistic in their statements about the likely course of HIV infection. Between 1983 and 1987, it was believed that only a minority of infected men would eventually develop AIDS. Between 1988 and 1992 this prognosis was adjusted to approximately 60 per cent.

Each brochure provided safe sex guidelines. As discussed above, until 1990 the primary message emphasized avoiding anal sex. Men who wanted to have anal sex were urged to use special condoms with the explicit warning that condoms were not 100 per cent safe. In the autumn of 1990, this focus on abstinence from anal sex was abandoned. Instead, brochures classified unprotected anal sex and oral sex with ejaculation as unsafe techniques and started to give information on condoms and condom use, leaving to the reader the choice between refraining from anal sex or having protected anal sex. In 1991 a brochure was published that was devoted exclusively to condoms and condom use.

Concurrent with these information brochures, small booklets were published in 1986, 1987, 1990, and 1992 that contained only the safe sex guidelines. Between 1988 and 1993, eight folders were printed for gay tourists about gay life in the Netherlands. Safer sex guidelines were also included in these folders. The Dutch Gay and Lesbian Association published a number of folders (in 1987, 1988 and 1992) that specifically targeted gay youth. Although these folders primarily addressed coming-out issues, each also included information about HIV and AIDS, as well as safer sex guidelines.

Brochures and folders were distributed through various channels. The majority of gay bars and discos in the Netherlands were supplied with a special rack to hold written HIV prevention materials, both the nationally published brochures as well as local folders and flyers. A widespread distribution network of volunteers, coordinated primarily by local chapters of the Dutch Gay and Lesbian Association or Municipal Health Services, looks after the supply of informational materials to these venues. A second major channel has been the safe sex promotion kits which were distributed by Safe Sex Promotion Teams (to be discussed later). Also, brochures and folders have been distributed to participants of several small group activities. The exact circulation figures are not known for the brochures, but generally, between 50000 and 100000 copies of each brochure were printed and distributed.

The autumn 1990 brochure and the concise 1990 version – containing only safe sex guidelines – were evaluated after they were published (De Kooning, 1992). In the first phase of this evaluation, prevention workers who contributed to the development of the brochures were interviewed and asked *post hoc* to reconstruct the intended goals and effects of the brochures. Subsequently, 31 gay men were sent the brochures and thereafter interviewed. These men were asked to evaluate the graphic design and the content of the brochures (for example the realism of certain behavioural recommendations) and, more specifically, to comment on whether the intended goals and effects – as stipulated by prevention workers – were covered by the design and content of the brochures. Both brochures received satisfactory ratings. In addition, respondents supplied several useful suggestions for improvement. The evaluation further highlighted the fact that it is hard to please every reader – which should not come as a surprise given the differences in background of a large target population. The length of the text and the tone of the language used were liked by some and disliked by others.

It is difficult to judge whether and to what extent brochures have influenced behavioural determinants and have changed the sexual behaviour of gay men, since research in this area has been scarce. A national cohort study involving 364 Dutch gay men who completed questionnaires once a year between 1986 and 1989 (De Vroome, 1994), showed that each year around 95 per cent of the cohort members reported having been in contact with AIDS education brochures. In general, the brochures received a high rating for usefulness. With respect to behaviour, the study showed that the frequency of contact with AIDS education brochures was significantly higher among men who consistently used condoms for anal sex, compared to men who never used condoms.

Posters

Posters have also been used as a means of drawing attention to safer sex messages. In the first poster campaign – in 1986 – two Robert Mapplethorpe photographs were used as background for safe sex messages. In 1988, a series of eight posters was published with one theme: 'Safe Sex. Keep it up.' This series used the work of famous Dutch photographers. By selecting diverse photographs, the developers of the campaign wished to acknowledge social variations in the gay subculture. This approach was repeated in 1991, when four different posters were published with the theme: 'Live Wild. Have Safe Sex.' Besides safer sex messages, posters have been used to announce small-group activities (to be described below), or to recruit volunteers for interventions. No data are available about the circulation of posters, nor about their effectiveness.

Other AIDS Information

At the beginning of the epidemic, articles on HIV and AIDS concerning gay men were regularly published in both *De Gay Krant* (a national bi-weekly gay newspaper), and *SEK* (the monthly magazine for members of the Dutch Gay and Lesbian Association). In 1984, both periodicals started to collaborate and published a new monthly periodical called *AIDS Info*, initially with a circulation of 40000 copies (later 60000). *AIDS Info* was targeted at gay men – including men living with HIV or AIDS – and it contained articles with recent news about a broad array of subjects, such as medical aspects of HIV and AIDS, HIV prevention, and policy aspects. Through its independent status it could be (and was) critical towards developments in HIV/AIDS prevention, treatment, and policy. The Ministry of Health subsidized the distribution. *AIDS Info* was enclosed in *De Gay Krant* and *SEK*. It was also distributed to gay bars and discos. The last issue of *AIDS Info* appeared in 1993. In 1994 it was re-launched as a bimonthly magazine named *LUST for LIFE* published under the responsibility of the SAD-Schorer Foundation.

A national cohort study (De Vroome, 1994) showed that *AIDS Info* reached many gay men in the cohort (from 79 per cent in 1986 to 97 per cent in 1989), and that it received the highest ratings (in terms of the usefulness of the information supplied) compared to a wide range of other HIV/AIDS-information sources. With respect to behaviour, this study showed that the frequency of contact with *AIDS Info* was a significant predictor of safer sex.

Small Group Activities

The first group activity that briefly addressed AIDS took place in 1984. It was a five-evening course for gay men on health issues in the broadest sense, including psychosocial aspects. Subjects addressed included STDs, alcohol and drugs, compulsive sex, and promiscuity. Besides trainers from the SAD, representatives from government health institutions – including psychologists from mental health centres – contributed to the course. After being piloted, it was agreed that the course would travel through the Netherlands. Support from regular health institutions in other regions, however, was limited. It was therefore transformed into a weekend course that was offered by the SAD and organized nationally. Over time, the focus of the weekend workshops has narrowed from health issues in the broadest sense, to AIDS and (un)safe sex. The initial workshop has been evaluated. With respect to behaviour change, this evaluation showed that 72 per cent of respondents did not have anal sex in the six-month follow-up period compared to 55 per cent in the six months preceding the workshop (Wennink, 1988). The course ran until 1988.

In 1987 and 1988 the SAD set up a workshop that was an adaptation of the Eroticizing Safe Sex Workshop designed by Gay Men's Health Crisis in

New York. The goals of the workshop were to strengthen positive attitudes towards safer sex as well as to improve negotiating skills with respect to safer sex. The SAD supplied trainers as well as materials (posters and brochures) for the recruitment of participants. A total of 65 workshops with 758 participants were organized nationwide. No process or outcome evaluation results are available. This workshop was succeeded by the Safe Sex Video Show 1.

The Safe Sex Video Show 1 was an intervention developed for small groups, guided by a video that contained information on HIV/AIDS and safer sex. The video also depicted several role plays in real life settings that addressed relevant issues like countering justifications for having unsafe sex, and reactions to meeting an HIV positive sex partner. In this video, education on safer sex included the message to refrain from anal intercourse. However, the video did offer a brief demonstration of condom use. The Safe Sex Video Show was moderated by two experienced trainers who discussed specific themes with participants (knowledge of risks, the consequences of risk information for individual behavioural decisions, and coping with barriers for safer sex). The aim was to create interaction between participants and to have them discuss safer sex, thereby inducing or strengthening group norms that favoured safer sex. From 1988 until 1990, 156 groups with slightly more than 3000 participants were reached nationwide.

No process or effect evaluation results are available. However, the large number of performances of the show suggests that the show was popular, and that it undoubtedly addressed the need for information about HIV/AIDS among gay men. In 1990, the Safe Sex Video Show 1 was succeeded by the Rubber Road Show.

The policy change with respect to the prevention message for gay men led in 1990 to the development of an activity that explicitly addressed condom use in anal sex. In its test phase, it was named The Condom Workshop. The primary goals were to promote the use of condoms when having anal sex, and to provide skill training in the proper use of condoms. Secondary goals were to provide adequate information about risks of anal sex, to discuss barriers to condom use, and to increase knowledge about condoms and condom use. The workshop was led by two trainers, and lasted approximately three hours. At the start of the workshop, participants were explicitly told that refraining from anal sex was the best way of avoiding HIV infection and that the workshop intended to promote (proper) condom use among men who would not or could not refrain from anal sex.

The format of the intervention was similar to the Safe Sex Video Show 1: it consisted of parts of its videotape, together with a talk show and condom use skills training. The Condom Workshop was evaluated through process evaluation as well as outcome evaluation using a pre-test/post-test design (eight workshops with a total of 69 participants; Hoekzema and Dingelstad, 1991). The outcome study looked at changes in knowledge, skills, attitudes and social norms with respect to condom use and sexual behaviours. There were significant changes between pre- and post-test on several items to do with knowledge, skills, attitudes and social norms. The report also described changes towards safer sexual behaviour at the second post-test (two months after the workshop), although no significance levels were provided. Participants were very satisfied with both the content of the training and the expertise of the trainers.

On the basis of this evaluation, the Condom Workshop was modified into The Rubber Road Show which was implemented nationwide. In 1990 and 1991, 35 shows were organized which attracted 446 participants. Participants were recruited through advertisements in a national newspaper and the gay press, and through flyers distributed among local chapters of the Dutch Gay and Lesbian Association. The Rubber Road Show was eventually incorporated in the Safe Sex Videoshow 2.

The Safe Sex Videoshow 2 was launched in 1991 under the name 'In The Heat of the Moment'. The small group format of the Safe Sex Video Show 1 was maintained. A new videotape was developed which was pre-tested by communication experts and health educators. The major differences from the previous video show were the content of the videotape and the way it was used in the programme. In the new videotape, additional topics were addressed such as coping with difficult sexual situations and preventing relapse. The video depicted a number of scenes that each led up to a moment when a decision had to be made to have safer sex or not. At that moment the video was stopped and the trainers discussed with the group what they would do in such a situation. After this discussion, the video showed one viable solution for handling the situation appropriately. In 1991 and 1992 there were 99 shows with 1680 participants. From 1993 until the present the programme has continued to be executed, albeit rather irregularly. The Safe Sex Video Show 2 has been sold to other countries, for example to France and England [2]

'In the Heat of the Moment' was accompanied by a process and effect evaluation that included 33 shows (De Kooning and Sandfort, 1993). The study evaluated effect variables before and immediately after the show (n = 352). A second post-test was conducted three months after the show (n = 166). Effect variables included knowledge, attitudes, self-efficacy, behavioural intentions, and behaviour. There were significant short- and long-term changes in some of the knowledge items, specifically related to risks of several sexual behaviours. Most items on attitudes, and self-efficacy did not show short- and long-term changes in the desired direction. Finally, there were hardly any changes in sexual behaviours between pre-tests and post-tests. The process evaluation showed that participants, on average, were very positive about the content of the show and the quality of the trainers. The majority of men reported that the show made them more aware of their attitudes towards safer sex, one-third of the men said that they could better distinguish safer from unsafe practices, and 20 per cent of respondents reported that participating in the show resulted in less anxiety about HIV infection risks.

Outreach Activities

In 1988, the first prevention project in cruising areas for gay and bisexual men was launched in Utrecht. In 1989 the project was extended to the other major cities in the Netherlands (Amsterdam, Rotterdam, and the Hague). The core activity of the project was to send trained volunteers to cruising areas where they spoke with men in these areas about the importance of safer sex. The major goals of the activity were to disseminate information on safer sex, to reinforce a social norm of safer sex in cruising areas, to provide visitors to cruising areas with solutions to overcome personal barriers to having safer sex in these areas, and finally, to refer visitors to organizations that offer information on HIV and AIDS (for example the AIDS Hot Line) or relevant services (for example condom sale). Based on a survey conducted among these volunteers which assessed their evaluation of the training they had received (Waldhober, 1990a), the intervention was further developed and implemented nationwide. In 1993, the Public Health Services in 15 cities and regions supported a Cruising Area Project.

The projects were supported on a national level by the SAD-Schorer Foundation, which provided materials to recruit volunteers (posters and flyers), extensive training for new volunteers, and, as of 1993, registration forms to be used by the volunteers for each conversation at cruising areas to keep track of the activity. Together with the registration form, a computer program for data entry and data analysis was supplied to project coordinators in each Public Health Service.

All Cruising Area Projects participated in a nationwide process evaluation in 1993 (De Jong, 1994). One part of the evaluation was based on the registration forms, and consisted of an overview of the number of conversations, the topics that were addressed in these conversations, characteristics of cruising area visitors, and self-reported sexual practices in cruising areas. The results show that in 1993 the 78 volunteers approached a total of 2684 men. Slightly more than 10 per cent of these men refused to talk. The topics most frequently addressed in conversations were: HIV/AIDS knowledge including misconceptions about sexual risks, intentions and barriers to having safer sex, and the availability of condoms. With respect to self-reported behaviour, the results show that 68 per cent of visitors had oral sex at cruising areas (77 per cent consistently safe), and that 30 per cent of visitors engaged in insertive and/or receptive anal sex (68 per cent consistently safe).

Since 1983 there have been several initiatives to reach gay men in bars and discos. From 1990 onwards, this outreach activity has become more structured through the creation of Safe Sex Promotion Teams (Waldhober, 1990b). A Safe Sex Promotion Team comprises three to six gay men who give shows at gay bars and discos as well as on special occasions with gay audiences. The act most usually consists of songs, dance, and cabaret with safer sex themes. All members of promotion teams were trained in performing the acts. In addition, they received extensive training in talking with gay men about safer sex after their show. They also distributed safer sex kits containing HIV prevention brochures and condoms. The primary goal of this activity was to support gay men who visited bars and discos with behavioural change towards safer sex, and with the maintenance of safer sex behaviour. Semi-professional artists were used first of all to ensure a high artistic quality of the acts, but also because it was believed that professional acts would increase the likelihood that bar owners would cooperate. Also, the use of performance was believed to be a better method to deal with emotional aspects of safer and unsafe sex. Finally, it was hoped that the active distribution of safer sex materials would reach men who had not been reached by previous safer sex brochures.

Between 1990 and 1994 the Safe Sex Promotion Teams made 229 appearances, reached an estimated 54 000 gay men, distributed over 23 000 safe sex kits, and had over 5000 conversations with gay men about safe sex (Van Stoppelenburg, 1995). The work of the Safe Sex Promotion Teams has not been evaluated in terms of its effects.

Future Directions

The end of 1992 is an important landmark in relation to HIV prevention among gay men in the Netherlands. It coincided with a period in which preparations were made to decentralize primary prevention budgets, including

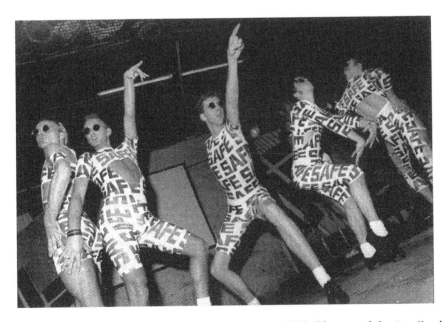

Figure 3.2 *A Safe Sex Promotion Team in action in 1991. Photograph by Jan Carel Warffemius, courtesy of the SAD-Schorer Foundation.*

those related to HIV prevention. Henceforth, budgets for HIV prevention would largely be transferred from national organizations to the local level, and thereafter local Municipal Health Services in the Netherlands became responsible for HIV prevention, including the development and implementation of prevention activities for gay men in their region. All HIV prevention professionals who worked at the national level in several organizations were placed within one organization, namely the SAD-Schorer Foundation. The Prevention Team of the SAD-Schorer Foundation is currently responsible for the development and publication of HIV education brochures. With respect to group activities, their task changed from programme development and programme execution to the provision of support for prevention workers in Public Health Services who are organizing HIV prevention for gay men at the local

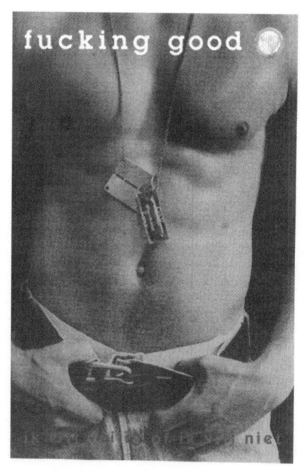

Figure 3.3 *A recent brochure (1994). Courtesy of the SAD-Schorer Foundation.*

level. This reorganization took considerable time since all parties involved had to get accustomed to their new tasks. Organizing adequate HIV prevention at the local level has become the major challenge for the coming years.

With respect to the content of HIV prevention, the focus is shifting towards gay population subgroups, like young gay men, male sex workers, and HIV positive men. There is also an increased focus on sexual behaviour within beginning relationships – especially among young gay men – since recent research has shown heightened levels of unprotected sex with steady partners within relatively short-lasting relationships.

Discussion

Between 1983 and 1993, HIV prevention for gay men in the Netherlands developed into a highly professional field. The fact that there was a strong involvement of gay men in HIV/AIDS policy organizations from the beginning of the epidemic has had several consequences. First of all, this situation permitted representatives of the gay subculture to directly influence prevention policy for gay men, and to contribute directly to intervention development. It further allowed swift responses to be given to changes and new developments in the gay subculture. On the other hand, most gay men involved in HIV prevention have received no training in health education or related disciplines. Therefore, it has taken time and training to develop interventions systematically, based on germane theories and using appropriate methods.

With respect to written materials, there has been a constant effort to inform and update the gay community about HIV/AIDS issues. The concurrent publication of background information on the one hand and materials that summarize the safer sex guidelines on the other hand, has aimed to meet differences in information needs. There now exists a relatively well functioning system to distribute these written materials.

The first group activity that was developed, focused on AIDS within a broader context of (sexual) health. Successive group activities have focused primarily on HIV and AIDS. The Safe Sex Video Show 1 successfully introduced the use of video fragments as a catalytic agent for introspection and discussion in groups. A video format was preserved in both follow-up activities. Over 5000 gay men have participated in these small group activities over the years.

Outreach work in cruising areas has evolved into an intervention that is planned and implemented by health educators and volunteers at the local level, supported by professionals at the national level who assist with recruitment, training, and evaluation. Safe Sex Promotion Teams have reached substantial numbers of gay men and have proven to be a very satisfactory method of disseminating HIV/AIDS information. Recently, two regions in the Netherlands have launched a programme that used the same format. Continuation of these types of outreach activities at the local level ensures that members of the gay community will continue to be informed about HIV prevention.

The wide range of AIDS prevention activities that were described in this chapter – ranging from information brochures to small-group interventions – was in most cases carefully planned. In most instances the intervention goals were made explicit, and development included expert consultation as well as careful pre-testing among target group members. Health education theorists have repeatedly stressed the need for careful and systematic planning if interventions are to be effective (Mullen, Green and Persinger, 1985; Kok, 1991). In general, one has to make sure that relevant determinants of behaviour are addressed by specific intervention methods. The identification of relevant determinants and effective methods emphasizes the indispensable role of theory in intervention development (Fisher and Fisher, 1992; Kelly and Murphy, 1992; Mullen *et al.*, 1995).

However, another vital component of the planning process consists of process and effect evaluations. Process evaluations provide information about the extent to which interventions were carried out as planned and may highlight unforeseen problems with the execution of interventions. Effect evaluations have to examine whether interventions led to changes in behavioural determinants and subsequently to changes of behaviour. Effect evaluations especially have unfortunately received considerably less attention within AIDS prevention intervention research in the Netherlands. Therefore, relatively little is known about the effectiveness of much of the work undertaken. New activities have usually been based on the experiences of those who carried out previous interventions, while evaluation has often been limited to process evaluation. The most likely explanations for the absence of effect evaluation research are time and financial constraints. Fortunately, the recent policy document of the Programme Coordination Committee for AIDS Research (PccAo) explicitly acknowledges this problem. Projects that include effect evaluations, as well as initiatives that focus on the effectiveness of new intervention methods, are now among the priorities on the research agenda for the next few years (PccAo, 1995).

The challenge for the coming years will be to maintain the high quality of HIV prevention for gay men that has been achieved by the continuous efforts of numerous professionals and volunteers in the Netherlands over the past decade.

Notes

1 In the Netherlands, Public Health Services are governed by a number of laws, most importantly the Collective Prevention Act. This Act stipulates that municipalities, either individually or jointly, should provide a Public Health Service. Thus, municipalities own, finance, and control a Public Health Service.

2   In England the videotape was seized by Customs because the scenes were considered to be too explicit; it took a while to convince them that the videotape was meant to be an educational tool.

References

ALGRA, Y. (1988) 'Jack-off parties, een nieuwe methode ter bevordering van de homo-emancipatie en ter voorkoming van AIDS', *Tijdschrift voor Seksuologie*, **12**, pp. 123–6.

FISHER, J.D. and FISHER, W.A. (1992) 'Changing AIDS-risk behavior', *Psychological Bulletin*, **111**, pp. 455–74.

HOEKZEMA, C. and DINGELSTAD, A. (1991) *De Condoomworkshop. Evaluatierapport naar Aanleiding van een Preventie-activiteit van de SAD over Condoomgebruik bij Mannen met Homoseksuele Contacten*, Master Thesis, Utrecht: Universiteit Utrecht.

DE JONG, M. (1994) *Het baanproject. Landelijke Evaluatie 1993*, Amsterdam: SAD-Schorerstichting.

VAN KALMTHOUT, M. (1993) *De Produktie van Voorlichtingsmateriaal over AIDS voor Homomannen*, Amsterdam: Buro GVO.

KELLY, J.A. and MURPHY, D.A. (1992) 'Psychological interventions with AIDS and HIV: Prevention and treatment', *Journal of Consulting and Clinical Psychology*, **60**, pp. 576–85.

KOK, G. (1991) 'Health education theories and research for AIDS prevention', *HYGIE*, **10**, 2, pp. 32–9.

DE KOONING, D. (1992) *Evaluatieonderzoek Aidsfolders 'Homoseks & AIDS' en 'Stand van Zaken'*, Utrecht: Universiteit Utrecht.

DE KOONING, D. and SANDFORT, TH.G.M. (1993) *Verslag Evaluatie-onderzoek Safe Sex Videoshow 2*, Utrecht: Universiteit Utrecht.

VAN DER LINDEN, J. (1984) *AIDS: An Information, Education, and Prevention Project in the Netherlands*, Paper presented at the European AIDS Conference, Amsterdam, 20–22 January 1984.

MULLEN, P.D., GREEN, L.W. and PERSINGER, G. (1985) 'Clinical trials of patient education for chronic conditions: a comparative meta-analysis of intervention types', *Preventive Medicine*, **14**, pp. 753–81.

MULLEN, P.D., EVANS, D., FORSTER, J., GOTTLIEB, N.H., KREUTER, M., MOON, R., O'ROURKE, T. and STRECHER, V.J. (1995) 'Settings as an important dimension in health education/promotion policy, programs, and research', *Health Education Quarterly*, **22**, pp. 329–45.

OUD, R. (1986) *Homocondoom. Een Onderzoek naar de Rol van het Condoom bij het Voorkomen van AIDS*, unpublished report.

PCCAO (1995) *Programma Aidsonderzoek 1995–1997*, Amsterdam: PccAo.

VAN STOPPELENBURG, E. (1995) *Eind-evaluatie Safe Sex Promotieteams*, Amsterdam: SAD-Schorerstichting.

DE VROOME, E.M.M. (1994) *AIDS-voorlichting onder Homoseksuele Mannen*.

Diffussie van Veilig Vrijen in Nederland (1986–1989), Doctoral Thesis, Amsterdam: Thesis Publishers.

WALDHOBER, Q. (1990a) *Op de Baan. Rapportage van een Onderzoek onder Medewerkers aan een Outreaching Voorlichtingsproject over AIDS en Veilig Vrijen onder Mannen met Homoseksuele Contacten*, Amsterdam: Bureau Onderzoek, Tekst & Uitleg.

WALDHOBER, Q. (1990b) *Safe Sex Promotie Teams. Rapportage van een Onderzoek naar een Outreaching Voorlichtingsproject in Homo-uitgaansgelegenheden over AIDS en Veilig Vrijen onder Mannen met Homoseksuele Contacten*, Amsterdam: Bureau Onderzoek, Tekst & Uitleg.

WENNINK, J. (1988) *Resultaten Enquête Deelnemers aan de SAD GVO-cursus AIDS, Gezondheid en Sexualiteit*, unpublished report.

VAN WIJNGAARDEN, J. (1984) *Evaluatie Beleidscoördinatie AIDS*, unpublished report.

DE WIT, J.B.F. (1994) *Prevention of HIV Infection among Homosexual Men. Behavior Change and Behavioral Determinants*, Doctoral Thesis, Amsterdam: Thesis Publishers.

DE ZWART, O. and SANDFORT, TH.G.M. (1993) *'Gebruik een Condoom of Neuk niet'. Een Kwalitatief Onderzoek naar de Wijze waarop de Nevenschikkende Boodschap Kan Worden Vormgegeven*, Utrecht: Universiteit Utrecht.

Chapter 4

AIDS among Injecting Drug Users in the Netherlands: The Epidemic and the Response

Erik van Ameijden and Anneke van den Hoek

This chapter describes, from an international perspective, developments in the magnitude of the drug user population in the Netherlands and the response of the government, the AIDS and HIV epidemic among injecting and non-injecting drug users in the Netherlands, AIDS prevention measures targeted at this group and their evaluation. With regard to prevention and evaluation, the emphasis is on Amsterdam, the only city with high reported HIV prevalence (30 per cent, compared to less than 12 per cent in other cities) where most evaluation studies have been performed. We conclude that the combination of preventive measures taken has been effective in slowing down the development of the HIV epidemic, although HIV transmission still occurs at a moderate level. It is not possible to say which of the measures taken have been the most effective.

The Drug Epidemic and the Response

An increase in hard drug use in the Netherlands started in the early 1970s, the main type of hard drug used being heroin, though polydrug use is common (heroin was often combined with amphetamines in the past, while presently it is often combined with cocaine).

Worldwide, three major policy orientations underlie most programmatic efforts to deal with recreational drug use and drug abuse. These are criminalization, medicalization, and harm reduction. Criminalization seeks to restrict access to psychoactive drugs by placing strict criminal penalties on the possession and sale of drugs and on the possession and distribution of needles and syringes. The sale of needles and syringes without medical prescription may also be prohibited. Medicalization defines the non-medical use of psychoactive drugs as a chronic and relapsing psychiatric or metabolic disease, and prescribes a treatment of the origin. Methadone maintenance, methadone detoxification, and various treatments based on psychiatric principles come into this category. By eliminating withdrawal symptoms, methadone maintenance can reduce the drive to obtain and inject heroin. When combined with other necessary social and psychological supports, methadone treatment can be an important factor in helping to stabilize drug users' lives. A third policy option is harm reduction. Harm reduction programmes may include needle and syringe exchange schemes, bleach distribution, and low-threshold methadone maintenance. Harm reduction programmes acknowledge the often intractable nature of drug use and the frequent propensity for relapse, and seek to reduce undesirable impacts on the individual and society that may result from drug using behaviours (Buning *et al.*, 1986; Brettle, 1991; Des Jarlais, Friedman and Ward, 1993). It is important to note that all three of these policy and programme options predate the discovery of HIV, and both drug treatment and harm reduction efforts have been modified in response to the HIV epidemic (Buning, Van Brussel and Van Santen, 1990; Coutinho and Hartgers, 1992), as described below.

The USA exemplifies a country where criminalization has been the principal policy and where harm reduction efforts are severely restricted by federal and state laws.

Australia, the United Kingdom, and the Netherlands have been leaders in harm reduction. In 1976 in the Netherlands, policies were implemented to separate the markets for and users of soft drugs (for example cannabis products) and hard drugs. Penalties on the possession and sale of soft drugs are smaller. For hard drugs a dual-track policy was adopted: dealing and trafficking are approached from a criminal standpoint, while the use of hard drugs is approached from a health viewpoint. Abstinence remains the first goal, but if a drug user is not able or willing to stop, social and medical care is provided. Though in the Netherlands the emphasis is on harm reduction, criminalization and medicalization also play a role.

Liberal drug policy in the Netherlands has not led to a high number of hard drug (heroin, cocaine, amphetamine) users per inhabitant and the proportion of injectors among drug users is relatively low. This may explain the relatively small impact of injecting drug users in the whole of the AIDS epidemic (see below).

In national prevalence studies, the number of opiate addicts in the late 1980s was estimated at 21 000–25 000 by Driessen (1990), at 15 000–20 000 by De Zwart (1989), and at 30 000 by Stichting Intraval (1995). In general, the number of hard drug users is difficult to estimate (Korf, Reijenveld and Toet, 1994) which may explain the variability in estimates. The number of injecting drug users (IDU) can be estimated to be 8000–12 000 in the Netherlands (population 16 million), which translates to a low rate per inhabitant compared to other European countries (WHO–EC Collaborating Centre on AIDS, 1994a).

As in many countries, most drug users live in the big cities. In Amsterdam, the largest city of the Netherlands (population 700 000), 7500 drug users were estimated to be resident in 1993 (Van Brussel, Van de Woude and Van Lieshout, 1993). This group consisted of 2400 Dutch drug users, of whom about 20–40 per cent inject; 1700 ethnic minority drug users (mainly Surinamese and Antillean people with Dutch nationality), of whom 5 per cent inject; and a very crude estimate of 3400 drug users with other nationality (mainly German and Italian), of whom 70 per cent inject. In total, there may be 2500 persons in Amsterdam who currently inject drugs, leading to an estimated 0.3 per cent of Amsterdam inhabitants being drug injectors. This figure is among the lowest compared to other cities in Europe and elsewhere (WHO Collaborative Study Group, 1993). This may be explained by the introduction of Chinese drug use rituals (chasing the dragon, that is heroin smoking), Surinamese/Antillean drug users having a taboo on the penetration of the skin, the high purity and low price of heroin, as well as fear of HIV and AIDS.

Whereas the number of drug users has not substantially changed over time in Amsterdam, there are some signs to suggest a decrease in parenteral administration of drugs. First, among new entrants to the Amsterdam cohort study (a large longitudinal study among injecting and non-injecting drug users), heroin smoking and cocaine freebasing have increased, though the decrease in injection has not been significant (Hartgers *et al.*, 1991). Second, among drug users newly entering methadone programmes, the proportion currently injecting was only 14 per cent in 1993 (Van Brussel, Van de Woude and Van Lieshout 1993). Last, the mean age of Amsterdam drug users in treatment has increased from 32.9 years in 1989 to 35.6 years in 1993 (WHO–EC Collaborating Centre on AIDS, 1994b). It is unclear whether this means that the scale of the hard drug problem is waning or whether the drug service is having difficulty in establishing contact with new, younger users, especially young persons from the second generation of ethnic minorities.

Comparably low figures have been found for Rotterdam (the second largest city, population 600000). Korf, Reijneveld and Toet (1994) judged the best estimate of the yearly number of opiate users to be about 4400 during 1988–90, whereas another study in 1995 estimated the lower bound of the yearly number of drug users in Rotterdam to be 3500, of whom about 50 per cent were injectors (Wiessing, Houweling and Koedijk, 1995).

In the Netherlands there has not been a crack epidemic as observed in the United States, shown to be strongly associated with the HIV epidemic. However, at present crack is available on the streets (Van Brussel, Van de Woude and Van Lieshout, 1993) and there are some indications of increasing use.

The AIDS Epidemic

The first IDU was diagnosed with AIDS in 1985 in the Netherlands. Through 1994, the cumulative AIDS incidence was 3474, of whom 73 per cent were gay men and only 10 per cent were IDUs. The proportion of IDUs among AIDS cases increased rapidly from 0 per cent in 1982 to 10 per cent in 1988, whereafter it has reached a plateau of about 13 per cent (Table 4.1) (Inspectie voor de Gezondheidszorg, 1995). This proportion is low compared to most other European countries; for instance, in Italy and Spain through 1994, 65 per cent of the cumulative number of AIDS cases were IDUs (WHO–EC Collaborat-

Table 4.1 AIDS diagnoses in the Netherlands by year of diagnosis and in two specific riskgroups, 1982–94

	Total n	Injectors n (%)	Heterosexuals n (%)
1982–84	55	0 (0)	1 (2)
1985	67	1 (1)	1 (1)
1986	136	6 (4)	4 (3)
1987	242	16 (7)	19 (8)
1988	325	34 (10)	16 (5)
1989	391	34 (9)	30 (8)
1990	416	41 (10)	34 (8)
1991	446	43 (10)	45 (10)
1992	516	55 (11)	49 (9)
1993	458	59 (13)	76 (17)
1994	432	54 (13)	86 (20)
Total	3474	343 (10)	361 (10)

Note that before 1982 no AIDS cases were identified and that especially in 1994 the number of AIDS cases may become somewhat higher because of reporting delay.

ing Centre on AIDS, 1994a). This low proportion is probably due to both the low number of IDUs and low HIV infection rates in the Netherlands. From 1993 onwards, more persons with AIDS are likely to be heterosexually infected than parenterally. Among Amsterdam inhabitants, 1603 people cumulatively have been diagnosed with AIDS through December 1994, accounting for half of all AIDS cases in the Netherlands (Bindels and Mulder-Folkerts, 1995). The distribution according to risk groups was not substantially different from the Netherlands as a whole: only 173 (11 per cent) of AIDS cases were IDUs and 94 (6 per cent) were heterosexual non-IDUs.

HIV Prevalence and Incidence among Injecting Drug Users

There is a large geographical variation in HIV seroprevalence levels among IDUs. About 30 per cent of IDUs in Amsterdam are infected, 10 per cent in Rotterdam and Zuid-Limburg (an area in the extreme south of the Netherlands, close to the borders of Belgium and Germany), and in other cities HIV prevalence rates are less than 3 per cent (Table 4.2). This variation is observed even for cities close to one another: Amsterdam, The Hague and Alkmaar are about 30 kilometres apart, the HIV prevalences being 28, 2 and 3 per cent, respectively. These variations are not explained by levels of self-reported risk behaviours, like the sharing of needles (Table 4.2). Explanatory factors may

Table 4.2 HIV prevalences and borrowing of used needles among injecting drug users in cities in the Netherlands

CITY/PLACE	YEAR STUDY	NUMBER STUDIED	HIV PREVALENCE	BORROWING NEEDLES*	REFERENCE
Amsterdam					
Cohort study	1985–88	251	34%	44%	Van den Hoek *et al.*, 1988
Methadone posts	1991	208	23%	na	Hartgers, Van Santen and Van Haastrecht, 1992
Street surveys	1990	199	37%	24%	Fennema *et al.*, 1993c
	1993	198	26%	18%	Fennema *et al.*, 1997b
Surinamese/Antillean	1992	29	17%	na	Fennema *et al.*, 1993b
Rotterdam, extreme problematic drug users	1985	29	3.4%	na	Barends, 1988
Survey Rotterdam	1995	492	11.6%	18%	Wiessing, Houweling and Koedijk, 1995
Den Haag, detoxification centre 'de Weg'	1988	56	1.8%	43%	Haan *et al.*, 1991
Survey Arnhem	1991/2	139	2.2%	42%	Wiessing, Houweling and Van den Akker, 1993
Survey Alkmaar	1991/2	74	2.7%	14%	Korf, Hes and Von Aalderen, 1992
Survey Deventer	1991/2	69	0.0%	8%	Wiessing, Houweling and Van den Akker, 1993
Survey Zuid-Limburg	1994	340	9.7%	19%	Wiessing, Houweling and Meulders, 1995

* during the previous 6 months before interview, among HIV positive and HIV negative drug users who have injected in the preceding 6 months.

include differences in needle sharing networks and selective mixing slowing down the transmission of HIV (Anderson, 1990). Also, HIV may have been introduced at different times in different communities. When HIV is introduced later in time, it is more likely that some risk reduction has taken place before this introduction, moderate levels of risk reduction being sufficient for a substantial slowing down of the HIV epidemic (Des Jarlais, 1994).

In general, HIV prevalences are highest in the south and lowest in the north of Europe. Compared to other European cities, HIV prevalence among Amsterdam IDUs is moderate-to-high (Richardson, Ancelle-Park and Papaevangelou, 1993). The migration of foreign HIV positive IDUs to Amsterdam may partly explain this high prevalence: in Amsterdam, the HIV prevalence among German and southern European IDUs is much higher than among Dutch IDUs (Van den Hoek *et al.*, 1988), but the incidence of new infections appears not to depend upon nationality (Van Ameijden *et al.*, 1992). Another explanatory factor for the high prevalence is that HIV had already spread before awareness of HIV and the adaption of preventive measures (HIV prevalence was already 30 per cent among members of these same groups in 1986).

As in many other cities worldwide (Des Jarlais, Friedman and Choopanya, 1992), HIV has rapidly spread among Amsterdam IDUs. Using stored sera of participants of the cohort study, the HIV incidence peaked around 1983 (Van Haastrecht *et al.*, 1991b). In this same cohort study, HIV incidence strongly declined thereafter, from 9.5 per cent per year in 1986 to 3.3 per cent in 1992 (Van Ameijden *et al.*, 1992). HIV incidence in Rotterdam has remained stable at 4 per cent per year from 1991 through 1994 (Wiessing, Houweling and Koedijk, 1995).

In Amsterdam, the introduction of HIV among IDUs appears to have followed that among homosexual men by about two years (Van Haastrecht *et al.*, 1991b). Because 20 per cent of male IDUs also have a history of sex with other men (Van den Hoek *et al.*, 1991), it was initially hypothesized that HIV was introduced in the IDU population by behaviorally homosexual injectors. However, recent findings show that the HIV strains circulating among IDUs and homosexual men in Amsterdam are genetically different, indicating that HIV was most probably introduced by IDUs who were infected in other countries (Kuiken *et al.*, 1993).

The cumulative HIV incidence has been estimated by projecting the ratio between the number of AIDS cases and the prevalence of HIV infection in the Amsterdam cohort to the number of AIDS cases in Amsterdam as a whole (Van Haastrecht *et al.*, submitted). Approximately 1280 IDUs have acquired HIV infection as of October 1994, of whom 204 have been diagnosed with AIDS, while about 270 had died pre-AIDS. Therefore, the HIV prevalence of IDUs residing in Amsterdam that were still alive and free of AIDS was estimated to be around 800 in 1995. Since the incidence of HIV-related deaths has exceeded the incidence of new infections in recent years, it was concluded that the HIV epidemic among IDUs in Amsterdam is declining. In the same study, the number of HIV positive IDUs living elsewhere in the Netherlands who do not yet have AIDS has been estimated as at least 600. Between 200 and 300 HIV positive IDUs are estimated to live in Rotterdam alone (Wiessing, Houweling and Koedijk, 1995).

Risk Factors for HIV Infection and HIV Risk Behaviours among IDUs

In common with other countries, HIV is mainly transmitted among IDUs in the Netherlands via injection with needles that have already been used by somebody else. Sexual transmission occurs infrequently, as is indicated by the HIV prevalences being below 1.5 per cent among non-injecting heterosexual drug users, both in Amsterdam and other cities (Van Ameijden *et al.*, 1994a; Korf, Hes and Van Aalderen, 1992; Wiessing, Houweling and Koedijk, 1995; Wiessing, Houweling and Meulders, 1995). The one exception is a group of Surinamese and Antillean heterosexual non-injecting drug users in Amsterdam: among 169 persons, 5.2 per cent were infected, though injecting behaviour and homosexual behaviour may have been underreported in the sample due to cultural stigmas associated with these behaviours (Fennema *et al.*, 1993b). Another indication for the infrequent sexual transmission of HIV is that of 66 drug users in the Amsterdam cohort study who seroconverted for HIV, only three had not recently injected, one of them being a homosexual man. Furthermore, sexual behaviours or STD infection were not identified as risk factors for HIV prevalence (Van den Hoek *et al.*, 1988) or HIV incidence (Van Ameijden *et al.*, 1992).

Another transmission route may be frontloading (Grund, Kaplan and Adriaan, 1990), that is dividing drugs using two syringes, although the HIV risk of frontloading seems low relative to needle sharing (Samuels, Vlahov and Anthony, 1991). Shooting galleries do not exist in the Netherlands. At these places, several IDUs rent and use the same needles and syringes, and this almost random mixing is highly efficient for the spread of HIV (Anderson, 1990).

In Amsterdam, Rotterdam and Zuid-Limburg, where HIV prevalence is relatively high (Table 4.2), a number of risk factors for HIV prevalence and needle sharing have been indentified (Fennema *et al.*, 1993c; Hartgers *et al.*, 1992a; Hartgers *et al.*, 1992b; Van den Hoek *et al.*, 1988; Paulussen *et al.*, 1990; Wiessing, Houweling and Koedijk, 1995; Wiessing, Houweling and Meulders, 1995). Risk factors for sexual risk behaviour (for example condom use) have, however, hardly ever been determined. In the Amsterdam cohort, predictors for the incidence of HIV infection have also been established (Van Ameijden *et al.*, 1992). In summary, analyses show that risk factors for HIV prevalence, incidence and needle sharing differ substantially, both between and within cities. Though such differences may partly be explained by differences in study samples and data collection, regional prevention policies should be based not only on an extrapolation of risk factors found in other areas. Differences within cities (even within the Amsterdam cohort study) in risk factors for HIV prevalence, incidence and needle sharing may be explained by many factors. For instance, HIV prevalence is dependent upon HIV incidence, migration, death, and initiation/cessation of injection, among other factors. Furthermore, HIV incidence is determined by injecting and sexual risk behaviour, mixing patterns (who shares with whom) and HIV prevalence (affecting the likelihood of sharing or having sex with an HIV positive person) (Van Ameijden, 1994).

The National Response to HIV and AIDS among IDUs

In this section the basic prevention policy choices in the Netherlands will be compared to those of other industrialized countries. Several countries, including the Netherlands, already had drug treatment and harm reduction efforts before the discovery of HIV. These programmes have been modified in response to the HIV epidemic, including making methadone more accessible and increasing the methadone dose to reduce frequency of injection, expanding informational and outreach campaigns, implementing needle and syringe exchange schemes or needle distribution to increase needle availability, and implementing bleach campaigns to increase needle hygiene.

AIDS prevention campaigns for IDU in the Netherlands have been initiated by drug clinics, the government and private initiatives (for example self-help organizations). A broad distinction can be made between information and education campaigns on safer drug use and sexual contacts, and the creation and expansion of facilities (methadone maintenance, needle exchange, condoms). There are programmes on the national (for example safe sex and information campaigns for the general public) and on the regional/local level (for example outreach targeted at specific groups).

To increase needle availability, the Netherlands has primarily opted for 1:1 exchange in order to prevent needle-stick accidents to the general public by keeping potentially infectious injection equipment off the streets (on a limited scale, some pharmacies also sell needles). Furthermore, through syringe and needle exchanges IDUs can be reached for HIV information/education and for referral to methadone treatment. In 1995 there were at least 58 cities with 122 needle exchange locations in the Netherlands (Mainline, 1995). In some other countries (such as France and Italy), the policy of choice has been needle distribution by the liberalization of syringe vending in pharmacies (Ingold and Toussirt, 1993). In countries with a strong record of criminalization of IDUs (such as the USA), not needle availability but needle cleaning (by the use of bleach) has been promoted in several cities.

Whereas some countries have a long history of prescribing methadone (United Kingdom, Switzerland, the Netherlands), others are in the middle of a process of expanding or developing methadone services (Spain, Germany,

Belgium) (Buning, 1994). By 1994, there were also European countries where the provision of methadone is very limited (France, Norway), or forbidden (Greece). A previous study gives a detailed comparison between methadone maintenance programmes in the Netherlands and other countries with regard to type of dispensing practices, dose- and time-limits for prescribing methadone, programme entry criteria, staffing, integration with other services, and urine testing (Gossop and Grant, 1991). Since the 1970s in the Netherlands, methadone has been regarded as a major preventive and treatment option, and since 1984 methadone has been distributed to a reasonably constant number of at least 12000 drug users (about 70 per cent of all heroin users), of which about 9000 are in maintenance and 3000 in withdrawal programmes (Driessen, 1990).

A last important example of differences between countries concerns HIV testing and counselling policy. Testing and counselling may not only reduce HIV risk (for example IDUs who test positive may reduce HIV risk in order not to infect others), but are also important for the appropriate timing of early treatment of HIV infection. The United States and Sweden are examples of countries where this measure is the cornerstone of HIV prevention. In the Netherlands it is available but not actively promoted, as there were initial serious doubts about the benefits of early treatment (which is changing now) and much weight has been given to the possible adverse effects of knowledge of HIV seropositivity (for example stress, anxiety, discrimination).

More information on Dutch prevention programmes for IDUs in an international perspective is given elsewhere (Van Ameijden, 1994; Van Ameijden, Van den Hoek and Coutinho, 1994; Van Ameijden *et al.*, 1994a; Van Ameijden *et al.*, 1994b; Van Ameijden *et al.*, 1995). In the following section, AIDS prevention in Amsterdam will be described in depth, as about one-third of all injecting and non-injecting drug users in the Netherlands reside there, and as a thorough evaluation of AIDS prevention measures targeted at IDUs has only been carried out in Amsterdam. Prevention in other parts of the Netherlands is comparable though less extensive.

Specific AIDS Prevention Measures for IDUs in Amsterdam

In Amsterdam, prevention measures all operate within the concept of harm reduction and participation in all programmes is voluntary. The Amsterdam methadone programmes have attracted considerable international attention. This programme is one of the oldest in the world and, although it was originally not aimed at AIDS prevention, it may also reduce injection frequency and needle and syringe sharing and includes an extensive care system with the ambulatory dispersion of methadone to heroin users. Via this system the Amsterdam Municipal Health Service aims to reach problematic drug users and special groups (drug using sex workers, people from other countries, users in prisons), general practitioners aim at 'regulated' drug users and the CAD (alcohol and drugs advice agency) mainly aims at a relatively small group of drug users who are willing to stop the use of hard drugs other than methadone and undergo urinalysis to control for use of drugs other than methadone (Reijneveld, 1992). There are three corresponding levels of treatment: at the lowest level is the methadone bus system, the middle level the methadone clinics and general practitioners, and the highest level the drug detoxification clinics (Coutinho and Hartgers, 1992). The low-threshold maintenance programmes are meant to contact as many drug users as possible. In practice, this means that the use of drugs other than methadone is permitted, one can easily leave and re-enter the programmes (there are no waiting lists) and methadone is given out at several places (also by mobile buses) (Buning, Van Brussel and Van Santen, 1990). As a result of this approach, it is estimated that 60 to 70 per cent of the drug users in Amsterdam are reached by the various types of programmes. Relatively low maintenance doses have been provided to try to stabilize drug users' lives and as soon as the client is willing to refrain from illegal drug use (which remains the first goal), the client can 'graduate' to other methadone programmes with a higher threshold. Because of the convincing evidence that higher dosages are necessary to reduce injecting behaviour, the mean dose has been increased from 40 mg in 1990 to 54 mg in 1993 (Van Brussel, Van de Woude and Van Lieshout, 1993). Other opiates (that is injectable morphine (Derks, 1990), dextromoramide (palfium)) have been provided to a few long-term drug users as an experiment.

Internationally, the first needle exchange programme was initiated in Amsterdam in 1985 at the instigation of a drug users' organization, the Junkie Union. In 1995, one million needles and syringes were provided, return rates being about 90 per cent. The absence of registration, the various locations at which to exchange equipment (14 in 1992, operated by governmental and non-governmental organizations, including methadone posts) and the large numbers of needles that can be exchanged, ensure a low threshold. At the 'Regenboog', an organization where 50 per cent of all needles are exchanged, sterilized water, alcohol swabs, ascorbic acid and spoons are sold at low prices. We crudely estimated that in the early 1990s about half of the necessary new needles were obtained via an exchange programme, while the remainder were bought in medical shops, some pharmacies, small shops in the red light district, on the streets or from dealers. In general, new injection equipment is relatively easy to obtain in Amsterdam. Frequent, long-term injectors in particular attend the exchange programmes (Hartgers *et al.*, 1992a). At night, when the exchanges are all closed, needles/syringes are sold on a small scale via a vending machine in which used equipment can be disposed of.

HIV testing and counselling have not actively been promoted in Amsterdam (see above), though there are anonymous (no registration) testing facilities in Amsterdam at the Municipal Health Service and at the STD clinics. Additionally, physicians may occasionally test IDUs for HIV infection. In the

Amsterdam cohort study among newly entering IDUs, the proportion who already had a prior HIV test result gradually increased from 29 per cent in 1989 to 59 per cent in 1994 (Langendam, Van Ameijden and Van den Hoek, 1995). Of 200 Amsterdam IDUs recruited on the streets in 1993 and who had never participated in the Amsterdam cohort study, 60 per cent had had a prior HIV test (Fennema, personal communication). In the cohort study itself, about 600 IDUs received their test results between 1985 and 1995 as a result of participating in the study. These figures may overestimate the proportion tested, as they are probably based on longer term and easily accessible injectors. Partner notification of partners of IDUs who tested HIV positive is not practised in Amsterdam (Bindels *et al.*, 1992). Only the contacts of heterosexual, non-injecting index patients are notified.

The information campaigns in Amsterdam offer a clear example of harm reduction. For instance, in leaflets (available in various languages) safe injection rules are given, but it is stressed that the injection of drugs is a risky method of drug administration. Furthermore, cleaning syringes by boiling for five minutes or rinsing with bleach are recommended *only* when new equipment is not available. In Amsterdam, bleach itself is not actively distributed. On a limited scale there are outreach activities, providing information and education (for example streetcorner workers).

As STDs are highly prevalent among Amsterdam IDUs and may facilitate the sexual transmission of HIV (Van den Hoek, Van Haastrecht and Coutinho, 1989), STD control is an important part of AIDS prevention. Condom use is promoted to prevent sexual transmission of both HIV and STD. With respect to STD, case finding, adequate diagnosis and treatment are important. The STD clinics in Amsterdam are operated by the Municipal Health Service and also have a low threshold: STD check-ups and treatments are free of charge, appointments are not necessary and any name may be used. Contact tracing is done for all STD clinic patients with gonorrhoea, early syphilis and chlamydial infection.

The general goal of the Passer-by and Prostitution Project (PPP, part of the Municipal Health Service) is to give social and medical care to drug using sex workers, illegal non-Dutch drug users and drug users who are not registered as an inhabitant of Amsterdam, these groups having a substantial overlap (Gemeentelijke Geneeskundige en Gezondheidsdient Amsterdam, 1993). For these groups, there is a restricted methadone policy, that is methadone is only given on medical indications or within the scope of repatriation. Next to this, examination and treatment for STDs and the prevention of unwanted pregnancies have a high priority. For STD management, until recently there was close collaboration with a special STD clinic for drug using sex workers (this clinic was closed in 1996 because the number of STDs diagnosed dropped dramatically). Methadone enables sex workers who have an STD to stop working for a while, and methadone could be withheld for drug using sex workers in methadone programmes who did not attend this clinic regularly. This special clinic in itself was also low-threshold (location in the centre of

Amsterdam, open every Wednesday evening, treatment regardless of illegality and insurance, free condoms available).

Evaluation of Preventive Measures Targeted at IDUs

The vast majority of evaluation studies performed in the Netherlands are observational. There have been no randomized trials and only a few small-scale experiments without a control group. As will be discussed, observational studies may suffer from several methodological shortcomings (Van Ameijden, 1994; Van Ameijden, Van den Hoek and Coutinho, 1994; Van Ameijden *et al.*, 1994a; Van Ameijden *et al.*, 1994b; Van Ameijden *et al.*, 1995). Another problem is that evaluation has tended to start only after the implementation of key interventions. Nearly all evaluation studies among drug users in the Netherlands have been performed in Amsterdam linked to the cohort study. Still, several generalizable conclusions can be drawn.

Evidence from Surveillance

Although causality cannot be established in surveillance studies, one source of compelling evidence for the effectiveness of AIDS prevention measures targeted at IDUs comes from Dutch cities where HIV prevalences among IDUs have remained very low despite the introduction of HIV (Table 4.2). In the absence of formal HIV prevention campaigns and knowledge of HIV/AIDS, many cities have shown an increase in HIV prevalence of 20 per cent or more within one year (Des Jarlais, Friedman and Choopanya, 1992). Prevention efforts appear most effective if implemented when HIV rates were still relatively low.

In cities with high HIV prevalence among IDUs, evidence for the effectiveness of prevention programmes is harder to establish using surveillance data. It is crucial that data on trends over time are available, which is only the case for Amsterdam. In Amsterdam, HIV prevalence remained stable at about 30 per cent from 1986 through 1992 among new entrants to the open cohort study, subjects being mainly recruited via methadone maintenance programmes and an STD clinic for drug using sex workers. HIV prevalence was already 30 per cent when AIDS prevention started. The annual HIV incidence strongly declined from 10 per cent in 1986 to 3 per cent in 1992 (Van Ameijden *et al.*, 1992). Self-reported injecting risk behaviour strongly diminished, both at the individual level (Van den Hoek, Van Haastrecht and Coutinho, 1989) and community-wide (Van Ameijden, Van den Hoek and Coutinho, 1994) level. In Amsterdam as a whole, acute hepatitis B among IDUs also declined (Van Haastrecht *et al.*, 1991a). In the cohort study, the incidence of seroconversion for hepatitis B and C virus remained stable and high at 10 per cent per year, though estimates were crude owing to small numbers (Van Ameijden *et al.*, 1993). Heroin smoking and cocaine freebasing increased in the later intake groups in the cohort, which may also have had a favourable preventive effect for the transmission of HIV (Hartgers *et al.*, 1991). However, the rate of initiation of injecting remained stable (Van Ameijden *et al.*, 1994b). The decrease in sexual risk behaviour was also large: the number of partners decreased and condom use increased, both with regard to sex worker (Van Ameijden *et al.*, 1994a) and non-sex worker partners (Van Ameijden, Van den Hoek and Coutinho, in press). Also, among drug using sex workers the incidence of self-reported (Van Ameijden *et al.*, 1994a) and diagnosed (Fennema *et al.*, 1997a) STDs declined.

Such surveillance studies may be subject to several potential sources of bias, but biases do not appear sufficient to explain the observed trends (Van Ameijden, 1994). Briefly, the main reason for our confidence that a risk reduction has occurred stems from the consistency of results across studies, in spite of using different outcome measures (HIV prevalence and incidence, injecting and sexual behaviour), different designs (individual follow-up, serial cross-sectional) and different study populations. For instance, the decrease in self-reported risk behaviours may be explained by an increase in socially desirable answering, but self-reported risk reductions were corroborated by objective outcomes (HIV incidence, STD incidence). Also, in several studies trends were determined using only intake visits in the cohort study, thereby eliminating the possible effect of participation in the cohort study itself on behaviour change and on socially desirable responses. Another example of possible bias is the exhaustion effect, that is IDUs with the highest risk behaviours quickly acquire HIV infection and ultimately die of AIDS, leaving a group with lower HIV incidence and risk behaviour. Substantial bias due to exhaustion appears unlikely as new participants are included in the cohort every year and as the rate of initiation of injection was high and stable within the cohort study (Van Ameijden *et al.*, 1994b), new injectors having the highest HIV incidence (Van Ameijden *et al.*, 1992). Another problem may be that the study population has changed in time; groups of HIV positive and negative IDUs are dynamic owing to the initiation and cessation of injection, mortality and migration. However, in most studies trends were statistically adjusted for changes in demographic characteristics and behavioral variables. In general, it is highly unlikely that the large declines in HIV incidence and HIV risk behaviours can be explained by these possible biases.

Apart from AIDS prevention measures targeted at drug users, there may be alternative explanations for the observed risk reductions. First, it may be that behavioral change is part of a long-term secular trend that started before the implementation of any programme (that is before 1985). With regard to needle sharing, this appears not to be the case, as sharing was highly prevalent in the early 1980s and acute hepatitis B started to decline only after 1985 (Van Haastrecht *et al.*, 1991a). Decreases in sexual risk behaviour and STD incidence may be part of a trend, as the incidence of gonorrhoea and syphilis were already decreasing before 1985 (Van de Laar *et al.*, 1990; Treurniet and Davidse, 1993). STD control programmes have existed for decades in the

Netherlands and the STD prevalence is extremely low now. A second alternative may be that, in the absence of formal prevention programmes, IDUs would also have reduced risk behaviour on their own initiative after learning about AIDS (for example via the 'lay press'). However, many other studies have shown that knowledge alone is not sufficient for a sustained and large behavioral change (Hartgers, 1992; Des Jarlais, Friedman and Choopanya, 1992). It appears that at the very least the means for behavioral change (sterile injection equipment, condoms) have to be present for IDUs to allow them to change their behaviour.

For these reasons we conclude that the combination of preventive measures taken in Amsterdam has slowed down the spread of HIV infection among IDUs.

It is important to recognize that the Amsterdam approach is no precondition for behavioral change. Other cities, including San Francisco, New York, Edinburgh and Geneva, with different prevention activities, have seen large risk reductions (Van Ameijden *et al.*, 1995). Even with the large decline, the HIV incidence within the Amsterdam cohort study in Amsterdam of two to three per 100 person years in 1995 is still high, and comparable to rates found in other studies.

Evidence from Studies Evaluating Specific Interventions

Since AIDS prevention resources are scarce it is critical to identify those interventions with the greatest likelihood of success. Table 4.3 summarizes findings from the Amsterdam studies in which an intervention was associated with an outcome. For details we refer readers to the original articles. In summary, strong evidence for effectiveness was found for HIV testing and counselling, some for needle and syringe exchange programmes, and none for methadone programmes. (Although methadone programmes may prevent new HIV infections, AIDS prevention is not a primary goal of these programmes.) At first sight, these weak results seem to contradict the above conclusion that the combination of measures is effective. The finding that both attenders and non-attenders of methadone and needle exchange programmes strongly reduced injecting risk behaviour, illustrates the complexity of evaluation of specific interventions (Van Ameijden, Van den Hoek and Coutinho, 1994). We think this is mainly caused by non-attenders not being an appropriate control group in the comparison with attenders owing to: 1) contamination of the control group (for example non-attenders may be provided with needles and AIDS information by attenders and norms and attitudes may have changed in general); 2) high availability of needles and syringes by means other than the needle exchange; and 3) self-selection bias (methadone and exchange programmes may have attracted relatively high-risk IDUs, for example exchanging seems to be determined by social and financial motives (Hartgers, Van Santen and Van Haastrecht, 1992).

Table 4.3 Summary of results of observational studies in the Amsterdam cohort study among drug users with regard to effectiveness of three AIDS prevention measures

Preventive measure:	HIV testing + counselling	Needle exchange programme	Daily methadone treatments	Reference
Outcome variable:				
HIV prevalence	na	na	–	Hartgers et al., 1992c
HIV incidence	na	+/–	–	Van Ameijden et al., 1992
Injecting risk behavior	˙+	+/–	–	Van Ameijden, Van den Hoek and Coutinho, 1994
Starting to inject	+/–	na	–	Van Ameijden et al., 1994b
Sexual risk behaviour with clients	++	na	–	Van den Hoek, Van Haastrecht and Coutinho, 1990; Van Ameijden et al., 1994a
Sexual risk behaviour, with private partners	++	na	na	Van den Hoek, Van Haastrecht and Coutinho, 1990; Van Ameijden, Van den Hoek and Coutinho, in press
Mortality before AIDS diagnosis	na	–	–	Van Haastrecht et al., 1996

Body of evidence for effectiveness for specific intervention:
– none; +/– little; + strong; ++ very strong; na not applicable/not done

In fact, the finding that non-attenders of intervention programmes also reduced HIV risk is exactly what one would expect from the concept of harm reduction, as this is a community-wide approach which can affect all IDUs. Intervention at the community level and the low threshold of services may provide an explanation for discordant results of evaluation studies in non-Dutch countries. For instance, the effectiveness of needle exchange can more easily be demonstrated in an area where needles are scarce. Also, one would expect methadone programmes to be more protective when there are a limited number of treatment slots, stringent entry criteria with waiting lists and enforced abstinence from drugs via random urine testing practices not implemented in the Netherlands.

In summary, the evaluation of specific measures appeared to be very difficult in Amsterdam with the data available. A more complete discussion of biases and other issues associated with this topic can be found elsewhere, both for Amsterdam and in general (Van Ameijden, 1994; Van Ameijden *et al.*, 1995; Booth and Watters, 1994).

Potential for the Spread of HIV from IDUs to the General Population

IDUs may be important for the spread of HIV to non-IDUs, as a substantial proportion of HIV infected and non-infected IDUs are heterosexually active (Hartgers *et al.*, 1992d; Van den Hoek, Van Haastrecht and Coutinho, 1990; Wiessing, Houweling and Koedijk, 1995). Vaginal intercourse is the most widespread sexual practice in all types of heterosexual relationships. Condom use varies with respect to the type of sexual partnership, from steady, to occasional, to sex for payment relations. In Rotterdam, 9, 53 and 79 per cent consistent condom use was reported, in each of these relationships respectively (Wiessing, Houweling and Koedijk, 1995).

Sexual behaviour surveys in several countries suggest a high potential for a further spread of HIV from IDUs to the non-drug using heterosexual population. In an early Amsterdam study among drug using prostitutes in 1989, of whom 30 per cent were HIV positive, 81 per cent had contracted one or more STD in the previous six months (Van den Hoek *et al.*, 1989). The presence of an STD may facilitate transmission of HIV and indicates HIV risk behaviour. Of HIV positive IDUs in Amsterdam, who were all aware of HIV serostatus, about 20 per cent put others at risk of HIV infection through unsafe sex (Hartgers *et al.*, 1992d), more than half of their sexual partners having never injected. In Rotterdam, of HIV positive IDUs, 12 per cent have a non-injecting steady partner and, in total, 42 per cent of HIV infected IDUs have unprotected sexual contact with one or more partners, though some of these partners may also be HIV positive and inject drugs (Wiessing, Houweling and Koedijk, 1995). In Zuid-Limburg comparable results were found (Wiessing, Houweling and Meulders, 1995).

Due to the larger number of clients compared to private partners, HIV transmission via sex work contacts may be relatively more important. For Amsterdam drug using sex workers, the mean number of unprotected client contacts was about 10 per month in 1992 and it was estimated that 25 men become infected with HIV each year via sex with these Amsterdam sex workers (Van Ameijden *et al.*, 1994a).

Despite this potentially high risk, there are no indications that IDUs contribute substantially to the HIV epidemic in the non-drug using, heterosexual population.

First, of the 3474 AIDS cases in the Netherlands diagnosed through December 1994, only 361 (10 per cent) were heterosexually infected with HIV and of these 361, only 9 per cent reported having had sex with an IDU (40 per cent originated, or had had a sexual partner, from an AIDS endemic country).

There is no evidence that the proportion infected via IDUs is increasing over time. The same picture is found for Amsterdam separately: 94 (6 per cent) of 1603 AIDS cases were judged to be heterosexually infected, and 14 per cent of these 94 reported sex with an IDU. Internationally, these percentages are relatively low. For instance, about 40 per cent of heterosexual AIDS cases in Italy were presumably infected via IDU.

Second, HIV surveillance in several non-IDU subgroups show low HIV prevalence rates. Among pregnant women in the Amsterdam region during 1988–91, 27 (0.12 per cent) of 22 165 were HIV positive, of whom 17 were of non-Dutch nationality (Bindels, Mulder-Folkerts and Boer, 1994). Of 213 male clients of female sex workers in Amsterdam, one (0.5 per cent) was HIV infected, this man having a history of homosexual behaviour (Van Haastrecht *et al.*, 1993). Among 201 female sex workers without a history of injecting drugs, three (1.5 per cent) were infected, who all originated from AIDS endemic countries (Van Haastrecht *et al.*, 1993). Among heterosexual attenders of the STD clinic in Amsterdam without a history of injection, HIV seroprevalence remained stable and below 1 per cent, and 20 of 23 HIV infected heterosexuals were not Dutch (Fennema *et al.*, 1995). In Rotterdam, heterosexual attenders of the STD clinic also exhibited an HIV prevalence below 1 per cent (Willems, Postema and Van der Meijden, 1993).

Thus, migration and travel seem to play a more important role in heterosexual transmission than sexual contacts with IDUs. This is in contrast with the perceived high levels of sexual risk behaviour of IDUs. A recent study in the Amsterdam cohort suggests a possible explanation (Van Ameijden, Van den Hoek and Coutinho, 1994). It appeared that sexual risk behaviour was too crudely studied. Though overall levels of risk remained high and stable with regard to non-clients, in specific high risk groups large sexual risk reductions were observed. For instance, condom use only increased strongly among IDUs who knew themselves to be HIV positive and among IDUs who knew themselves to be negative but who had had a known HIV positive partner. Apart from condom use being highest in highest risk relationships (non-random condom use), partner choice appeared to be selective (non-random mixing): injectors more often had injecting partners, HIV positives more often had HIV positive partners, and so on. This so-called like-with-like mixing strongly diminishes the risk for further sexual transmission of HIV within IDUs and from IDUs to the population more generally (Anderson, 1990).

Discussion

Because of methodological shortcomings of evaluation studies, proof of a causal effect of specific preventive measures is not available. Carefully constructed, controlled studies that include random assignment could, theoretically, produce findings that permit direct attribution of causal effect. In reality, such studies are nearly impossible to implement, as they are expensive, take a long time to complete and are subject to other logistical, ethical and methodo-logical problems. Therefore, it is important not to wait for such proof before implementing prevention programmes, the rationale being that several combi-nations of programmes are effective and that HIV can rapidly spread in the absence of such interventions.

Because of drawbacks linked to the evaluation of specific measures, sur-veillance may be a superior means of providing insight into the effectiveness of intervention efforts. Serial cross-sectional studies are capable of measuring the effects of complex, multifaceted interventions that seek to impact on entire communities. To make a careful interpretation of surveillance data possible, data-collection has to be started before the implementation of interventions and a large variety of outcome variables have to be used, including data on the composition of IDU populations, changes in various risk and drug using prac-tices, infection rates, the demographics of the IDUs sampled, mortality, mor-bidity, migration and population sizes.

Even in communities with relatively rich AIDS prevention activities, and among many well informed individuals who have received drug treatment, HIV testing and counselling and who have easy access to sterile needles and syringes, risk behaviour has not been eliminated. This is best illustrated by HIV seroconversion within the Amsterdam cohort in spite of the high use of needle exchange programmes (42 per cent obtained needles exclusively via exchanging), methadone maintenance (61 per cent reported daily treatments), HIV testing and counselling, and a high level of knowledge on HIV/AIDS (Van Ameijden *et al.*, 1992). A substantial residue of risk still remains: in Amsterdam, while HIV incidence has stabilized at two to three per 100 person years, 20 per cent of IDUs still report borrowing used needles in a six-month period. There may therefore be some level of risk behaviour that cannot be prevented by existing measures which may stem from a variety of environmen-tal, life-situational and psychological factors. Further risk reduction may not be possible without new and more rigorous interventions. However, a more optimistic view is that a prolonged period of time is required before the ultimate effect of preventive measures is reached. Preliminary data show that decreases in injecting risk behaviour have levelled off and reached a plateau.

In high HIV prevalence areas, such as Amsterdam, it appears difficult to achieve risk reduction of a magnitude that is sufficient to significantly reduce HIV prevalence. However, at present the number of AIDS and non-AIDS deaths among HIV positive Amsterdam IDUs exceeds the number of IDUs newly infected with HIV. Nevertheless, because of the episodic and relapsing nature of drug use and risk behaviour, efforts need to be sustained. This applies in both low- and high-prevalence areas. With regard to extension of Dutch AIDS prevention measures targeted at IDUs, possibilities include short, medium, and long-term strategies.

A short-term, low-cost policy can be the improvement of existing preven-tion programmes with regard to service delivery and their contact with drug users. Existing measures may be made more efficient when they are targeted at high risk groups. For instance, in Amsterdam new injectors have been found to be at highest risk of acquiring HIV infection and there appears to be a high rate of recruitment of new injectors. Therefore, it is very important that educational and other interventions are suitable both for new recruits and for those with a long history of drug injection. New injectors might be reached via the methadone and syringe exchange programmes when the threshold is kept low, although outreach may also be necessary.

A medium-term policy is to implement new prevention measures, which will often be more expensive than improving existing programmes. In the Netherlands, HIV testing and counselling is possible but not actively promoted. However, the strongest indications for effectiveness were found for this intervention, for lowering levels of both sexual and injecting risk behaviour (Van Ameijden *et al*, 1995; Langendam, Van Ameijden and Van den Hoek, 1995). Therefore, more active testing may lead to a reduction in parenteral and sexual transmission of HIV, both within IDUs and from IDUs to the population. Via contact tracing, non-IDUs can be identified who are infected by sexual contact with IDUs, thereby preventing further HIV transmission.

A substantial number of IDUs who are in methadone maintenance continue to inject heroin and/or cocaine. This is one of the reasons why in 1995 the National Health Council's Committee on Medicinal Intervention in Drug Addiction advised the Dutch Minister of Health to initiate an experiment for the prescription of heroin to 300 to 500 drug users at three to five sites. This only concerns heavily addicted persons with a long history of drug use who are not willing or able to refrain from drug use. This may lower HIV risk because of stabilization of drug users' lives, lowering the injection frequency in risky settings, and reducing the need to sell sex in order to be able to purchase heroin.

We do not recommend the distribution of bleach to clean used syringes in the Netherlands, an area where needle availability is high. Bleach appears difficult to use in practice and there are no indications for field effectiveness (Van Ameijden *et al*., 1995).

A long-term strategy is the prevention of initiation into drug injecting and encouraging current injectors to cease the practice. Unfortunately, this appears difficult. In Amsterdam, high and stable rates of initiation into injecting have been found, despite HIV education, methadone treatments and HIV testing and counselling. Among Amsterdam drug users who had stopped injecting for one year or more, 70 per cent had started injecting again at five years of follow-up (Van Ameijden *et al*., 1994b). It is crucial for the future course of the HIV epidemic among IDUs to develop methods to reach new initiates into injection with prevention activities, to prevent initiation of injecting among non-injectors, and to promote the cessation of injection. Prevention of drug use itself is a broader goal. This should start in early adolescence or childhood. However, there has always been and there will probably always be a group of individuals in the population who use drugs. Also, it may be that large-scale community changes are necessary to prevent drug use, because of its multiple linkages with family situation, poverty, unemployment and homelessness.

As the eradication of drug injecting is an unlikely outcome and HIV prevalence rates are expected to remain high in several areas in the next decade, prevention targeted at sexual behaviour change and STD control remain important. Though presently there are no indications of a major and/ or growing heterosexual HIV epidemic in the Netherlands, the sexual transmission of HIV both among IDUs and from IDUs to their non-IDU sexual partners may well increase. The continued monitoring of HIV prevalence among non-drug using heterosexual populations with a high HIV risk, such as STD patients, will therefore remain important.

References

VAN AMEIJDEN, E.J.C. (1994) *Evaluation of AIDS prevention measures among drug users: the Amsterdam experience*, Doctoral Thesis, Amsterdam: Universiteit van Amsterdam.

VAN AMEIJDEN, E.J.C., VAN DEN HOEK, J.A.R. and COUTINHO, R.A. (1994) 'A substantial decline in injecting risk behaviour among drug users in Amsterdam from 1986 to 1992, and its relationship to AIDS-prevention programs', *American Journal of Public Health*, **84**, pp. 275–81.

VAN AMEIJDEN, E.J.C., VAN DEN HOEK, J.A.R. and COUTINHO, R.A. (in press) 'Large declines in sexual risk behavior with non-commercial partners among heterosexual injection drug users in Amsterdam, 1989–1995', *American Journal of Epidemiology*.

VAN AMEIJDEN, E.J.C., VAN DEN HOEK, J.A.R., VAN HAASTRECHT, H.J.A. and COUTINHO, R.A. (1992) 'The harm reduction approach and risk factors for HIV seroconversion in injecting drug users, Amsterdam', *American Journal of Epidemiology*, **136**, pp. 236–43.

VAN AMEIJDEN, E.C.J., VAN DEN HOEK, J.A.R., MIENTJES, G.H.C. and COUTINHO, R.A. (1993) 'A longitudinal study on the incidence and transmission patterns of HIV, HBV and HCV infection among drug users in Amsterdam', *European Journal of Epidemiology*, **9**, pp. 255–62.

VAN AMEIJDEN, E.J.C., VAN DEN HOEK, J.A.R., VAN HAASTRECHT, H.J.A. and COUTINHO, R.A. (1994a) 'Trends in sexual behaviour and the incidence of sexually transmitted diseases and HIV among drug using prostitutes, Amsterdam 1986–1992', *AIDS*, **8**, pp. 213–21.

VAN AMEIJDEN, E.J.C., VAN DEN HOEK, J.A.R., HARTGERS, C and COUTINHO, R.A. (1994b) 'Risk factors for the transition from non-injecting to injecting drug use and accompanying AIDS risk behaviour in a cohort of drug users', *American Journal of Epidemiology*, **139**, pp. 1153–63.

VAN AMEIJDEN, E.J.C., WATTERS, J.K., VAN DEN HOEK, J.A.R. and COUTINHO,

R.A. (1995) 'Interventions among injecting drug users: do they work?', *AIDS*, **9** Supplement A, pp. s75–s84.

ANDERSON, R.M. (1990) 'The significance of sexual partner contact networks for the transmission dynamics of HIV', *Journal of Acquired Immune Deficiency Syndrome*, **3**, pp. 417–29.

BARENDS, W. (1988) 'Routinematig HIV-onderzoek in een Rotterdams methadonprogramma', *Medisch Contact*, **43**, pp. 58–60.

BINDELS, P. and MULDER-FOLKERTS, D. (1995) 'AIDS-patiënten gemeld in Amsterdam: Kwartaal overzicht nummer 23', *AIDS-surveillance Amsterdam*, Amsterdam: GG & GD.

BINDELS, P.J., MULDER-FOLKERTS, D.K. and BOER, K. (1994) 'The HIV-prevalence among pregnant women in the Amsterdam region (1988–1991)', *European Journal of Epidemiology*, **10**, pp. 331–8.

BINDELS, P.J.E., HENQUET, C.J.M., VAN DEN HOEK, J.A.R., LEENTVAAR-KUIJPERS, A. and COUTINHO, R.A. (1992) 'Het waarschuwen van huidige en vroegere seksuele partners van met HIV geïnfecteerde personen: is de tijd er rijp voor?', *Nederlands Tijdschrift voor de Geneeskunde*, **136**, pp. 933–7.

BOOTH, R.E. and WATTERS, J.K. (1994) 'How effective are risk-reduction interventions targeting injecting drug users?', *AIDS*, **8**, pp. 1515–24.

BRETTLE, R.P. (1991) 'HIV and harm reduction for injecting drug users', *AIDS*, **5**, pp. 125–36.

VAN BRUSSEL, G.H.A., VAN DE WOUDE, D.H. and VAN LIESHOUT, S.J.M. (1993) 'Werkt het Amsterdamse sociaal-medische drugshulpbeleid?', Jaarbericht van de drugsafdeling GG & GD waarin opgenomen de jaarcijfers '93, Amsterdam: GG & GD, Sector GGZ.

BUNING, E.C. (1994) 'Methadone in Europe', *International Journal of Drug Policy*, **5**, pp. 221–5.

BUNING, E.C., VAN BRUSSEL, G.H.A. and VAN SANTEN, G. (1990) 'The methadone by bus project in Amsterdam', *British Journal of Addiction*, **85**, pp. 1247–50.

BUNING, E.C., COUTINHO, R.A., VAN BRUSSEL, G.H.A., VAN SANTEN, G.W. and ZADELHOFF, A.W. (1986) 'Preventing AIDS in drug addicts in Amsterdam', *Lancet*, **i**, p. 1435.

COUTINHO, R.A. and HARTGERS, C. (1992) 'AIDS and drug abuse treatment: the value of methadone maintenance', *Current Opinion in Psychiatry*, **5**, pp. 426–9.

DERKS, J. (1990) *Het Amsterdamse morfine verstrekkingsprogramma: een longitudinaal onderzoek onder extreem problematische druggebruikers*, Doctoral Thesis, Utrecht: Universiteit Utrecht.

DRIESSEN, F.M.H.M. (1990) *Methadon Verstrekking in Nederland*, Utrecht: Bureau Driessen.

FENNEMA, J.S.A., VAN AMEIJDEN, E.J.C., COUTINHO, R.A., VAN DOORNUM, G.J.J., HENQUET, C.J.M. and VAN DEN HOEK, J.A.R. (1993a) 'HIV prevalence among clients attending a sexually transmitted diseases clinic in Amsterdam: the potential risk for heterosexual transmission', *Genitourinary Medicine*, **69**, pp. 23–8.

FENNEMA, J.S.A., VAN DEN HOEK, J.A.R., HUISMAN, J.G. and COUTINHO, R.A. (1993b) 'HIV-prevalentie onder Surinaamse en Antilliaanse druggebruikers in Amsterdam', *Nederlands Tijdschrift voor de Geneeskunde*, **137**, pp. 2209–13.

FENNEMA, J.S.A., VAN AMEIJDEN E.J.C., VAN DEN HOEK, J.A.R., VAN DEN AKKER, R. and COUTINHO, R.A. (1993c) 'De HIV-prevalentie bij intraveneuze druggebruikers in Amsterdam: een onderzoek op straat', *Tijdschrift voor de Sociale Gezonheidszorg*, **71**, pp. 267–72.

FENNEMA, J.S.A., VAN AMEIJDEN, E.J.C., HENQUET, C.J.M., VAN DOORNUM, G.J.J., COUTINHO, R.A. and VAN DEN HOEK, J.A.R. (1995) 'HIV-surveillance op een polikliniek voor seksueel overdraagbare aandoeningen in Amsterdam, 1991–1994: lage en stabiele prevalentie onder heteroseksuele bezoekers', *Nederlands Tijdschrift voor de Geneeskunde*, **139**, pp. 1595–8.

FENNEMA, J.S.A., VAN AMEIJDEN, E.J.C., COUTINHO, R.A. and VAN DEN HOEK, J.A.R. (1997a) 'Clinical sexually transmitted diseases among HIV-infected and non-infected drug-using prostitutes', *Sexually Transmitted Diseases*, **24**, pp. 361–71.

FENNEMA, J.S.A., VAN AMEIJDEN, E.J.C., VAN DEN HOEK, J.A.R. and COUTINHO, R.A. (1997b) 'Young and recent-onset injecting drug users are at high risk for HIV', *Addiction*, **92**, pp. 1457–65.

GEMEENTELIJKE GENEESKUNDIGE EN GEZONDHEIDSDIENST AMSTERDAM (1993) *Passanten en Prostitutie Project: Sociaal Verslag, Jaarcijfers/verrichtingen 1992*, Amsterdam: GG & GD, Sector GGZ.

GEMEENTELIJKE GENEESKUNDIGE EN GEZONDHEIDSDIENST AMSTERDAM (1994) *Methadonverstrekking in Amsterdam in 1993: Jaaroverzicht van de Centrale Methadon Registratie*, Amsterdam: GG & GD, Sector GGZ.

GOSSOP, M. and GRANT, M. (1991) 'A six country survey of the content and structure of heroin treatment programmes using methadone', *British Journal of Addiction*, **86**, pp. 1151–60.

GRUND, J.P.C., KAPLAN, C.D. and ADRIAAN, N.F.P. (1990) 'The limitations of the concept of needle sharing: the practice of frontloading', *AIDS*, **4**, pp. 819–21.

HAAN, H.A., VAN DEN HOEK, J.A.R., VAN HAASTRECHT, H.J.A., VAN DER MEER, C.W. and COUTINHO, R.A. (1991) 'Relatief lage HIV prevalentie onder druggebruikers ondanks riskant spuitgedrag', *Nederlands Tijdschrift voor de Geneeskunde*, **135**, pp. 218–21.

VAN HAASTRECHT, H.J.A., VAN DEN HOEK, J.A.R., BARDOUX, C, LEENTVAAR-KUIJPERS, A. and COUTINHO, R.A. (1991a) 'The course of the HIV epidemic among intravenous drug users in Amsterdam, the Netherlands', *American Journal of Public Health*, **81**, pp. 59–62.

VAN HAASTRECHT, H.J.A., VAN DEN HOEK, J.A.R., MIENTJES, G.H.C. and

COUTINHO, R.A. (1991b) 'Did the introduction of HIV among homosexual men precede the introduction of HIV among injecting drug users in the Netherlands?', *AIDS*, **6**, pp. 131–2.

VAN HAASTRECHT, H.J.A., FENNEMA, J.S.A., COUTINHO, R.A., VAN DER HELM, T.C.M., KINT, J.A.P.C.M. and VAN DEN HOEK, J.A.R. (1993) 'HIV prevalence and risk behaviour among prostitutes and clients: migrants at increased risk for HIV infection', *Genitourinary Medicine*, **69**, pp. 251–6.

VAN HAASTRECHT, H.J.A., VAN AMEIJDEN, E.J.C., VAN DEN HOEK, J.A.R., MIENTJES, G.H.C., BAX, J.S. and COUTINHO, R.A. (1996) 'Predictors of mortality in the Amsterdam cohort of HIV-positive and HIV-negative drug users', *American Journal of Epidemiology*, **143**, pp. 380–91.

VAN HAASTRECHT, H.J.A., BINDELS, P.J.E., VAN DEN HOEK, J.A.R. and COUTINHO, R.A. (submitted) 'Estimating the size of the HIV-epidemic among injecting drug users in Amsterdam'.

HARTGERS, C. (1992) *Risk behavior among injecting drug users in Amsterdam*, Doctoral Thesis, Amsterdam: Universiteit van Amsterdam.

HARTGERS, C., VAN SANTEN, G.W. and VAN HAASTRECHT, H.J.A. (1992) 'De HIV-prevalentie onder druggebruikers die methadon verstrekt krijgen bij de drugsafdeling van de GG & GD te Amsterdam', *Tijdschrift voor de Sociale Gezondheidszorg*, **70**, pp. 275–9.

HARTGERS, C., VAN DEN HOEK, J.A.R., KRIJNEN, P., VAN BRUSSEL, G.H.A. and COUTINHO, R.A. (1991) 'Changes over time in heroin and cocaine use among injecting drug users in Amsterdam, the Netherlands, 1885–1989', *British Journal of Addiction*, **86**, pp. 1091–7.

HARTGERS, C., VAN AMEIJDEN, E.J.C., VAN DEN HOEK, J.A.R. and COUTINHO, R.A. (1992a) 'Needle sharing and participation in the Amsterdam syringe exchange program among HIV-seronegative injecting drug users', *Public Health Reports*, **107**, pp. 675–81.

HARTGERS, C., VAN DEN HOEK, J.A.R., COUTINHO, R.A. and VAN DER PLICHT, J. (1992b) 'Psychopathology, stress and HIV-risk injecting behaviour among drug users', *British Journal of Addiction*, **87**, pp. 857–65.

HARTGERS, C., VAN DEN HOEK, J.A.R., KRIJNEN, P. and COUTINHO, R.A. (1992c) 'HIV prevalence and risk behavior among injecting drug users in "low-threshold" methadone programs in Amsterdam', *American Journal of Public Health*, **82**, pp. 547–51.

HARTGERS, C., KRIJNEN, P., VAN DEN HOEK, J.A.R., COUTINHO, R.A. and VAN DER PLICHT, J. (1992d) 'HIV risk behavior and beliefs of HIV-seropositive drug users', *Journal of Drug Issues*, **22**, pp. 833–47.

VAN DEN HOEK, J.A.R., VAN HAASTRECHT, H.J.A. and COUTINHO, R.A. (1989) 'Risk reduction among intravenous drug users in Amsterdam under the influence of AIDS', *American Journal of Public Health*, **79**, pp. 1355–7

VAN DEN HOEK, J.A.R., VAN HAASTRECHT, H.J.A. and COUTINHO, R.A. (1990) 'Heterosexual behaviour of intravenous drug users in Amsterdam: implications for the AIDS epidemic', *AIDS*, **4**, pp. 449–53.

VAN DEN HOEK, J.A.R., VAN HAASTRECHT, H.J.A. and COUTINHO, R.A. (1991)

'Homosexual prostitution among male drug users and its risk for HIV infection', *Genitourinary Medicine*, **67**, pp. 303–6.

VAN DEN HOEK, J.A.R., COUTINHO, R.A., VAN HAASTRECHT, H.J.A., VAN ZADELHOFF, A.W. and GOUDSMIT, J. (1988) 'Prevalence and risk factors of HIV infections among drug users and drug using prostitutes in Amsterdam', *AIDS*, **2**, pp. 55–60.

VAN DEN HOEK, J.A.R., VAN HAASTRECHT, H.J.A., SCHEERINGA-TROOST, B. and COUTINHO, R.A. (1989) 'HIV infection and STD in drug addicted prostitutes in Amsterdam: potential for heterosexual HIV transmission', *Genitourinary Medicine*, **65**, pp. 146–50.

INGOLD, F.R. and TOUSSIRT, M. (1993) 'Transmission of HIV among drug addicts in three French cities: implications for prevention', *Bulletin on Narcotics*, **45**, pp. 117–34.

INSPECTIE VOOR DE GEZONDHEIDSZORG (1995) *AIDS in Nederland: Tweede kwartaal 1995*, Ministerie van Volksgezondheid, Welzijn en Sport, Rijswijk.

DES JARLAIS, D.C. (1994) 'Cross-national studies of AIDS among injecting drug users', *Addiction*, **89**, pp. 383–92.

DES JARLAIS, D.C., FRIEDMAN, S.R. and CHOOPANYA, K. (1992) 'International epidemiology of HIV and AIDS among injecting drug users', *AIDS*, **6**, pp. 1053–68.

DES JARLAIS, D., FRIEDMAN, S.R. and WARD, T.P. (1993) 'Harm reduction: a public health response to the AIDS epidemic among injecting drug users', *Annual Reviews of Public Health*, **14**, pp. 413–50.

KORF, D., HES, J. and VAN AALDEREN, H. (1992) *Waar Je Mee Omgaat; AIDS Risico's in Alkmaarse Drugscenes*, Alkmaar: Brijder Stichting.

KORF, D.J., REIJNEVELD, S.A. and TOET, M.P.H. (1994) 'Estimating the number of heroin users: a review of methods and empirical findings from the Netherlands', *International Journal of the Addictions*, **29**, pp. 1393–1417.

KUIKEN, C.L., ZWART, G., BAAN, E., COUTINHO, R.A., VAN DEN HOEK, J.A.R. and GOUDSMIT, J. (1993) 'Increasing antigenic and genetic diversity of the V3 variable domain of the HIV envelope protein in the course of the AIDS epidemic', *Proceedings of the National Academy of Sciences of the United States of America*, **90**, pp. 9061–5.

VAN DE LAAR, M.J.W., PICKERING, J., VAN DEN HOEK, J.A.R., VAN GRIENSVEN, G.J.P., COUTINHO, R.A. and VAN DE WATER, H.P.A. (1990) 'Declining gonorrheoa rates in the Netherlands, 1976–88: consequences for the AIDS epidemic', *Genitourinary Medicine*, **66**, pp. 148–55.

LANGENDAM, M., VAN AMEIJDEN, E.J.C. and VAN DEN HOEK, J.A.R. (1995) 'HIV-testen en counselen in Amsterdam: kenmerken van niet eerder op HIV geteste injecterende druggebruikers', *Tijdschrift voor de Sociale Gezondheidszorg*, **73**, pp. 354–9.

MAINLINE, (1995) 'Landelijk overzicht spuitenomruil', *Mainline*, **5**, 2, pp. 30–1.

PAULUSSEN, T.G.W.M., KOK, G.J., KNIBBE, R.A. and CRAMER, A. (1990)

'Determinanten van aan AIDS gerelateerde risicogedragingen van intraveneuze druggebruikers', *Tijdschrift voor de Sociale Gezondheidszorg*, **68**, pp. 129–36.

REIJNEVELD, S.A. (1992) 'Ambulante methadonverstrekking in Amsterdam; een gedifferentieerd systeem?', *Tijdschift voor de Sociale Gezondheidszorg*, **70**, pp. 592–8.

RICHARDSON, C., ANCELLE-PARK, R. and PAPAEVANGELOU, G. (1993) 'Factors associated with HIV seropositivity in European injecting drug users', *AIDS*, **7**, pp. 1485–91.

SAMUELS, J.F., VLAHOV, D. and ANTHONY, J.C. (1991) 'The practice of "frontloading" among intravenous drug users: association with HIV-antibody', *AIDS*, **5**, p. 343.

STICHTING INTRAVAL (1995) *Drugs binnen de grenzen*, Groningen: Stichting Intraval.

TREURNIET, H.F. and DAVIDSE, W. (1993) 'Trends in de frequentie van sexueel overdraagbare aandoeningen in Nederland', *Nederlands Tijdschrift voor de Geneeskunde*, **137**, pp. 1457–61.

WHO COLLABORATIVE STUDY GROUP (1993) 'An international comparative study of HIV prevalence and risk behaviour among drug injectors in 13 cities', *Bulletin on Narcotics*, **45**, pp. 19–46.

WHO–EC COLLABORATING CENTRE ON AIDS (1994a) 'AIDS-surveillance in Europe', Quarterly report no. 44, WHO–EC Collaborating Centre, Saint-Maurice, France, December.

WHO–EC COLLABORATING CENTRE ON AIDS (1994b) 'Surveillance of AIDS/HIV in Europe, 1984–1994. European centre for the epidemiological monitoring of AIDS', WHO–EC Collaborating Centre, Saint-Maurice, France.

WIESSING, L.G., VONDEWINKEL, B. and HOUWELING, H. (1992) *Surveillance van HIV-infecties onder druggebruikers; een haalbaarheidsstudie in Deventer*, Rapport nr. 441002001. Bilthoven/Utrecht: RIVM/NIAD.

WIESSING, L.G., HOUWELING, H, VAN DEN AKKER, R. (1993) *HIV-infecties en risicogedrag onder druggebruikers in Arnhem*, Rapport nr. 528910003, Bilthoven/Arnhem: RIVM/Dienst welzijn en volksgezondheid.

WIESSING, L.G., HOUWELING, H. and KOEDIJK, P.M. (1995) *Prevalentie en risicofactoren van HIV-infectie onder druggebruikers in Rotterdam*, Rapport nr. 213220001, Bilthoven: RIVM.

WIESSING, L.G., HOUWELING, H. and MEULDERS, W.A.J. (1995) *Prevalentie van HIV-infecties onder druggebruikers in Zuid-Limburg*, Rapport nr. 214230001, Bilthoven: RIVM.

WILLEMS, P.W.J.M., POSTEMA, E.J. and VAN DER MEIJDEN, W.I. (1993) 'HIV prevalentie en risicofactoren voor infectie bij bezoekers van de SOA-polikliniek behorend bij het AZR-Dijkzicht', presented at First national conference on STD in the Netherlands, Veldhoven.

DE ZWART, M.W. (1989) *Alcohol, Tabak en Drugs in Cijfers*, Utrecht: NIAD, afdeling Onderzoek.

Chapter 5

Sex Work and HIV in the Netherlands: Policy, Research and Prevention

Ine Vanwesenbeeck and Ron de Graaf

The days when combating STDs was seen as equivalent to combating prostitution are long gone, but sex workers (and, to a lesser extent, their clients) are still often considered in need of special attention in the context of STD prevention. Everywhere, the advent of AIDS has given a new spirit to preventive interventions targeted at sex workers, the measures being either repressive, investigative or supportive. This chapter deals with the research and policy directed at sex workers and their clients in the Netherlands 'since AIDS'. In our discussion, we limit ourselves to heterosexual sex work. We will start with a description of sex work in the Netherlands: its legal and social status, the different forms and the people involved. Next, we will consider studies of sex workers and clients on issues related to HIV and we will discuss prevention activities, aimed at sex workers and their clients, that have been conducted during the last decade. Finally, we will address the question of what needs to be done in terms of sex worker policy and preventive activities in the future.

The Legal and Social Status of Sex Work in the Netherlands

Many consider the Netherlands a pioneer in liberal attitudes towards sex work. They have seen or heard about the red light district in Amsterdam and assume that sex work is all perfectly permissible and respectable in the Netherlands. Some Dutch authors have also portrayed the country as a forerunner when it comes to attitudes towards sex work (for example Belderbos and Visser, 1987; Boutellier, 1991). But are they right to do so?

Let us first look at the legal situation. In most European countries it is not illegal for individual women to engage in sex work. However, the organization and pursuit of sex work are formal legal offences practically everywhere. This is the situation in the Netherlands as well. Nevertheless, large differences exist between the European countries in the activities formulated under the common denominator 'prohibition of organization'. In the Netherlands, this bears on 'making a profession or habit of causing or encouraging indecent acts by others' (Art. 250bis, Dutch Penal Code) and 'living off the earnings of a prostitute' (Art. 432), while in countries such as Sweden, the United Kingdom,

France and Belgium, laws on organization also encompass renting premises for the purpose of sex work and public advertising for sex work activity. Regulations such as these can make it very difficult for sex workers to organize their work and lives. This is the case to a much lesser extent in the Netherlands. Other measures such as the registration and medical examination of sex workers are not mandated by law in the Netherlands, as they are in Austria, Greece and certain parts of Germany (see Alexander, 1993).

Large differences exist between different European countries in the fierceness with which prostitution laws are enforced. The Netherlands is known as one of the least repressive countries for sex work. Brothels, clubs and escort services are widely tacitly condoned and window and street sex work is tolerated in specific districts. France or Britain on the other hand, offer examples of more repressive regimes. Soliciting is illegal everywhere and sex workers are routinely arrested and fined. Laws against procuring are enforced against sex workers' families and against sex workers who work together or share a flat, it being often taken for granted that one lives off the earnings of a sex worker when one lives with her. Still, varying forms of tacit condoning and toleration can be seen in all European countries. Since condoning is mostly limited to certain geographical areas, or to certain forms of sex work, a policy of condoning is often a policy of regulation, even if the activities being regulated are formally against the law.

Considering the relatively mild legal restrictions put on sex workers and the reticence of Dutch authorities to enforce the law against prostitution, it can be concluded that the Dutch policy is indeed a relatively liberal one. However, the straightforward acceptance and decriminalization of sex work appears to be unattainable in the Netherlands. One of the reasons the Netherlands has often been looked (down) upon as a 'mecca' for sex work, is that for about a decade it seemed very likely that the prohibition statements would be deleted from the Criminal Code and that a policy was going to be adopted in which, under certain conditions, the organization of sex work could be legal business. However, in November 1993 proposals for such a law reform ultimately came up for vote in parliament but did not receive enough political support. The reform proposals were withdrawn and the situation remained as it was. Experts in the field maintain that in the end moral considerations as well as the inability to properly distinguish sex-work-as-free-choice from sex-work-under-force, are the prime reasons for the legalization process to have taken this turn (Visser, in press). If the distinction was made at all, sex work by immigrant women was all too easily and opportunistically taken as an equivalent of sex-work-under-force.[1]

Moreover, the social status of sex workers would not have changed dramatically with a legal shift. It is true that, in the Netherlands, sex work is openly discussed as possibly 'another form of work' by the public at large and in the media, and experts and authorities can hardly ever be caught making stigmatizing or denigrating remarks about sex work. It has been argued that, for the Netherlands as opposed to other countries, the appearance of AIDS has not led to a revival of the traditional forms of moralism (Mooij, 1993) or a 'moral panic' targeting homosexual men and female sex workers. Dutch attitudes seem to be rather lenient and 'matter-of-fact'. However, the open and liberal character of public discourse contrasts with widespread ambivalent or even negative private opinions and behaviour. Having listened to many sex workers describing their experiences of negative social reactions, one cannot maintain that the Dutch population fully accepts them or their work, much less respects them for it. At best, sex workers are met with a kind of compassionate awe for what they have to go through. Openly claiming a liberal attitude towards sex work is one thing, but unequivocally and unproblematically practising this attitude when dealing with sex workers, is another. Negative public opinion apparently exists alongside 'Dutch leniency'. On closer examination, ambivalence towards sex work and stigmatization of sex workers seems, perhaps more than elsewhere, camouflaged by a liberal discourse.

However, it has to be said that Dutch feminists and sex workers are among the strongest advocates of decriminalization in Europe. The radical feminist view of sex work as inherently opposing female human rights is considered too one-sided by most Dutch feminists. No longer are solely negative consequences attached to sex for payment. The wishes of sex workers to be recognized as professional workers are also widely acknowledged. The pro-sex work view is also strongly advocated by some of the sex workers themselves who have been organized in 'The Red Thread' since 1985. In collaboration with some American advocates of the decriminalization of sex work the First World Whores' Congress was organized in Amsterdam in 1985, and Dutch women were closely involved in the organization of the second one in Brussels in 1986 (Pheterson, 1989). One might say that as far as a feminist movement can exert influence on the position of sex workers, Dutch feminists have been an important force in enhancing their social status in the Netherlands.

We must conclude, however, that neither this substantial societal force nor the relatively liberal policies have so far succeeded in bringing about a radically different legal status for sex workers. Moreover, the general moral climate toward sex work does not seem to be substantially better than in other countries, perhaps only less openly negative or hostile. Even if the argument remains that working as a sex worker in a comparatively free, liberal, condoning and rich country is relatively comfortable, the Dutch sex workers' situation differs only in degree, not substantially from that of their colleagues in other countries.

Forms of Sex Work

Sex work has many different faces in the Netherlands. Street sex work, where soliciting takes place on the public road, is one of the most visible forms. An estimated 80 per cent of the street sex workers are illicit drug users (Van der Helm *et al.*, 1995). Street sex workers are self-employed, but sometimes finance the drug needs of their partners. The earnings per contact in this kind of sex work are relatively low.

Window sex work (which hardly exists outside the Netherlands and Belgium) is also a public form: soliciting of clients takes place from behind a window. As in street sex work, the contact is especially directed towards sex. Verbal communication with the client is limited, partly because of the fact that a large number of the window sex workers may not be fluent in the local language. Window sex workers work relatively independently. They hire a room for about 100 guilders for an afternoon or evening from a proprietor who interferes minimally with their activities.

Sex clubs are private and more business-like, and sex workers work less independently here. Clients and the sex workers socialize first in a private space which includes a bar. In general, these sex workers hand over 40 to 60 per cent of their earnings to the owner. Contact with the client lasts considerably longer than in street or window sex work and is directed not only towards sexual gratification. Part of the contact is conversation prior to the sexual contact. Brothels are very similar to clubs. However, a brothel operates on a smaller scale, with generally fewer sex workers at work and usually there is no bar. The client is expected to make his choice from the available sex workers as soon as he arrives. There is little conversation or socializing. Usually, the proprietor receives less than half of the sex worker's earnings.

In escort sex work, sex workers can recruit clients independently or via an intermediary agency by means of advertisements placed in national, regional or local daily or weekly newspapers. Sometimes escort sex work also originates from a club. The contact takes place in the client's house or in a hotel. Compared to other forms, the aspect of sex work is less obviously present, partly because the contact takes place on the client's territory. Home sex work, lastly, resembles escort sex work in regard to its home atmosphere and personal character, and clients being solicited by means of advertisements. The difference is that the contact takes place in the home of the sex worker instead of the client's house or hotel. The sex worker works on her own, decides her own working hours, and no money has to be paid to a proprietor. The National Committee on AIDS Control (NCAB) estimates that, in heterosexual sex work, 30 per cent of the sex workers work in both clubs and brothels, 30 per cent in windows, 10 per cent in streets, and 30 per cent at home or as escorts (NCAB, 1988/1990).

The People Involved

It is extremely difficult to assess the size of the population involved in sex for payment. In the Netherlands, the total number of sex work places for female sex workers is often estimated at 20–25000 (Visser, in press). It may be assumed that the number of women occupying them either full- or part-time is higher. Taking a number of 20 000 working places occupied by one woman as a starting point, one can calculate the number of men visiting sex workers. Research has shown that sex workers have an average of 80 commercial contacts per month and that clients pay for sex an average of 20 times per year (De Graaf *et al.*, 1992; Alary, 1993). Thus, the estimate of 20 000 sex workers leads to an estimate of 960 000 clients per year, which is approximately 16 per cent of the Dutch male population of 16 years and older. However, national surveys, asking about engaging in sex for money, invariably show a much lower percentage. In the most recent national study, 2.8 per cent of 500 18–50-year-old heterosexual men reported having had contact with a sex worker in the previous year (Van Zessen and Sandfort, 1991). Even when this percentage is corrected to 4 per cent to allow for under-reporting, the same figures as used above would lead to an estimated number of only 10 000 sex workers (De Graaf, 1995), quite a difference from the number presented earlier. The truth must be somewhere in between. The NCAB has decided to adopt a wide margin and estimate there are 15–20 000 people working in sex work in the Netherlands (NCAB, 1988/1990).

Because of the internationalization of sex work, the ethnic composition of the sex worker population has changed considerably in the last few decades. Before 1970, almost all of the sex workers in the Netherlands were white and Dutch, with the exception of a few Surinamese and Antillean women. Later, the list became more varied. Initially, women from South-east Asia came to Holland, particularly from Thailand and the Philippines. Then they came from Africa, especially Ghana, and then from Latin America, particularly from Colombia and the Dominican Republic. Latin American women currently constitute the largest group among the foreign sex workers in the Netherlands. Furthermore, Surinamese, Antillean, Indonesian, Moluccan, and to a lesser degree Moroccan and Turkish women work in sex work. And since the disappearance of the Iron Curtain there has been a flood of East European women arriving in the country. This group in particular is strongly increasing in number.

In the middle of 1985, 30 to 40 per cent of the sex workers working in Amsterdam were of non-Dutch origin, an estimated 40 to 50 per cent of whom were in the Netherlands illegally (Brussa, 1989). Brussa estimated that, depending on the type of sex work, 30 to 60 per cent of the sex workers in the Netherlands were of non-Dutch origin. An important characteristic of these women is that they are very mobile, both in their own countries and internationally. Moreover, they come from areas of the world were HIV is already present, at least to some extent, among the heterosexual population, or they have already worked in regions where this is the case (Koenig, 1989). These characteristics suggest a high need for STD/HIV monitoring and prevention among both sex workers and their clients.

Prevalence of HIV Infection among Prostitutes and Clients

At the beginning of the AIDS epidemic, research in Amsterdam indicated no evidence of HIV infection among 84 non-injecting drug using sex workers who were recruited at STD clinics and through club doctors (Coutinho and Van der Helm, 1986). These results and those from later Dutch studies do not differ from other studies in Western countries. HIV prevalences among sex workers who do not inject drugs are zero or very low, and those among sex workers who inject are substantial, dependent on the HIV prevalence among those with whom they share injection attributes (Day, 1988). Injecting drugs with contaminated needles, having private partners who themselves inject, and originating from AIDS endemic areas are the most important risk factors for HIV infection among sex workers in Western countries.

Among injecting drug users (IDUs) in Amsterdam (1985–87), a group in which 83 per cent of the women were sex workers, 28 per cent were HIV positive (Van den Hoek *et al.*, 1988). As in other Western countries, in the Netherlands large regional differences exist in HIV prevalence among IDUs and the sex workers among them (Wiessing *et al.*, 1995). A longitudinal study in Amsterdam among non-IDU heterosexuals who visited STD clinics is one of the few studies in Western countries in which HIV prevalence among sex workers' clients is reported (Hooykaas *et al.*, 1989). At enrolment in this study, none of the 114 sex workers and 64 clients were infected. During the follow-up period, one sex worker who had injected drugs before 1982 seroconverted, as well as one client who had sex with sex workers who injected drugs. In later research in Amsterdam at STD clinics and workplaces of sex workers, three of 201 non-IDU sex workers and one of 213 clients were infected (Van Haastrecht *et al.*, 1993). The three sex workers had recently come to the Netherlands from AIDS endemic countries; the client had had homosexual contacts in the past. This study is part of European HIV prevalence research among sex workers (1990–91), from which it appears that 35 of 110 (31.8 per cent) sex workers who injected drugs and 11 of 756 (1.5 per cent) non-IDUs were HIV-positive (Alary, 1993). Infection among non-IDUs was associated with sub-Saharan African origin, inconsistent condom use, previous ulcerative STD, and the use of petroleum-based lubricants.

Protective Behaviour and its Determinants among Sex Workers and Clients

Research in 1985 indicated that condom use among 84 non-drug-using sex workers working in Amsterdam was relatively low; 48 per cent used them regularly and 52 per cent less frequently (Coutinho and Van der Helm, 1986). Later studies indicate increased condom use. For example, in a cohort study (1987–89) among heterosexuals an increasing trend in consistent condom use between their first and third visits to an STD clinic among sex workers (from 73 to 80 per cent) and clients (from 43 to 57 per cent) was found (Hooykaas *et al.*, 1991a). A later study (1991) conducted at an STD clinic and at places of sex work in Amsterdam indicated that 66 per cent of the sex workers and 56 per cent of the clients consistently used condoms (Van Haastrecht *et al.*, 1993). In that study it was found that sex workers who did not always use condoms, compared to consistent users, reported more clients, worked more days per week, had lived in the Netherlands more often for less than three years, had financially supported others more often, and had fewer other legal sources of income. These characteristics showed a strong correlation with Latin American origin. Among clients, inconsistent condom use was associated with a higher number of sexual contacts, relatively more contacts with Latin American sex workers, having been born outside the Netherlands, and lower income and educational levels. Clients recruited into the study at places of sex work reported a discernibly higher consistent condom use than clients recruited at STD clinics. For sex workers, the opposite was true. It might be that clients go to STD clinics if they have had unprotected sex and might have contracted an infection, while sex workers are more likely to have themselves routinely checked, even if they have not had unsafe contact.

Longitudinal research (1986–92) conducted in Amsterdam among injecting drug users indicates an increase from 36 to 66 per cent in consistent condom use among the individual sex workers from their first to their eighth visit (Van Ameijden *et al.*, 1994). A cross-sectional increase in condom use at intake was seen, from 21 per cent in 1986 to 58 per cent in 1991. Conforming to this increase, the number of self-reported STDs in this study decreased. The greatest behavioural change was among HIV-infected IDUs: at intake they reported a lower degree of condom use than non-infected women, but this difference disappeared in the course of time. In addition, it appeared the shorter the stay of non-Dutch sex workers in Amsterdam, the more often STDs were reported. This might imply that working in sex work for a short time is associated with less condom use. The increases in self-reported condom use among IDU and non-IDU sex workers and clients which were seen in these different studies are confirmed by the decrease in the incidence of various STDs found among sex workers in the period 1984–90 (Treurniet and Davidse, 1993).

In a recent study of factors influencing sex workers' protective behaviour, 127 respondents working in different settings were interviewed extensively (Vanwesenbeeck *et al.*, 1994). In the previous year, 81 per cent always used condoms. Among these sex workers three protection styles could be identified. Risk-takers regularly and unselectively worked without a condom. They tended to be born outside the Netherlands, worked under the highest financial pressure, had the highest job stress (most clients, fastest work routine) and the lowest job satisfaction. The work was very negatively evaluated, and was seen as the only way to make money. They did not see themselves as professionals. They used drugs more frequently, and had the most psychosomatic complaints. They had experienced the most severe abuse and violence, both off and on the job. Consistent condom users had a moderately positive, but essentially businesslike attitude to the work. They saw it as a job and strove for professionalism. They worked under relatively low financial pressure. Their work rhythms can be described as relaxed; they worked the fewest hours and had the lowest number of clients. A positive attitude towards the work brings about an abundance of supportive (symbolic, hygienic) motivations for consistent condom use which relate to the wish to fit the work into positively formulated codes of behaviour. Selective risk takers abstained from using condoms selectively and occasionally. They also worked under relatively low financial pressure. However, they were more likely to define professionality in terms of 'a good service' than in terms of a 'professional detachment'. Their less businesslike attitude can be seen in the fact that they valued some emotional attachment to (regular) clients, and they did not completely rule out their own sexual pleasure during work. Sexual or emotional desires may lead them to have unprotected sex with one or a few (regular) clients. From this study it can be concluded that sex workers' protection behaviour can be understood in the context of personal histories and the significance the work has for them.

Finally, some studies only dealt with clients' protective behaviour. Among samples of the general Dutch and Amsterdam population, clients' inconsistent condom use in the preceding year was low (9 per cent) (Van Zessen, 1991) or non-existent (Veugelers *et al.*, 1992). Van Mens (1989) found that 75 per cent of 136 clients recruited by means of advertisements always used condoms in the preceding year. Age did not influence condom use. Men with a private regular sexual partner used condoms with sex workers more often than men without such a partner. Men's perception of a sex worker as 'neat and clean', and their trust in a sex worker to whom they often went, did play a role in not using a condom. In a quantitative study among 559 Dutch clients recruited by ads in newspapers and interviewed by phone, which provided the anonymity many clients demand, 14 per cent did not always use condoms in the previous year (De Graaf *et al.*, 1997). The determinants of condom use among these men were examined on the basis of previous qualitative research among 91 clients, which showed that their preventive behaviour was particularly related to the meaning of, and the motivation towards, their commercial contacts (Vanwesenbeeck *et al.*, 1993). The study among the 559 clients showed that, compared to consistent condom users, inconsistent users were less highly educated, had twice as many contacts with sex workers, and had more contacts with sex workers they visited regularly. They were either more emotionally motivated to visit sex workers than were consistent condom users, or exhibited a stronger need for sexual variation. Their visits to sex workers were more often compulsive (they experienced these visits as something over which they had no control and which they would prefer to stop), they had a more negative attitude towards prostitution in general, they evaluated condoms more negatively, they had a higher personal efficacy to achieve unsafe contacts, and they had a higher general risk assessment, commensurate to their behaviour. Consistent protection behaviour was not only intrinsically motivated: a minority of men reporting safe sex only, did not use condoms because they themselves wanted to, but because sex workers insisted upon it.

Sex Work Networks and the Potential Spread of HIV

Two studies (1990–91 and 1993) show that sex work in the Netherlands consists of different segments which are reasonably independent of each other (De Graaf *et al.*, 1992; De Graaf *et al.*, 1996). Sex workers seemed to change the places in which they work. However, they did not frequently move from one type of sex work to another because of the specific individual (dis)advantages of the types. Only 18 per cent of 127 sex workers had changed type in the preceding year, but were not arbitrary in their choices. Women moved primarily in and out of brothels and clubs, or between these and window sex work. There was hardly any exchange between street sex work and other types. Working in more than one type at a time was also not reported. Approximately half of the (91 and 559) clients in both studies had used only one type in the last year; 80 per cent used one or two types. Clients therefore did not make arbitrary use of different sorts of sex work. Personal preference played a role, as well as financial resources. Only 3 per cent of the clients reported unsafe sex in two or more types, indicating that there is very little 'bridge-forming' between the different types. The prevalence of different STDs in different types of sex work shows evidence for the segmentation of sex work networks. Among Latin American window sex workers and their Turkish and Moroccan clients, other STD infections are found than among IDU street sex workers and their clients (Van de Laar *et al.*, 1991; Prins *et al.*, 1994).

In the two above-mentioned studies, different levels of condom use between the different types of sex work were found (De Graaf *et al.*, 1992; De Graaf *et al.*, in press). Condoms were most frequently used in clubs and brothels, but less often in street sex work (especially among IDU sex workers and their clients), in window sex work involving Latin American sex workers and their Moroccan and Turkish clients, and in home and escort sex work. Other studies have also shown that minority ethnic clients engage in unsafe sex more often (Hooykaas *et al.*, 1991b; Van Haastrecht *et al.*, 1993). It is important to the potential spread of HIV that Turkish and Moroccan men usually go only to window sex workers who are not Dutch. One of the reasons is that they usually have a low income and these women charge low prices. Considering the relatively low frequency of condom use and the high degree of partner change within this limited group, network formation with a high density is possible. The fact that some (non-IDU) Latin American and African women who work in window sex work are HIV-infected, means that there is a potential for the spread of HIV in this type of sex work. The relatively low use of condoms in street sex work may also contribute to a further spread of HIV, because many of the IDU sex workers, who mainly work on the streets, are already infected. The relatively low number of clients per home and escort sex worker, and the phenomenon of the steady client which occurs frequently in these types of sex work, imply that despite the relatively high frequency of unsafe contacts, the absolute number of unprotected sexual acts with different partners is decidedly lower, than in window or street sex work. This means that future spread of HIV in these latter types of sex work is less likely.

It can be concluded that fear of the entire sex work circuit as the focus of HIV infection is not justified. On the basis of the information about the extent of segmentation in sex work, and the degree of risk behaviour in the various types, it is justified to focus educational campaigns on special groups of sex workers and clients.

The Organization of Prevention Activities

In 1988, the NCAB explicitly recommended to national and local governments dealing with AIDS policy for sex work, not to try to stop people selling and buying sex, but to encourage them to have safer sex. The committee warned that repression of a particular form or aspect of sex work will always have a knock-on effect on other forms and that stringent regulations will have the most adverse effects on the most vulnerable groups of sex workers. It stated that involuntary measures would not only be ineffective, but also counter-productive and it strongly advised against mandatory HIV testing and the registration of sex workers (NCAB, 1988/1990). These recommendations have been taken to heart by those responsible for prevention policy aimed at people involved in sex work: no repressive measures have been taken, and on the whole prevention activities have been educative, facilitative and supportive.

Generally speaking, prevention programmes are carried out through the Municipal Health Services, who take the leading role in coordinating and implementing regional and local activities (Van der Helm *et al.*, 1995). However, not all Municipal Health Services see prevention activities targeted at sex workers or clients as a priority. In addition to the municipal health workers, different sorts of low-threshold services are in place in the larger cities. These are often equipped with their own outreach field workers. The Dutch Foundation for STD Control acts as the national coordinating and supporting body for HIV/STD prevention, including in sex work.

Some provisions and services, targeting sex workers and clients for STD prevention, amongst others, have their origins in the 1970s and are still in place. They are needed all the more since the AIDS epidemic. Additional, more specific programmes, interventions and education materials have been developed more recently as a response to new prevention needs. Research findings such as those described above have strengthened awareness among educators that prevention needs to be geared to specific subpopulations in sex work and must be sensitive to their specific conditions, behaviour and attitudes in order to be successful. This awareness has by now been translated into a number of well-tailored education materials and intervention programmes. Below, we will first discuss some of the 'older', more general (although by no means omnipresent) services, such as outreach fieldwork and living rooms in streetwalker districts. Then we will describe the more recent materials and interventions, as they have been developed for the sex worker population in general and for specific subpopulations (injecting drug using sex workers, migrant sex workers and (migrant) clients).

Outreach Fieldwork

In many cities and surrounding regions in the Netherlands, social workers and health educators, predominantly from the Municipal Health Services, visit sex workers on their working sites. Fieldworkers often spend an afternoon or an evening in the red light district, brothels and clubs some three or four times a week. Traditionally, they provide women and brothel owners with information on STDs and STD prevention, and inform them of the consulting hours and routines at the Municipal Health Services. They maintain the link between the sex work circuit and the health service. Because of the ever changing composition of the sex worker population, and the now even more urgent context of AIDS, their work is never done. Fieldworkers can keep a close eye on changes and developments in the field. They also often function as persons of confidence for sex workers in a variety of areas, and, if necessary, can make referrals to appropriate helping agencies. In addition, they also have a function signalling abusive situations, which they can report to the police. In particular, migrant women are also given information on where to go in the case of trafficking, exploitation or abuse in any other way, such as the Foundation against Trafficking Women. Migrant women particularly may need encouragement in seeking help from the vice squad, because in their countries of origin the police are often not to be trusted.

Huiskamers in streetwalker districts

Until the 1970s, streetwalking was against the law everywhere in the Netherlands, although it was to be found in a good number of places. When hard drug use increased and both heavy drug using sex workers and drug dealers appeared on the streetwalking scene, the situation in a number of large cities worsened dramatically. The idea was hit upon to create 'zones of tolerance', where sex work could be better controlled (among others, in terms of neighbourhood nuisance) and where sex workers could more easily be reached for all sorts of interventions. Sex workers feel relatively safe in zones of tolerance since here they can work in a more relaxed way and negotiate more freely with clients because they do not have to be on the look-out for the police all the time. This also strengthens solidarity between sex workers, and greater condom use. The 'zones of tolerance' were provided with *huiskamers*, a house or sometimes a large bus where sex workers can take a rest, wash themselves, have a cup of coffee and buy some food. There are paid professional staff in these *huiskamers*, as well as volunteers, clergymen and student workers. More recently, doctors are regularly present and provide the women with STD check-ups and other medical advice. Condoms are made available at very low costs and, although all *huiskamers* have a policy against injecting drugs on the premises, most of them do provide new syringes and needles in exchange for used ones. By now, *huiskamer* projects have been set up in seven large Dutch cities.

The *huiskamers* vary to the degree in which they develop special activities for women (and transsexuals and transvestites) around the issue of STD/HIV prevention. Some, for instance, regularly organize workshops around safer sex and other themes, while others limit themselves to the provision of basic services: a roof, a rest, something to eat, someone to talk to, and information if requested.

The National Prevention Campaign for Sex Work

In 1990, a national campaign targeted at the whole sex work circuit, 'Safe Sex Sure', was launched by the Foundation for STD Control. It aimed, among other things, at reinforcing and promoting safer sex, including sex work, as something that is socially normal. Materials were developed for female sex workers, brothel owners and clients. All materials were produced in close cooperation with members of the target group, carefully pre-tested, and distributed in clubs, brothels and among independently working sex workers by Municipal Helath Services fieldworkers and social workers, drug counsellors and the sex workers' union.

For female sex workers, an illustrated magazine called *Safe Sex at Work and at Play* was developed containing detailed information about HIV and STD prevention, contraception, gynaecological testing, and safer injecting drug use. Tips are given on how to negotiate for safer sex and where to go for HIV-related counselling and treatment. In addition, a small, decorative case has been designed with a condom and a trial-size tube of lubricant. Health educators could present women with these packets and thus had the opportunity to discuss the possibilities of safer sex at work and at home and to emphasize the importance of using water-based lubricants.

For brothel owners, a brochure called *Safe Sex is Sound Business* was developed with advice on safe house policy and on hygienic working conditions. Posters and cardboard stand-up displays with an erotic photo and with the slogan 'Safe Sex Sure' printed in seven languages were also distributed. Space was kept available for sex work businesses to add their own logo or advertisement. Process evaluation has shown that these materials are widely known about and used. All materials, for sex workers as well as for brothel owners, are now being revised and updated.

Specific Policy Toward Drug Using Sex Workers

It is estimated that about 80 per cent of sex workers working the streets are heavy users, and injectors, of illicit drugs (Van der Helm *et al.*, 1995). Certainly not all of the injecting drug using sex workers are reached (well enough) though the living rooms and the activities that take place there. In order to improve HIV prevention involving injecting drug using sex workers, to facilitate their receptiveness to preventive messages, and to make preventive messages more acceptable to them, the Foundation for STD Control has turned to peer-support in addressing this group. So far, two 'experience-experts' (ex-sex workers and ex-IDUs) have been trained to work as prevention workers. They work from the *huiskamers* in Rotterdam and Nijmegen, and give attention both to safer sex and safer drug use. In close cooperation with these experience-experts, several brochures have been developed, in which the information links well with the subculture and daily reality of injecting drug using sex workers. They provide general information on STDs, HIV and AIDS, sexual techniques and condom use, and safer injecting drug use. In one brochure, interaction with clients is discussed. Another one deals with the issue of safer sex in private life and a third one is especially designed for partners of injecting drug using sex workers. All brochures have been translated into French, German and English and posters have been designed to draw attention to their existence.

In Amsterdam, relatively many IDUs in sex work come from outside the Netherlands, for instance from Germany, and are without a legal permit to stay. They are not admitted to the large-scale Amsterdam methadone programme (which provides methadone to 2250 drug users every day, Van der Helm *et al.*, 1995), because it is the official policy of the city not to make treatment available for illegal IDUs. However, for over eight years, a special out-patient clinic for sex workers and non-Dutch people, the 'Prostitutie en Passanten Polikliniek' (PPP), has treated the many problems these groups deal with pragmatically. STD/HIV counselling, needle exchange, condom supply, check-ups on STDs and other infectious diseases, birth control measures and general medical checks are given high priority. Medical care is given free. If necessary (on medical grounds), methadone is prescribed. Severe psychosocial problems, often connected to sex work can, however, only marginally be attended to. The PPP clinic has continuously tried to repatriate patients, on a voluntary basis, to their home countries where, it is hoped, more fundamental drug treatment can be given and a reintegration into society can be assisted. Thus, in the context of a repressive policy, the PPP clinic tries to minimize health risks. In order to reach their target group, nurses and doctors are also available at set hours during the evening and night-time.

Specific Policy Towards Migrant Sex Workers

The education and information materials developed for the national campaign have been made available in other languages besides Dutch. The magazine *Safe Sex at Work and at Play* is also available in English, German and Czech, and the hand-outs with basic information have been translated for women from different countries in Central and Eastern Europe. For women who speak Spanish (mainly from Latin America), an education brochure in the form of a cartoon has been developed, called *Trabajo y Salud* (work and health). Additionally, for migrant women with lower reading abilities, audio cassettes in English, Spanish and Akan (a Ghanaian language) have been produced by the Municipal Health Service of Amsterdam. On the cassettes, basic information on HIV/STD transmission and prevention is interspersed with music. The information has to be continuously adapted to the changing composition of the population and to the needs of the specific groups. Only recently it has become clear, for instance, that relatively many sex workers from Eastern Europe badly need to be educated about contraception, in addition to receiving information about STD/HIV prevention.

The Foundation for STD Control has also developed peer-support projects for Latin American sex workers. Nine Latin American former sex workers have been trained and now, in collaboration with health workers, educate and give condom demonstrations for sex workers in six big cities. In Rotterdam, in addition, a Brazilian transvestite communicates prevention messages with her colleagues. The Latin American peers call themselves Mensajeras de Salud (health messengers). They can break down barrriers and can empathically address women in an emotional language that has a much higher chance of really being heard. In Amsterdam, where an estimated 70 per cent of window sex workers are from outside the Netherlands, an 'intermediary' (that is field-worker annexe coordinator), fluent in Spanish, has been working with migrant sex workers since 1992.

In trying to respond to the increasing mobility of migrant sex workers internationally, a concerted project for migrant sex workers, called TAMPEP (Transnational AIDS/STD prevention among Migrant Prostitutes in Europe Project), is being coordinated by the Mr A. de Graaf Foundation in Amsterdam (a national institute for research and policy on sex work). The other countries participating are Italy, Germany and Austria. TAMPEP advocates an approach in which STD and HIV/AIDS prevention is embedded in a broader framework of general health promotion. Within that framework, it is the objective to develop, in collaboration with migrant sex workers, more effective strategies and new materials for facilitating contact with the target group. During the first year of activities, several experimental outreach research and intervention projects in different regions were conducted, and a working methodology has been developed which can be adapted to the variety of situations which confront sex workers. Cultural mediators and peer educators are two important professional roles in this methodology. In their contacting, educating, training and supporting of migrant sex workers, they make use of materials in different languages that have been produced as a tool to improve the health and social conditions of migrant sex workers.

Local Initiatives Addressing Sex Workers

Besides these more specifically tailored interventions, a few additional, local initiatives have been developed for broader groups in the Netherlands. The Red Thread, for instance, has developed a sticker for window sex workers on which it says 'I work with'. After the stickers were handed out in the beginning of the 1990s, a large number of windows in the red light district in Amsterdam could be seen decorated with them, alerting clients to condom use as early in the negotiation process as possible. For women working the streets, brochures have been compiled with advice on safer sex and how to negotiate it with clients. A brochure called *Skilled in love and self-defence. Hints and Tricks for Street Prostitutes* has been developed by sex workers and health workers in Utrecht, and another one called *When the street is your job* by street workers and social workers in Rotterdam. These brochures not only help individual women to protect themselves efficiently against various risks, but have also been found to stimulate solidarity and feelings of collegiality among women who often see each other as rivals.

Another initiative is the health consulting hour for sex workers. In several cities the Municipal Health Service organizes these special hours for sex workers, which are ambivalently enjoyed by sex workers, because apart from being a well-tailored service they are also seen by many as an especially stigmatizing moment: being at the Municipal Health Service at those hours means you are in sex work! However, since 1991 in Alkmaar, the Municipal Health Service has taken these consulting hours to the window sex work area every two weeks. That way, women could be recruited on the spot. While initially being a specific STD and HIV-related service, women could also ask the doctors at the Municipal Health Service about more general health problems. And, whereas it was initially financed by several temporary grants, since 1994 it has become a joint venture between the Municipal Health Service and the window proprietors in the area, and has thereby been able to become a structural provision.

Specific Policy Towards Clients

All materials displayed at clubs and brothels are also designed to address clients. The positive, accepting tone of these messages, as for instance in 'be welcome to it and have it safely', are meant to enhance clients' positive attitudes towards sex for money, since it was found that positive attitudes towards sex and sex work are a prerequisite for 'playing the game by the rules', for having respect towards sex workers and for willingness to use a condom (Vanwesenbeeck *et al.*, 1993, 1994; De Graaf *et al.*, 1997). This relaxed tone is also struck during the 'condom hand-out actions' that are being organized by the Foundation for STD Control a couple of times a year in several areas with street and window sex work. Clients are spoken to about visiting sex workers and using condoms, while being offered a free condom with directions for use. Sex workers have reported that these actions 'on the spot' support and strengthen them in their safer sex negotiations with clients. A special brochure for clients of window sex workers is also produced. Since some of the clients are of a non-Dutch origin (for example Turkish or Moroccan), education is being conducted in collaboration with Educators Own Language (Voorlichters Eigen Taal, VET'ers).

Some of the staff of the living rooms for street sex workers have developed initiatives of their own. In Utrecht, for instance, clients were enticed to a discussion about condom use with the offer of a free snack. In another local initiative in Amsterdam, mime shows about condom use were held from behind a window in the red light district, while VET'ers talked about safer sex to clients in the streets and handed out condoms and flyers. One of the most playful preventive actions was conducted around World AIDS Day in 1990 at 18 different locations in Amsterdam. Around the town could be seen walking an unprotected 'penis', seven actors, an enormous condom, an old limousine, and an ambulance. The actors involved talked about safer sex with the largely male audience and everyone was given a condom.

The Future

In its policy plan for national STD/AIDS prevention activities in sex work 1996–98, the Foundation for STD Control observes that, in the past years, more clients and sex workers have been reached with prevention messages, because these have been better tailored to behaviour and background of specific target groups in sex work. However, continued attention to the sex work circuit is needed for different reasons, the Foundation asserts. First, the circulation of sex workers is high and the number of migrant sex workers is increasing, as well as the diversity of countries of origin and the number of languages and subcultures. Many migrant sex workers are not reached by the present network of health educators. The changing dynamics of sex work can be seen in the recent increase in sex workers, premise owners and intermediaries who come from the former East block. Second, the frequency of commercial contacts is high and a demand for unsafe sex (still) remains. Registration figures in non-curative STD control institutions show that sex workers and their clients are at relatively high risk for STD infections and that HIV seroprevalence among IDUs is rising. Many of the latter have insufficient knowledge of the interplay between STD and HIV, and their social situation is invariably bad. And, last but not least, the whole sex work trade is 'on the move'. Sex worker, brothel owner and client organizations, together with the Mr A. de Graaf Foundation, are developing initiatives for a self-regulation of the trade. The Ministry of Justice is again making plans for legalization of sex work. For all these reasons, prevention activities should be continued, extended and adapted to changing contexts. Additionally, they should be embedded in the more general process linked to the 'normalization' of sex work (Stichting SOA Bestrijding, 1996).

However, prevention activities in sex work are bound to fail if insufficient attention is given to the conditions under which they can indeed have their intended effects. This calls for differentiated policies, since sex work is a complex phenomenon and differences between sex workers, not only in terms of origin, are large. For a certain group of sex workers, social, psychological and economical conditions are often such, that a purely technical explanation about STDs, sexual techniques and condom use will not be enough to ensure the realization of preventive behaviour. Simple messages are unlikely to improve conditions for the most vulnerable group of women in sex work, who, forced by circumstances, mangled by traumatic experiences, and weakened and undermined by their consequences, may be inclined to submit to demands for unsafe sex (Vanwesenbeeck *et al.*, 1995).

Reasoning from this point of view, interventions on the demand side of the market for sex for money may be more promising than those on the supply side. It is absolutely crucial that prevention interventions involving clients be continued, fine tuned and extended. Messages should reinforce a positive image of sex work, of the professionality of sex workers and of safer sexual practices. Messages should also seek to address the aggressive (sexual) behaviour of clients and try to fight it, because it has been shown that aggressive behaviour by clients strongly associates with sex workers' low well-being and high risk (Vanwesenbeeck, 1994). Legal and punitive measures should be used against employers whose organizing activities involve deception, threats, extortion, or violence towards women. Sex workers have to be able to work of their own accord and under their own control in order to practise safer sex. For that and other obvious reasons, effective strategies against criminal practices forcing women into sex work should be developed on both a national and international level.

Sex workers themselves must be addressed as well, of course, in terms of measures that increase the possibility for preventive messages to take effect. Sex workers who feel and act like professionals and who are relatively well off, may be in need only of measures to improve their position as workers and to increase their control over the organization of sex work. The legalization of sex work and the recognition of sex workers' rights as workers are first crucial steps in this context. However, additional interventions are needed for more vulnerable groups of women, those grappling with severe economic need, violent life histories, social isolation and little support, or all of these. Migrant women and injecting drug using women are relatively often among this group. Interventions here should aim to create 'safety nets' wherever possible. Sites where women work in an 'unorganized' way should be targeted for more protection, which means that the availability of zones of tolerance and *huiskamers* has to be assured and extended. Programmes like TAMPEP, that address sex workers' STD/HIV risk and preventive behaviour in the wider context of their general health and well-being, deserve extension and wider replication.

Concrete initiatives to provide for the financial need of the most vulnerable women are hardly feasible in the short term. To some extent, we have to rely on general emancipation processes and policies which aim at strengthening women's social and economical position in the long run. However, particularly for those women whose drug dependence related financial necessity pushes them to sex work, one concrete measure could be to control more effectively the drug supply. Some experimental drug dispensing programmes in Liverpool and Amsterdam have already proven feasible and successful when carried out under strict conditions (Karsten, 1993). The municipality of Amsterdam is at the moment developing plans to test the free supply of heroin in the new Amsterdam zone of tolerance. It is irrational and shortsighted to deny women who regularly use illicit drugs a properly controlled source of supply.

While clients should be targeted more with educational messages, the more vulnerable prostitutes should be targeted mainly with provisions to enhance their interactional power. In AIDS prevention, it is important for outreach workers to take note of the experiences and cognitions of different groups of sex workers and their clients more than at present. People are more receptive to information if they see it is relevant to them and geared to their life-style, inhibitions and priorities. Interventions need continuous fine tuning and adaptation. Besides its obvious successes, the history of STD/HIV prevention in sex work in the Netherlands has shown that it is not easy to meet the needs of a marginalized group in negative circumstances, not least when the social well-being and risk of that group is influenced by numerous motives, emotions and (ir)rationalities other than health considerations.

Notes

1   The final version of this chapter was received in January 1997. By the time this book went to press, a new parliamentary debate about deleting the prostitution prohibition statements from the Penal Code was in advanced progress. A change in the law, offering local governments the possibility to employ a policy in which prostitution can be considered legal business under certain conditions, is to be expected by the end of 1998.

References

ALARY, M., for the European Working Group on HIV Infection in Female Prostitutes (1993) 'HIV infection in European female sex workers: epidemiological link with use of petroleum-based lubricants', *AIDS*, **7**, pp. 401–8.

ALEXANDER, P. (1993) *International Survey of the Status of Prostitution*, Internal Report, Geneva: World Health Organization.

VAN AMEIJDEN, E.J., VAN DEN HOEK, J.A.R., VAN HAASTRECHT, H.J. and COUTINHO, R.A. (1994) 'Trends in sexual behaviour and the incidence of sexually transmitted diseases and HIV among drug-using prostitutes, Amsterdam 1986–1992', *AIDS*, **8**, pp. 213–21.

BELDERBOS, F. and VISSER, J.H. (Eds) (1987) *Beroep: Prostituée*, Utrecht: SWP.

BOUTELLIER, J.C.J. (1991) 'Prostitution, criminal law and morality in the Netherlands', *Crime, Law and Social Change*, **13**, pp. 201–11.

BRUSSA, L. (1989) 'Migrant prostitutes in the Netherlands', in G. PHETERSON (Ed.), *A Vindication of the Rights of Whores*, Seattle: Seal Press.

COUTINHO, R.A. and VAN DER HELM, TH. (1986) 'Geen aanwijzingen voor LAV/HTLV-III onder prostituées in Amsterdam die geen drugs gebruiken', *Nederlands Tijdschrift voor Geneeskunde*, **130**, p. 508.

DAY, S. (1988) 'Prostitute women and AIDS: anthropology', *AIDS*, **2**, pp. 421–8.

DE GRAAF, R. (1995) *Prostitutes and their Clients; Sexual Networks and Determinants of Condom Use*, Doctoral Thesis, Wageningen: Ponsen & Looijen.

DE GRAAF, R., VAN ZESSEN, G., VANWESENBEECK, I., STRAVER, C.J. and VISSER, J.H. (1992) 'Condom use and sexual behaviour in heterosexual prostitution in the Netherlands', *AIDS*, **6**, pp. 1223–6.

DE GRAAF, R., VAN ZESSEN, G., VANWESENBEECK, I., STRAVER, C.J. and VISSER, J.H. (1996) 'Segmentation of heterosexual prostitution into various forms: a barrier to the potential transmission of HIV', *AIDS Care*, **8**, pp. 417–31.

DE GRAAF, R., VAN ZESSEN, G., VANWESENBEECK, I., STRAVER, C.J. and VISSER, J.H. (1997) 'Condom use by Dutch men with commercial heterosexual contacts: determinants and considerations', *AIDS Education and Prevention*, **9**, pp. 411–423.

VAN HAASTRECHT, H.J.A., FENNEMA, J.S.A., COUTINHO, R.A., VAN DER HELM, T.C.M., KINT, J.A.P.C.M. and VAN DEN HOEK, J.A.R. (1993) 'HIV prevalence and risk behaviour among prostitutes and clients in Amsterdam: migrants at increased risk for HIV infection', *Genitourinary Medicine*, **69**, pp. 251–6.

VAN DER HELM, TH., BIERSTEKER, S., VAN MENS, L. and VAN DEN HOEK, A. (1995) 'The Netherlands', in EUROPEAN INTERVENTION PROJECTS AIDS PREVENTION FOR PROSTITUTES, *Europap 1994 Final Report*, Gent: Europap Coordination Centre.

VAN DEN HOEK, J.A.R., COUTINHO, R.A., VAN HAASTRECHT, H.J.A., VAN ZADELHOFF, A.W. and GOUDSMIT, J. (1988) 'Prevalence and risk factors of HIV infections among drug users and drug-using prostitutes in Amsterdam', *AIDS*, **2**, pp. 55–60.

HOOYKAAS, C., VAN DER PLIGT, J., VAN DOORNUM, G.J.J., VAN DER LINDEN, M.M.D. and COUTINHO, R.A. (1989) 'Heterosexuals at risk for HIV: differences between private and commercial partners in sexual behaviour and condom use', *AIDS*, **3**, pp. 525–32.

HOOYKAAS, C., VAN DER LINDEN, M.M.D., VAN DOORNUM, G.J.J., VAN DER VELDE, F.W., VAN DER PLIGT, J. and COUTINHO, R.A. (1991a) 'Limited changes in sexual behaviour of heterosexual men and women with multiple partners in the Netherland', *AIDS Care*, **3**, pp. 21–30.

HOOYKAAS, C., VAN DER VELDE, F.W., VAN DER LINDEN, M.M.D., VAN DOORNUM, G.J.J. and COUTINHO, R.A. (1991b) 'The importance of ethnicity as a risk factor for STDs and sexual behaviour among heterosexuals', *Genitourinary Medicine*, **67**, pp. 378–83.

KARSTEN, C. (1993) *Female Hard Drug-users in Crisis. Childhood Traumas and Survival Strategies*, Utrecht: NIAD.

KOENIG, E.R. (1989) 'International prostitutes and transmission of HIV', *Lancet*, **i**, pp. 782–3.

VAN DE LAAR, M.J.W., SLEUTJES, M.P.M., POSTEMA, C.A. and VAN DE WATER, H.P.A. (1991) 'Seksueel overdraagbare aandoeningen bij allochtone bevolkingsgroepen; een oriënterend onderzoek', *Nederlands Tijdschrift voor Geneeskunde*, **135**, pp. 1542–7.

VAN MENS, L. (1989) 'De invloed van de vrij veilig campagne op condoomgebruik bij prostituanten', *Maandblad Geestelijke Volksgezondheid*, **44**, pp. 774–86.

MOOIJ, A. (1993) 'Aids en de machteloosheid van het oude moralisme', *Psychologie en Maatschappij* , **65**, pp. 353–66.

NCAB (1988/1990) *AIDS en Prostitutie*, Amsterdam: NCAB.

PHETERSON, G. (Ed.) (1989) *A Vindication of the Rights of Whores*, Seattle: Seal Press.

PRINS, M., BINDELS, P.J.E., COUTINHO, R.A., HENQUET, C.J.M., VAN DOORNUM, G.J.J. and VAN DEN HOEK, J.A.R. (1994) 'Determinants of penicillinase producing Neisseria gonorrhoeae infections in heterosexuals in Amsterdam', *Genitourinary Medicine*, **70**, pp. 247–52.

STICHTING SOA-BESTRIJDING (1996) *Beleidsplan Preventie van AIDS/SOA in de Prostitutie. 1996 tot en met 1998*, Utrecht: Stichting SOA-Bestrijding.

TREURNIET, H.F. and DAVIDSE, W. (1993) 'Trends in de frequentie van seksueel overdraagbare aandoeningen in Nederland', *Nederlands Tijdschrift voor Geneeskunde*, **137**, pp. 1457–61.

VANWESENBEECK, I. (1994) *Prostitutes' Well-being and Risk*, Amsterdam: VU University Press.

VANWESENBEECK, I., DE GRAAF, R., VAN ZESSEN, G., STRAVER, C.J. and VISSER, J.H. (1993) 'Protection styles of prostitutes' clients: intentions, behavior, and considerations in relation to AIDS', *Journal of Sex Education and Therapy*, **19**, pp. 79–92.

VANWESENBEECK, I., VAN ZESSEN, G., DE GRAAF, R. and STRAVER, C.J. (1994) 'Contextual and interactional factors influencing condom use in heterosexual prostitution contacts', *Patient Education and Counseling*, **24**, pp. 307–22.

VANWESENBEECK, I., DE GRAAF, R., VAN ZESSEN, G., STRAVER, C.J. and VISSER, J.H. (1995) 'Professional HIV risk taking, levels of victimization, and well-being in female prostitutes in the Netherlands', *Archives of Sexual Behavior*, **24**, pp. 503–15.

VEUGELERS, P.J., VAN ZESSEN, G., SANDFORT, TH.G.M., CORNELISSE-CLAASSEN, T.M. and VAN GRIENSVEN, G.J.P. (1992) 'Seksualiteit en risicogedrag van Amsterdamse mannen', *Tijdschrift voor Sociale Gezondheidszorg*, **70**, pp. 87–94.

VISSER, J. (in press) 'Prostitutiebeleid: terug bij af?', in *De Emancipatie van de Prostitutie*, Utrecht: Humanistisch Studiecentrum Nederland.

WIESSING, L.G., HOUWELING, H., MEULDERS, W.A.J., CERDÁ, E., JANSEN, M., VAN LOON, A.M. and SPRENGER, M.J.W. (1995) *Prevalentie van HIV-infecties onder Druggebruikers in Zuid-Limburg*, Bilthoven: RIVM.

VAN ZESSEN, G. (1991) 'Huidig seksueel gedrag', in G. VAN ZESSEN and T. SANDFORT (Eds), *Seksualiteit in Nederland; Seksueel Gedrag, Risico en Preventie van AIDS*, Amsterdam: Swets & Zeitlinger.

VAN ZESSEN, G. and SANDFORT, T. (1991) *Seksualiteit in Nederland*, Amsterdam: Swets & Zeitlinger.

Chapter 6

AIDS Prevention for Migrants in
the Netherlands

Loes Singels

From the start of the Dutch AIDS prevention programme, migrants were considered a priority group, in need of targeted prevention efforts. Since the middle of the 1970s, when the number of migrants to the Netherlands started to increase, it had been noted that, because of linguistic and cultural barriers, these groups were not usually well informed by health education campaigns aimed at the Dutch public in general. In order to ensure that the entire population, including migrants, was well informed about HIV/AIDS, the National Committee on AIDS Control (NCAB) set up a specific Migrants AIDS Prevention Project. It is important to stress that epidemiological evidence was not the reason for starting targeted prevention activities in the Netherlands. There were no indications that minority groups were more affected by HIV/AIDS than the indigenous Dutch population. The fact that mobility can be an important factor in the spread of AIDS was, however, an additional reason for organizing targeted AIDS prevention. Migrants can arrive from countries with a relatively high incidence of HIV, and often remain in close contact with relatives and friends living in the country of origin.

By setting up a specific Migrants Project, the Netherlands together with countries like Norway and Switzerland, developed a coherent policy for AIDS prevention among the migrant communities from an early stage. In many other European countries, migrants did not become a target group until much later, or not at all.

In this chapter, the aims and the activities of the Migrants Project, the results from related scientific research conducted by others, and the recent developments and the plans for the future will be described. First, some information will be presented about the numbers and backgrounds of the various migrant communities in the Netherlands, and about the general principles of health education for these groups, which had been set up several years before the start of the AIDS epidemic. AIDS prevention for migrants was built on these principles embedded in existing health care structures.

Numbers and Backgrounds of Migrants

Migrants have been coming to the Netherlands for many years, and for various reasons. As in most Western European countries, the main migration movements consist of people from former Dutch colonies, labour migrants, asylum seekers and refugees. In 1995, officially, there were 799842 migrants living in the Netherlands, making up 5.1 per cent of the total Dutch population (Centraal Bureau voor de Statistiek, 1995). If the second generation migrants are included, the total number of migrants living in the Netherlands comes to 2.6 million people (about 17% of the total Dutch population). It is estimated that an additional 50000 migrants are not registered because they do not yet have a permit to stay, or because they came into the country illegally.

People from former colonies have been migrating to the Netherlands since World War Two. About 200000 people came from Indonesia during the period from 1945 to 1949, the year this country became independent. These migrants had Dutch nationality and most of them spoke the Dutch language. They assimilated within Dutch society and are usually no longer regarded as 'migrants'.

Migrants from the Moluccas on the other hand, who came in great numbers to the Netherlands in 1951, when their island became part of the Republic of Indonesia, were placed in specific reception centres. Even though most Moluccan migrants have now left these centres, they are still much more regarded as a separate ethnic group, some of them still holding on to their ideal of one day returning to a free Moluccan country. About 50000 Moluccans live in the Netherlands today.

People from the former Dutch colony of Surinam have been migrating to the Netherlands since the beginning of the 1960s. In 1975, just before this country became independent, there was a large influx of these migrants. Today about 260000 Surinamese people live in the Netherlands. From the Dutch Antilles, formally still a part of the Dutch Kingdom, about 90000 people migrated to the Netherlands. Both Surinam and Antillian people migrated in search of better working and educational opportunities and to escape from the deteriorating economic situation at home (Schumacher, 1987).

From the 1960s, labour migrants came to live in the Netherlands. These were at first invited by large industrial companies. Later on, migrants came on their own initiative. At first, only men came to the Netherlands. Since about 1975, they have been joined by their families. Most labour migrants come from Mediterranean countries. In the beginning many people came from countries like Italy, the former Yugoslavia, Spain and Portugal. Later, larger numbers came from Turkey and Morocco; today these two groups are among the largest migrant groups. Approximately 240000 Turks and 195000 Moroccans live in the Netherlands.

Finally, asylum seekers from various countries (Iran, Iraq, Vietnam, Sri Lanka, Somalia, the former Yugoslavia, parts of Central and sub-Saharan Africa) came to the Netherlands, requesting refugee status. As in other Western European countries, the number of asylum seekers has increased enormously since the 1980s. Whereas in the beginning of the 1980s a few thousand asylum seekers came to the Netherlands every year, in 1994 this number increased to 50000. Because of this increase the Dutch reception policy has changed. Only people who can prove they are escaping from war, violence and personal persecution for reasons of race, religion or political conviction will be granted a refugee status.

Regarding migrants, the Dutch government now applies the so-called policy of 'discouragement'. New migrants can only come into the country within the framework of reunification of families and marriage with spouses from the country of origin. The prospect is that for the foreseeable future fewer people will migrate to the Netherlands than during the past three decades.

Unlike the situation in some other countries, the composition of the Dutch population cannot be regarded as a 'melting pot'. Instead, a number of distinguishable ethnic groups live together, some more, some less assimilated within Dutch society. The expression 'migrants' will be used here when referring to all these different groups of migrants, ethnic minorities and refugees. The expression 'communities' will be used to refer to a group of people with the same ethnic background. It does not necessarily imply that this group is united or coherent.

Health Education for Migrants

In the Netherlands as elsewhere, migrants are clearly not a homogeneous group. There are great differences in their cultural and religious background, and their command of the Dutch language. Furthermore, the educational and socio-economic status they had in their home country will vary. This status is usually connected to the reason why they migrated: refugees are, for instance, generally higher educated people compared to labour migrants from Turkey and Morocco. Nevertheless, there are similarities in the way many if not all of these communities differ from the general Dutch public. First of all, their living and working conditions are usually more severe. Factors like hard physical labour, bad housing conditions, low income and the stressful effects of migration influence the health of migrants. Furthermore, these communities differ from the Dutch regarding the way health care services are used. Many migrants do not use all the facilities available, partly because they do not know about their existence, partly because they are not familiar with these kinds of services. Culturally formed habits of health seeking behaviour and expectations about medical care play an important role in the way facilities are used and appreciated. Pregnant migrant Moroccan women from rural areas, for instance, are used to being assisted by traditional midwives, who exercise special rituals to protect the woman during the delivery. Such women may be reluctant to use professional pre- and postnatal care in the Netherlands, because they consider this kind of medical care irrelevant and unnecessary (Bartels, 1987).

Health care professionals have not always known how to deal with specific migration-related health problems. They also experienced communication problems, not only because of differences in language, but also because of differences in cultural background, ideas, expectations and behaviour concerning health care.

In order to tackle this complex set of problems, general health education for ethnic minorities has been conducted by both governmental and non-governmental organizations. In 1976, the National Health Education Office for Migrants was founded, financed by the government. This office developed programmes aimed at both migrants and health care professionals. Migrants were informed about the services available (both physical and mental care) and about preventive behaviour. On the other hand, health care professionals were informed about the cultural backgrounds of the ethnic minority communities.

To diminish communication problems, free interpreter services have been made available by the government. Approximately 700 interpreters are available, speaking more than 85 languages. They can be asked to assist health care professionals both in person or by telephone. This service is, however, not frequently used by health care professionals, because they consider it too time-consuming. The above mentioned insights and principles concerning health education for migrants form an important backcloth against which to understand the work of the Migrants AIDS Prevention Project.

Objectives of the Migrants Project

The general starting point for AIDS prevention for the Dutch public was adopted for the Migrants Project: AIDS prevention should be focused at the target group as a whole, rather than at people specifically at risk. Consequently, the Migrants Project aimed at providing *all* members of the migrant communities with relevant AIDS prevention information in order to raise awareness and to increase levels of knowledge. Additionally, the project aimed to stimulate migrant organizations to become involved in AIDS prevention, in order to create a climate of opinion that would enable the subject of AIDS to be discussed.

Support for these objectives derived from the few available data at the beginning of the project. An early research study among 183 Turkish and 213 Moroccan men and women, carried out in Amsterdam, supported indications from workers in the field that these communities were not well informed about the exact routes of transmission and the necessary means of prevention (Cornelissen-Claasen and De Vree, 1989). Furthermore, there were indications that some members of several ethnic communities had the idea that AIDS did not concern them. This idea was connected to the conviction that they were not vulnerable to infection from HIV as long as they lived according to their cultural/religious rules and regulations. These 'official' rules imply for the Muslim communities, for instance, that sexual intercourse is permitted only in the context of marriage and that homosexual contacts are not allowed. Consequently, many members of minority ethnic groups had the idea that AIDS did not concern them and, on the other hand, that AIDS was a taboo subject, not to be openly discussed.

Indications from field workers also indicated that, even if migrants do speak Dutch, they can still miss the point of a health education message if they are not familiar with the images used. In the very first AIDS campaign for the Dutch general public, for instance, leading parts were played by 'a flower and a bee'. The reference to sexual intercourse implicit in such imagery – so obvious for the Dutch – was not recognized by most members of migrant communities. As a result some gained the impression that AIDS could be transmitted by insects.

It was therefore decided to take into account the cultural backgrounds of particular ethnic groups, to use the native language as much as possible, and to use specific migrant information channels, like migrant media and community networks, for disseminating AIDS-related messages.

Working Method and Structure of the Migrants Project

The aim of the Migrants Project was to develop a coherent prevention programme. This programme would entail the initiation, coordination and stimulation of prevention activities. These tasks were carried out by a coordinator, with support from an advisory board. The main institutions for general health education, including the Foundation for STD Control and Municipal Health Services, were represented on this board. These institutions subsequently carried out the prevention activities. Financial support for these activities, especially for the development of methods and materials, was made available by the government and by the AIDS Fund.

The project was placed within the structure of the NCAB, and the project's policy working plans were integral parts of the Dutch National AIDS Policy. The annually established working plans were used as a reference standard by the AIDS Fund to make decisions on requests for financial support for prevention activities, submitted by the executing institutions.

In 1995 the government decided to discontinue the NCAB. Since then the Migrants Project has been a part of the Netherlands Institute for Health Promotion and Disease Prevention (NIGZ). In this Institute all expertise on health education for ethnic minorities is brought together.

From 1990 onward, the issue of AIDS and migrants has also been addressed regularly in international settings. The coordinator of the Migrants Project collaborates closely with other European countries and with countries of origin to exchange information and models of good practice. This networking was initiated by the European AIDS and Mobility Project (Van Duifhuizen, 1991).

Target Groups

Several criteria have been employed for selecting target groups. Priority has been given to the largest migrant communities and to communities with a relatively isolated position within Dutch society. Communities with large differences in culture and language, compared to the Dutch general public, have been prioritized. Activities first started with people from Turkey, Morocco and the former colonies Surinam and the Dutch Antilles. Later, in 1991, activities were set up for smaller migrant communities, including Moluccans, Cape-Verdians and other sub-Saharan Africans, refugees and asylum seekers.

During the course of the Migrants Project, target groups have been redefined. Special programmes have been set up for subgroups within the target groups, such as drug users and school drop-outs, because they were difficult to reach by the regular programmes aimed at migrants. Since 1994, women of different migrant communities have been considered a separate target group. Peer educators reported that many of these women experienced feelings of helplessness, not knowing what to do, for example, when their sexual partners had sex with other people. A new method, including training in assertiveness in order to teach women to discuss safe sex with their partners, was considered necessary and is now being developed.

Cooperation with Migrant Organizations

A few migrant groups in the Netherlands, including Moluccans and Africans, have taken the initiative to set up community-based organizations for AIDS prevention. In 1994, for instance, the African Foundation of AIDS Prevention and Counselling (AFAPAC), was established to provide information and support for sub-Saharan Africans living in the Netherlands. Until then, only a few targeted activities had been developed for members of this community.

The aim of the Dutch Migrants Project to involve migrant organizations in AIDS prevention has been less successful with Turkish, Moroccan, Surinam and Antillian communities. The fact that the AIDS policy for migrants is enacted through (semi)governmental structures may have been an obstacle for creation of these organizations. The need to become involved is obviously less urgent when the National Programme includes activities for these specific groups. Furthermore, most existing migrant organizations in the Netherlands are more focused on issues like education and labour than on health.

AIDS Prevention in Practice: Main Projects

The main prevention projects for migrants include peer education, telephone helplines and a mass media campaign.

Peer Education

In 1989, a course was developed to train peer educators to provide information in face-to-face contacts. In 1990 the first peer educators, mainly men and women from Turkey, Morocco, Surinam and the Dutch Antilles, were ready to carry out educational activities for groups of compatriots. Today about 90 peer educators from 10 different ethnic communities are available. Within a period of three years, approximately 40000 migrants have been reached this way, mostly in coffee houses, community centres, mosques or at large cultural events (Van Haastrecht, 1995).

Peer education was chosen as an educational method because of the advantage that the education could be given orally and in the native language. This choice was closely linked to the tradition of disseminating information orally in many migrant communities, and also because of the relatively high level of illiteracy among certain target groups. Also, a peer educator is likely to share the cultural habits and beliefs and therefore knows how to discuss adequately 'difficult' subjects like sexuality and homosexuality. Furthermore, it was expected that peer educators could serve as exemplary models, making it clear that AIDS does concern a specific community as well. In practice this proved to be an important asset. However, there were also indications that peer educators were not fully accepted as professional educators by all members of the target groups. Some participants, mostly male, make this clear by questioning the knowledge of the peer educators, stating that they would prefer a doctor as an educator.

Peer educators are quite often approached for support in assisting people getting an HIV-test or advising about the psycho-social problems faced by people living with HIV/AIDS. It is hard for peer educators to respond to these requests, since they are not trained to do this. These questions can be considered as important indications that counselling activities carried out by the regular health care services do not always function well for the migrant communities. Alerting the coordinator of the Migrants Project to these requests is in fact another important task of the peer educators.

Telephone Helplines

In addition to the Dutch AIDS Helpline, telephone helplines were set up for Turkish and Moroccan people in 1990, and for Chinese people in 1993. The aim of this service was to offer members of these communities the opportunity to obtain free information about AIDS in their native languages anonymously. This plan could not be carried out to full satisfaction due to several practical problems. For the Moroccan helpline no suitable employees could be recruited. The Turkish line functioned for about two years, staffed by peer educators who were present two days a week. An average of four people called on each of these days. In the opinion of the NCAB, this number was not sufficient to justify the costs of employment and therefore it was decided to discontinue this service in 1994. For Chinese people the service was never put into effect at all. As a result, the role of all three helplines has been restricted to supplying information about AIDS on audio cassettes. At the time of writing, an average of 200 people call each line every month.

Since 1993, funding has been made available to staff these helplines on special occasions like World AIDS Day by educators from the respective migrant groups. This service is then widely advertised in the migrant media and generally well used. Fifty-nine Turkish, 111 Moroccan and 69 Chinese people called the Helpline on World AIDS Day in 1995. Compared to earlier years, a shift can be noticed in the kinds of questions asked, from factual questions about AIDS to more personal questions, giving an indication of the problems migrants encounter with regard to AIDS. Some callers, for instance, have reported negative experiences with pre- and post-test counselling. Others say they would like to be tested but are afraid to see a doctor. One Moroccan caller took the opportunity to talk to the peer educator about his HIV positive status, about which he had not dared to tell anyone, not even his wife.

Mass Media Campaigns

To support small-scale activities like peer education and to create a supportive environment for migrants affected by HIV/AIDS, a one-year mass media campaign titled 'AIDS Concerns Everyone' started in December 1995 for people from Turkey, Morocco, Surinam and the Dutch Antilles. The campaign strategy consisted of a mix of media, including television, radio, newspapers, leaflets, posters and helpline services. Members of the target groups were involved in the production and pre-testing of all materials.

The radio programmes for the Turkish and Moroccan communities were produced within the context of another project, 'Translating the AIDS Message Across Europe'. In cooperation with the United Kingdom, France and Italy these programmes aimed to promote greater awareness of telephone helplines as part of World AIDS Day activities. Even though different countries work within different policy frameworks, it proved profitable to exchange experiences and expertise. By working together it was possible to develop programmes more efficiently and also to reach more members of the relevant target groups.

Although the campaign has not yet been evaluated, reports by peer educators give the impression that there is great interest in the campaign and that the issue of AIDS is frequently discussed. There has also been a widespread distribution of relevant materials. Many local migrant radio stations have been prepared to cooperate and broadcast the radio programmes offered to them. The printed materials produced were sold out within two weeks.

Research

Until now, few studies of the AIDS-related knowledge, behaviour and beliefs of different migrant communities have been conducted. Only a few research projects, mainly qualitative studies focusing on subgroups within some communities, have been carried out. In 1993 and 1994, qualitative research on the sexual behaviour of Turkish, Moroccan and Surinam men was carried out by the University of Amsterdam (Everaert and Lamur, 1993; Van Gelder and Lamur, 1993; Lamur and Terborg, 1994). The purpose of these studies was to identify the strategies used to minimize risk. Forty-six Moroccan, 35 Turkish and 26 Surinam men were interviewed. Findings suggested that most respondents knew about HIV and AIDS, but also reported misconceptions about both means of transmission and prevention strategies. Members of all three groups thought, for instance, that people with AIDS could easily be identified by their appearance and that therefore it was easy to identify a non-infected partner. Some Surinam men also thought that AIDS could be cured by traditional Surinam herbal treatments.

The researchers concluded that the sexual behaviour of the majority of respondents could be considered risky since they failed to use condoms consistently. Research among the Turkish and Moroccan men showed that about a third of respondents had been at risk of HIV infection. Many respondents showed much resistance to the use of condoms because they consider condoms not 'natural' and because using condoms is seen as a sign of infidelity or of having sexual contacts with sex workers. The approach used by the Migrants Project is supported by the recommendations of these researchers who concluded that education on AIDS should take into account traditional beliefs and that efforts to change behaviour should be closely linked to traditional habits.

Other studies affirm that migrant men are involved in unsafe sexual behaviour. Compared to Dutch men, Turkish and Moroccan men have relatively more often unsafe sex with street sex workers, many of whom are drug injectors, and window sex workers. These sex workers, who are mostly of Latin American or African origin, reported that they had frequently had unsafe sexual contacts with Turkish and Moroccan men (De Graaf, 1995).

Studies of the prevalence of STDs show that Turkish and Moroccan men have a relatively higher prevalence of STDs than Dutch men. In some cities about a third of the male clients at STD clinics are migrants, mainly from Turkey and Surinam (SOA Stichting, 1993). This difference could be partly explained by the proposition that migrant men are more likely to use the free services offered by STD clinics, rather than visiting their general practitioner. Yet, in Amsterdam it has been noted that compared to several years before, the percentage of Dutch clients declined from 76 per cent in 1982 to 63 per cent in 1992. It was also noted that migrant men are more often infected in sex worker contacts. Since 1989, male clients of STD clinics have been asked if they go to sex workers. Twenty per cent of all STDs appear to have been transmitted in sex worker contacts. Among Turkish and Moroccan men this figure is 65 per cent (De Graaf, 1995).

The studies presented in this section report on qualitative data from a very small part of the migrant communities and some (analyses of) figures of STD clinics. No funding has been made available to investigate knowledge, attitudes, beliefs and behaviours of the larger migrant communities. Also, there exists little information about the effects of targeted prevention efforts for ethnic minorities carried out so far. This lack of information is a major hindrance for the development of the future policy of the Migrants Project.

Epidemiology

Although epidemiological evidence was not a significant factor leading to the setting up of targeted AIDS prevention activities for migrants, there has, however, since 1995, been a slight increase in the proportion of non-Dutch people with AIDS, compared with previous years. In 1991 about 20 per cent of all registered people with AIDS did not have Dutch nationality. A large proportion of these came from the USA, Canada and other Western European countries (about 12 per cent). By 1995 the total number of non-Dutch people with AIDS had risen to 24 per cent, due to an increase of patients from sub-Saharan Africa and the Caribbean.

Compared to Dutch people with AIDS, more non-Dutch people have been infected by heterosexual contact. Out of the total of those reported as being infected by heterosexual contact, 26 per cent came from a country with a high HIV prevalence and another 15 per cent have had a sexual partner from these countries (Gras, 1995).

Future Priorities

By setting up a specific Migrants Project, a coherent policy has been developed for AIDS prevention among migrant communities in the Netherlands. Prevention strategies, methods and materials have been developed, mainly in conjunction with these same communities. In general, the chosen policy seems to have functioned well. A large number of activities have been carried out by national and local institutions. It is, however, not possible to give accurate information about the achievements of these activities, since their effects have not been systematically evaluated.

At present it is considered important to continue targeted AIDS prevention for migrants living in the Netherlands. A few changes in the choice of aims, however, will be necessary. The results of the few small-scale research projects conducted among migrant communities indicate that even though respondents are aware of AIDS, they still engage in unsafe sexual behaviour. Therefore, it is considered important to shift the emphasis in AIDS education from raising awareness to changing attitudes and behaviour.

The main priority for the near future is to link AIDS prevention to general health education and health promotion, by incorporating AIDS into other issues like family planning and sex education. The reason for this choice is twofold. First, it is expected that members of migrant communities who are not interested in AIDS prevention *per se*, perhaps because they think that AIDS does not concern them, can be better reached this way. Second, in this way the AIDS policy for migrants can be adjusted to get it in line with recent developments in government policy. During the last couple of years, less money has been available for developing and executing AIDS prevention projects, both for the general public and for migrants. Institutions carrying out health education more generally have been urged by the government to conduct AIDS prevention within their standard policies and budgets. Because of this development, migrants risk being excluded from AIDS prevention programmes. Ensuring that special attention continues to be given to this target group is an important and continuing task for the Migrants Project.

The gradual increase in the number of infected migrants will have a growing impact on health care institutions. An investigation carried out by the NCAB in 1993 showed that health care professionals seem to find communication with migrants especially difficult when matters of sexuality or death are involved (NCAB, 1993). The interpreters available are not always well trained in these matters. Furthermore, health care professionals reported that many infected migrants tend to find themselves isolated from their relatives and friends. Since AIDS is still not openly discussed in several of the migrant communities, those affected may be afraid to talk about the problems that confront them or if they do, are very often blamed and neglected. Education within the health care setting, aimed at both the patients and the professionals, is therefore a new priority for the Migrants Project. For migrants with HIV/AIDS new styles of health promotion need to be developed to supply information on the progress of the disease and the kinds of care available. Such education needs to be carried out in the native language, addressing both the patient's and family members' concerns. In addition, support systems aimed at encouraging contact among infected migrants will be set up. Concurrently, health care professionals are to be trained in working with this group of patients, learning how to cope with the specific problems.

Finally, a comprehensive research project to collect data on knowledge, attitudes and behaviour among migrants and to evaluate the effects of the targeted prevention campaigns carried out so far, is of great importance. The lack of this kind of data is the main bottleneck in the development of a future policy for AIDS prevention among migrants in the Netherlands.

Loes Singels

References

Bartels, E. (Ed.) (1987) *Het Paradijs is onder de Voeten van de Moeders. Verloskundige Zorg aan Marokkaanse Vrouwen in Nederland*, Amsterdam: Vrije Universiteit.

Centraal Bureau voor de Statistiek (1995) *Allochtonen in Nederland*, Rijswijk: CBS.

Cornelissen-Claasen, T.M. and De Vree, R.M.M. (1989) *AIDS Voorlichting aan Turken en Marokkanen*, Sektor Onderzoek en Statistiek, Gemeente Amsterdam.

Van Duifhuizen, R. (1991) *AIDS and Mobility: The Impact of International Mobility on the Spread of HIV and the Needs and Possibility for AIDS/HIV Prevention Programmes*, Amsterdam: NCAB.

Everaert, H. and Lamur, H.E. (1993) *Alles wat Geheim is, is Lekker: Seksuele Relaties en Beschermingsgedrag onder Turkse Mannen*, Amsterdam: Het Spinhuis.

Van Gelder, P. and Lamur, H.E. (1993) *Tussen Schaamte en Mannelijkheid: Seksuele Relaties en Beschermingsgedrag onder Marokkaanse Mannen*, Amsterdam: Het Spinhuis.

De Graaf, R. (1995) *Prostitutes and their Clients; Sexual Networks and Determinants of Condom Use*, Doctoral Thesis, Wageningen: Ponsen & Looijen.

Gras, M. (1995) *Etniciteit en het Risico op HIV/AIDS*, Amsterdam: PccAo.

Van Haastrecht, P. (1995) *Jaarverslag 1994, Project Voorlichters Eigen Taal*, Rotterdam: GGD.

Lamur, H.E. and Terborg, J. (1994) *Risicoperceptie en Preventiestrategiën; Creools-Surinaamse Bezoekers van een Rotterdamse SOA-poli*, Delft: Euburon.

NCAB (1993) *Migranten en AIDS*, Amsterdam: NCAB.

Schumacher, P. (1987) *De Minderheden: 700.000 Migranten Minder Gelijk*, Amsterdam: Van Gennep.

SOA Stichting (1993) *Registratie Niet-curatieve SOA-bestrijding*, Utrecht: SOA Stichting.

Part 2

Policy Issues

Chapter 7

The Decisive Role of Politics:
AIDS Control in the Netherlands

Janherman Veenker

In the Netherlands, public problems which involve a conflict of interests are usually addressed with the help of an advisory body consisting of experts, the parties concerned and the government. This tried and tested approach is used both in times of crisis – such as the sudden emergence of AIDS – and for issues which require a continuous consideration of different interests – such as the reimbursement system for health care.[1] In the case of infectious disease control there is an extra impetus to set up a consultative structure, as no central body is solely responsible for this in the Netherlands. Responsibility is shared by several national authorities and city councils. This concerted approach of mutual advice, consultation and cooperation in the Netherlands is often described as 'coordination'. Since this term clearly means more than simply coordination as a tool for effective organization, I will use the term 'concerted coordination' to describe the processes at work.

Although concerted coordination is functionally necessary and in fact may help to bring about a supportive political climate, in itself it is not enough to create effective policy. This is even more true when a policy has to be innovative and may come in conflict with traditional values and vested interests. As was clear from the start, AIDS always held the potential to cause controversy. For an AIDS policy to be effective, therefore, the right political conditions needed to be established and maintained.

In this chapter I will describe how this has been done, what problems had to be faced and how far these problems could be solved. I will do so roughly chronologically. My conclusion will be that in the case of AIDS, positions taken by government and in Parliament have been decisive in determining AIDS policies in the Netherlands.

The Development of an Advisory Structure

To create an effective structure by which to respond to the AIDS crisis, the national advisory and consultative tradition was extensively used. The development of AIDS policy in the Netherlands can be divided into three periods, following the different coordinating structures that functioned over time: 1983–87 – National AIDS Policy Coordination Team; 1987–95 – National

Committee on AIDS Control (NCAB); 1995 onwards – Netherlands AIDS Fund.

Each of these three periods can be characterized more or less by the areas of AIDS policy that received the most attention and energy. Between 1983 and 1987 the foundation was laid for public information and prevention. The second period was dominated by concern for legal and ethical issues, especially the first four years between 1987 and 1991. From the late 1980s onward, issues of care and treatment came to the foreground, until by about 1995 they began to dominate AIDS policy. Epidemiological developments over this period were as follows. In 1983 a total of 24 persons was diagnosed with AIDS; in 1987 the cumulative total of AIDS diagnoses was 500. This figure had risen to 2078 by 1992 and 3609 by halfway through 1995.

The National AIDS Policy Coordination Team originated out of a succesful cooperation between gay (health) activists and Amsterdam health officials. The chairman, Hans Moerkerk, was both. Eventually the team consisted of 10 members representing prevention and education on STDs and drugs; gay and lesbian (service) organizations; bloodbanks; and Amsterdam and national health authorities. The AIDS Coordination Team started its work in September 1983. The government gave official approval by funding the post of National AIDS Coordinator in January 1984, Jan van Wijngaarden, and sending an official observer to the AIDS Coordination Team on behalf of the State Secretary of Health.

When in 1985 the State Secretary of Health reported to the Second Chamber of the States General[2] (hereafter 'Parliament') about AIDS for the first time, his report relied heavily on the groundwork laid by the AIDS Coordination Team.

> the report introduces a range of tools and points of departure, which would later be developed and implemented: the policy choice of an integrated approach to the medical, psychosocial and legal consequences of AIDS; the implicit choice of a specific AIDS prevention policy; implementation of AIDS prevention based on cooperation with the groups involved, making individual responsibility a point of departure; the explicit choice of integrating care and support into the existing sector of care organizations; the importance of scientific research and well coordinated policy making; combatting undesirable social consequences. (Reinking, 1993, p. 24).

In this first debate, the constructive and agenda-setting influence of the young coordination structure can very clearly be seen.

In the second report on AIDS to Parliament (July 1987) the coordination structure was upgraded and better focused. The NCAB was institutionalized as a formal advisory committee to the government. A wide range of medical, ethical and juridical expertise was added. Representation from persons with haemophilia and persons with HIV was added; participation from the gay and lesbian community was limited.

The new advisory structure implied that the government would take a more active and visible role. The then State Secretary of Health, Dick Dees,[3] highlighted this as follows: 'By now the issue of AIDS has developed into a grave problem area of public health with a clear political dimension' (Kamerstukken 19218 nrs 8–9, 1987, p. 28). When asked by Parliament what he meant with this political dimension, he answered that political decision making was required to establish priorities in funding to combat serious and terminal diseases, referring to AIDS in comparison with cancer and cardiovascular diseases. 'Moreover in the combat against AIDS fundamental values can be at stake (e.g. infringement of someone's privacy; restrictions on travelling abroad). Conflicting interests in these areas have to be balanced out at the political level' (Kamerstukken 19218 nr 12, 1988, p. 24).

During its eight years of existence, the NCAB issued about 90 pieces of advice and recommendations. These formed the basis for reports to Parliament and subsequent Parliamentary discussion. They also had a profound influence on the implementation of AIDS policies. By law, new advisory comittees, formally established by the government, can only exist for four years. This period may be extended with another four years in exceptional circumstances. The NCAB was positively evaluated in 1991 and its mandate was extended until 1995 because of the uncertainties surrounding AIDS. In 1995, the committee was disbanded. Most of its responsibilities were transferred to the AIDS Fund. This fund was established in 1985 to carry out private fund-raising for the fight against AIDS. In 1994, in order to make the most appropriate use of the funding available, the government decided to delegate responsibility for a large part of its spending on AIDS prevention, care and innovation to the AIDS Fund. The AIDS Fund develops an annual AIDS Policy Plan which is submitted to the Minister of Health[4] for approval.

The Initial Step: Securing Safe Blood Products

Decisions to safeguard blood and blood products are generally seen as the start of AIDS coordination in the Netherlands. In the second half of 1982, it became clear to a small group of experts and others involved that measures had to be taken regarding the blood supply. Although there was no certainty, the signals that an infectious agent was carried on through blood products were too strong. A closed meeting was held in January 1983, attended by health officials, representatives of the blood banks, of the haemophilia organization and of organizations of gays and lesbians. Decisions were made in the spring of 1983 (Coppoolse, 1988; Spijkerman, 1986; Tillemans, 1988).

There was a clear conflict of interest. The blood banks wanted to exclude all homosexual donors. The gay and lesbian movement wanted to avoid stigmatization and a witch-hunt against homosexuals. A compromise was reached with the help of the haemophilia organization and Amsterdam health officials. This compromise was founded on the realization that it would be technically impossible to exclude all homosexual donors. Who is to know for sure that no accepted donor is homosexual? This meant that voluntary cooperation by homosexual donors was necessary; homosexual donors would be urged to withdraw voluntarily. This message became part of the first information campaign for homosexual men, undertaken in Amsterdam in the spring of 1983. Blood banks contributed substantially to the budget for this campaign (Van Wijngaarden, 1989).

Supposedly most homosexual donors indeed withdrew voluntarily. There is, however, no way to be sure about this, since it is unknown how many behaviourally homosexual donors there were to begin with. Discussion about the voluntary withdrawal policy never really ended, even though there remained broad agreement between all parties involved. Over time some individual homosexual donors felt they had not been at risk for HIV infection and demanded to be allowed to donate blood. Some people with haemophilia rejected these demands and indicated that they felt a serious lack of solidarity.

The policy of voluntary withdrawal was not limited to behaviourally homosexual men. All individuals at risk of being HIV-infected were asked to do the same (for example persons who had had sex with a resident of a country where HIV is endemic). This was necessary because testing donated blood for antibodies is not sufficient to identify all infected blood. There is a window period after infection, during which no antibodies can be shown. Therefore for most categories of persons who are asked to refrain from donating blood, a period was stated during which they should not have engaged in behaviour that put them at risk for an HIV infection. As long as the behaviour concerned occurred before that period, they could safely donate blood (for example when the sex with a resident of a country where HIV is endemic occurred more than two years before the present donation). Such a period, however, was not stated for behaviourally homosexual men. As a result, behaviourally homosexual men became the only persons who were requested to withdraw as a category, instead of on the grounds of individual behaviour. On one occasion when the guidelines for blood banks regarding HIV prevention were being updated, the NCAB advised the exclusion only of men with homosexual contacts within a period of two years before donation. This advice was ignored by the blood banks, who decided to persist in totally excluding behaviourally homosexual men.

Besides this policy of voluntary exclusion, other measures had to be taken to secure the safety of the blood supply and blood products, after they became technically possible. The most important measure was the heat treatment of blood products, so as to inactivate HIV (and other infectious agents). Limited, but inconclusive information about heating as a means whereby to inactivate HIV was already available in 1983. The procedure became standard in 1985, but was not implemented at that time in every blood bank. Blood banks in the Netherlands work regionally and are to a large extent autonomous as long as the government has not issued formal directives. Heat treatment only became obligatory nationwide in 1988. A formal complaint against the government's apparent inertia regarding the procedures to secure safe blood products was filed with the 'Nationale Ombudsman'[5] in 1994 by the haemophilia organization. In 1995 the Ombudsman concluded that the Ministry of Health had ignored scientific information about the heat treatment of blood products and had failed to make it obligatory in time (De Nationale Ombudsman, 1995). The debate whether or not the government really should be blamed is still going on (Cohen, 1996). In the meantime the government has decided to allow each infected person with haemophilia compensation of Dfl 200000. It is interesting to note that the Nationale Ombudsman did not support every complaint by the haemophilia organization. In his opinion no government directive was needed, where responsible organizations and health officials had put adequate procedures into action on their own account. These included measures taken with regard to the exclusion of possibly infected donors.

The Political Necessity to Address the General Public

After initial activities to secure the safety of the blood supply, AIDS policy became mainly a policy of information and prevention. Between spring 1983 and spring 1987, prevention activities were directed towards groups at risk, not at the public at large. Until 1986, the available epidemiological data did not indicate that the general population was seriously at risk. The AIDS Coordination Team developed a policy towards the general public which it described as 'active-passive'. This consisted of making information available upon request, through folders and a telephone hotline run by volunteers. Good use was made of free publicity (AIDS Coordinatie Team, 1986). Methodologically and epidemiologically, it was not felt necessary to change this 'active-passive' policy and to address the general public directly.

In 1986/87 political pressure resulted in a change of information policy on AIDS. After the 2nd International Conference on AIDS conference in Paris in June 1986 and the London Summit Meeting of EC government leaders in December 1986, it became clear to politicians and government leaders that heterosexual transmission of HIV was possible (Van Wijngaarden, 1987; Groeneveld, 1989). For the first time widespread public unrest surfaced, which made the active dissemination of information to the general public necessary. The subsequent political pressure can be traced back to questions in Parliament in the autumn of 1986 and a formal consultation of the AIDS Coordination Team by the State Secretary of Health on 15 December 1986 (Letter by the State Secretary of Health to the Chairman of the Second Chamber, 1 April 1987, nr. DGVGZ/AGZ/BGZ–301608). The available budget for public information and prevention activities was quadrupled (at least) and the staff of several organizations involved was enhanced. The information activities of the AIDS Coordination Team were to be supervised by several committees, all chaired by the former head of the National Information Service ('Rijksvoorlichtingsdienst'), Gijs van der Wiel, at that moment the most prestigious official involved in AIDS policy.

The information and prevention workplan for 1987 was prepared by the AIDS Coordination Team, but published by the new NCAB. It announced the start of mass media campaigns, but at the same time extensively resumed the objections against information campaigns towards the general public. These objections included claims that:

- information and prevention work targeted at 'risk groups' will be epidemiologially more effective since HIV spreads from these risk groups to the population in general;
- the levels of fear among the general public may rise, which may contribute to stigmatization; and
- the costs are too high.

Additionally both the AIDS Coordination Team and the new NCAB felt that there was no epidemiological necessity to advise the general public to change its sexual behaviour.

This difference in view between the government and the AIDS Coordination Team was resolved by developing two separate general public campaigns. In spring 1987, a high profile information campaign was held, using the mass media. The AIDS Coordination team felt secure enough to support it, after pre-tests showed that the risk of panic and stigmatization was very low (Rozendaal, interview with Van Wijngaarden, 1995). In the autumn of that same year, a lower profile safe sex[6] campaign was held. These two separate campaigns have been held every year since then. Over time the information campaign was changed into a campaign that stresses understanding and solidarity. Starting in 1995, the safe sex campaigns target STDs in general (see Chapter 2 in this book).

The NCAB did not support the safe sex campaigns wholeheartedly. Some members continued to feel they were epidemiologically unnecessary and even dangerously confusing. In 1989, one of the former members of the AIDS Coordination team, Roel Coutinho, then vice chairman of the NCAB, expressed his doubts publicly (Coutinho, 1989). Having taking so public a position against a core feature of the AIDS information policy, it was inevitable he should resign from the NCAB.[7]

Sexual Values 'Defused' as a Potentially Dangerous Political Issue

When asked in 1987 by Parliament if his AIDS policy could be considered well balanced, given the fact that monogamy as a means of prevention got so little attention, the State Secretary of Health insisted that monogamy was mentioned.

> The experience with STD control however taught us that the promotion (by the Government) of a monogamous lifestyle has no effect with persons whose lifestyle is not monogamous. They will experience this message as moralizing and shut themselves off from further information. The information therefore tries to achieve realistic changes in behavior in a pragmatic and non-moralizing way, with respect for everyone's sexual views. (Kamerstukken, 19218 nr 12, 1988, p. 1)

This exchange of views in Parliament illustrates that by 1987 information and prevention activities were depoliticized to a large extent. This was achieved by a careful policy not to offend conservative Christian views within the population (Rozendaal, interview with Gijs van der Wiel, 1995).

This policy of not giving unnecessary offence became part of an overall strategy. Potentially controversial items, such as instructions on how to use condoms, or explicit affection/eroticism/sex between men, were tested first. Subsequently some distance was created between the government finance and the actual product. This was achieved by having television materials produced independently from the government, broadcasting them late at night, targeting them strictly to groups at risk, and so on. In the campaigns officially endorsed by the government, sexually explicit information was initially limited to printed material. The introduction of condoms, erotic contact between men, and so on, on television and on public billboards was gradually achieved, only after more and targeted activities had met no public or political resistance (Rozendaal, interview with Gijs van der Wiel, 1995).

All this does not mean that no conflicts arose with regard to sexual values. This became especially clear when it was decided to provide information about AIDS in high schools. After one year of preparation, the Dutch Educational Television (NOT) began a series of four nationally broadcast television programmes in October 1988. Both the national organizations of Catholic and Protestant school boards, who had been informed but not consulted about the contents,[8] objected publicly and fiercely against these programmes. They felt that too much stress was put on safe sex at the expense of abstinence. They also felt that the language used and the images shown were not in accordance with Christian values. Questions were asked in Parliament; the responsible Secretary of State for secondary education was embarrassed (Letter by the State Secretary for Education and Science to the Board of Councils for Protestant Christian Education, 11 November 1988, nr. VO/AL/BE–669.386). The incident threatened to become a direct political attack on government AIDS policy as such. Because of their constitutional rights[9] denominational schools, which form about two-thirds of all primary and secondary education, have a political influence that easily surpasses that of the churches they are affiliated with. The constitutional position of denominational schools also makes it extremely difficult to defuse a conflict of values politically (for example in Parliament), since the government has no final authority in the matter, but will be criticized instead for putting itself in such a vulnerable position.

The conflict was not allowed to become an openly political one, however. It was addressed in a closed, special meeting (25 November 1988), chaired by the earlier mentioned Gijs van der Wiel. Every effort was given to find some common ground. While all recognized the necessity of educating secondary pupils on AIDS, there was no consensus about the contents of such education. The national organizations of Catholic and Protestant school boards succesfully claimed separate budgets to develop their own materials, which were to be more value oriented and less sex oriented than the existing materials. The NCAB on the other hand, who feared that prevention efforts might become too diverse and confusing, negotiated succesfully that all materials would be developed under joint coordination. During 1989, three separate new educational 'packages' were developed, within a broad coordination structure. Eventually, the Catholic organizations decided not to publish their own material after all. A survey among 900 Catholic schools showed that only 175 would be interested in using these separate materials (*Katholiek Nieuwsblad*, 29 September 1989), and for the others existing materials were acceptable.

One year later, at a joint press conference (30 November 1989) two packages of educational materials were presented, one developed with general support by educational organizations of public and Catholic denomination, one developed by Protestant organizations. To emphasize that both packages were considered adequate from the perspective of AIDS prevention, the press conference was supported by all relevant national educational organizations and the NCAB. Since then, all schools have had a choice between materials developed for schools in general and materials developed specifically for Protestant schools.

The Dominant Political Discussion: Testing and Its Consequences

While monogamy and sexual values were not politicized, another issue was allowed to become the subject of intense political debate: testing and its consequences.

Testing policy was and is a fundamental aspect of the approach towards HIV/AIDS. The central question in a large number of recommendations made by the NCAB was the acceptability of the HIV test in certain situations. Associated with this was the question whether it would be acceptable to link certain consequences to a person's serostatus. (NCAB, 1995, p. 20)

During the time of the NCAB, Parliament formally discussed AIDS policy three times.[10] Conflicts of interest in relation to testing policy dominated these debates. The most important subjects were testing as part of the acceptance procedure for life insurance, testing as part of the medical examination for personnel recruitment, and anonymous and involuntary testing as part of HIV prevalence surveys (see also STG, 1992).

The tone of the Parliamentary debate had been set by the second government report on AIDS presented in 1987. In this report it was proposed to allow testing only after informed consent and with guarantees that the person involved had the choice whether or not to know the results. A clear personal request and a clear medical indication were to be prerequisite in every case. A policy of widespread testing, thereby violating privacy and the possibility of careful individual decision making (given the then many negative consequences of a positive result), was rejected on the grounds that there was no effective treatment, and that HIV cannot be transmitted through everyday social contact. Testing as part of a prevention strategy was also rejected, since a negative test result would not diminish the need for safe behaviour and might create false feelings of safety. In fact the privacy risks related to too casual a testing policy were considered detrimental to prevention, since people might become less receptive to information and education (Reinking, 1993).

The fact that the first recommendation by the NCAB concerned the accessibility of life and disability insurance is a signal of the seriousness of the debate at that time (December 1987). Experts and interest groups[11] felt that insurance companies could not just single out HIV-infected persons as an uninsurable risk. Screening on social risk factors via questions such as 'Are you a single man over 30, living in Amsterdam?' and routinely demanding an HIV antibody test based on social risk factors, was felt to be discriminatory and an unwarranted infringement of privacy. Between 1986 and 1988, informal and confidential meetings of representatives of insurance companies and interest groups were held, mediated first by the AIDS Coordination Team, later the NCAB. These meetings eventually resulted in a formal code of conduct, adopted voluntarily by the insurance companies. The code limits routine testing to life and (private) disability insurances to applications over an amount of NLG 300000 (approximately $175000). Testing for an insurance application under that amount only takes place when, after a positive answer is given to the question whether you have been treated for STDs or have used drugs intravenously, subsequent medical enquiries show that the STD was anal gonorrhea or unsterile needles were used when drugs were taken intravenously (Kamerstukken 19218 nr 51, 1992). It should be noted that Parliament has followed the proceedings very carefully and requested to be updated in detail by the Minister of Justice (Kamerstukken 19218 nr. 10, 1988; Kamerstukken 19218 nr. 41, 1990). In parallel, Parliament opened a discussion on prognostic testing for genetic risk factors when applying for a life insurance. In his report of January 1990, the Minister of Justice informed Parliament that the insurance companies had adopted a code of conduct regarding prognostic testing for genetic risk factors similar to that regarding HIV/AIDS.[12]

Testing on HIV as part of the medical examination for personnel recruitment was rejected by the government in 1990 (Kamerstukken 19218 nr. 40, 1990). The government refused, however, to initiate legislation, but preferred to rely on self-regulation by employers and their organizations, along the same lines as the insurance companies. Since this has not happened yet, Parliament is at the moment discussing new legislation on this matter. The proposed legislation aims to prohibit all prognostic medical examinations for both personnel recruitment and insurances and limit medical examinations to the actual requirements of certain jobs only. As for AIDS and HIV infection the proposal incorporates the existing code of conduct.[13]

In 1989, the National Health Council proposed to begin periodical, anonymous HIV seroprevalence surveys among the general population. This provoked a passionate debate. The NCAB considered the epidemiological necessity not pressing enough to change the policy of informed consent regarding HIV testing. In 1990, the State Secretary of Health supported this opinion, and rejected the proposal for anonymous general population seroprevalence surveys (Kamerstukken 19218 nr. 39, 1990). A system of HIV surveillance has been developed that takes place on the basis of surveys with informed consent at out-patient STD clinics in Amsterdam and Rotterdam, among pregnant women in Amsterdam, and among drug users in a number of cities (NCAB, 1995).

The Political Conditions for Innovation

Concerted coordination was indispensable in creating effective AIDS policy in the Netherlands, but it was not the decisive factor. Advisory and consultative structures simply helped to create the political conditions that made innovative AIDS policy possible. More decisive, however, was a clear determination politically to handle AIDS in a competent and innovative way. This political determination became visible in 1987 when the government, backed by Parliament, weighed the necessity to address public anxiety higher than the policy developed through earlier concerted coordination. By subsequently 'defusing' the potential political danger of a discussion on sexual values, room was made for a political debate on issues of privacy and individual rights in relation to testing and a possible HIV positive serostatus. The need for the government to take decisive responsability also became clear in the lapse in the introduction of heat treatment for blood products. In this case parties involved could come far through a coordinating structure, but not far enough. Faster, more effective measures (that is earlier obligatory introduction of heating procedures) would have meant a direct intervention by the government itself, for which at the time the political basis apparently was insufficient.

That it was politically possible for the government to take such a relatively innovative position lay to some extent in the nature of the AIDS crisis as it unfolded in the 1980s. It was almost self-evident that AIDS would force innovation in the areas of prevention, care, treatment, research and legislation. The political background offers some important additional explanations. At the beginning of the 1980s in the Netherlands broad social consensus existed on the need for emancipation of gay men and lesbian women. Unconnected (and probably more fragile and disputed), a similar consensus existed on the need for harm reduction as the main approach of the use of recreational drugs. This consensus in both areas of public concern had been hard to achieve and was still considered vulnerable. The government was therefore active in both areas. The expertise of the gay and lesbian community was welcome at every level of AIDS policy, as was the case with drug users and their service organizations (STG, 1992). This expertise was to a large extent activist in character and brought with it its own human rights agenda.

Another important coincidence was the fact that the Netherlands formally adopted a new Constitution in 1983. This Constitution – developed through the 1970s and reflecting many progressive views of that period – begins in article 1 with a clear prohibition of discrimination and secures in articles 10 and 11 the protection of privacy and the integrity of the human body. Most of these new constitutional rights had yet to be worked into legislation, for which AIDS offered an urgent and undisputed impetus (NCAB, 1995).

These were supportive aspects of the political background. There was also an important inhibiting factor. At the beginning of the 1980s, Dutch health care policy was chiefly aimed at controlling costs. This has remained so during the 1980s and 1990s. It meant that extra, usually temporary, funding had to be made available for AIDS, most usually for a period of three or four years at the most. AIDS policy in these areas therefore has mostly been *ad hoc* and too often 'management by crisis'. Given the financial constraints, and continuous political stalemates regarding the financing of health care, the AIDS field has demonstrated some remarkably effective lobbying.

Sometimes the development of AIDS policies conflicted with vested interests. Often common ground could be found, as was the case in the conflict with the denominational schools. Or a deal could be struck pending more final measures, as happened with the insurance companies. The fact that genuine interest and concern existed at the highest political level, however, has been crucial for the quality of the AIDS policy in the Netherlands, and the extent to which it could be developed.

Notes

1 Under Dutch law, health costs are covered by a system of universal coverage, combining national and private health insurance, on the basis of contributions from both employers and employees. As a consequence,

health insurance in relation to HIV/AIDS did not (have to) become a political issue.

2 The Second Chamber of the States General is the only part of the Dutch Parliament directly elected by the citizens. It has final responsibility for determining legislature and public expenditure; it elects the prime minister, ministers and state secretaries.

3 Dick Dees chaired the Netherlands AIDS Fund until 1997.

4 Health as an area of government responsibility was in the 1980s part of the Ministry of Welfare, Health and Culture. A Secretary of State was responsible for the 'health portfolio'. In 1994, the Ministry changed into the Ministry of Health, Welfare and Sport and a Minister became responsible for the 'health portfolio'.

5 As a last resort, besides other formal procedures of complaint and appeal, the public can complain about any act of the authorities to the 'Nationale Ombudsman' – an institution that originates in Sweden. The 'Ombudsman' (by law) investigates the complaint independently, has access to all relevant information and can demand cooperation by the authorities. His results are published openly. He has no other competences beyond impartial investigation (for example to sanction or punish). His conclusions, however, tend to have immediate political impact.

6 In many countries it is customary to speak of 'safer sex' campaigns. In the Netherlands this has never been the case. All prevention activities have deliberately been targeted towards 'safe sex'.

7 In addition, Coutinho also criticized the rejection by the government of general, anonymous HIV seroprevalence surveys – proposals which he supported. He objected that AIDS policies risked being dominated by moral, ethical and political opinions, instead of the actual reality of the matter.

8 In itself this was, as far as I can trace back through the original dossiers, a genuine mistake out of inexperience of the NCAB and the project coordinators.

9 These constitutional rights secure total independence regarding educational content combined with full public funding.

10 Extended Committee Meetings (UCV) out of Parliament were held on 25 April 1988, 18 June 1990, 1 June 1992.

11 Since then organized in a platform, co-founded by the Dutch Gay and Lesbian Association (NVIH COC): Breed Platform Verzekeringen (Broad Platform Insurances).

12 Insurance companies have the right to exclude persons from a life-insurance on medical grounds. This had always been the case for people with haemophilia, until treatment became possible. HIV threatened to bring back total uninsurability. In 1992 Government and insurance companies agreed to establish a mutual guarantee fund for people with haemophilia. This means that they may now take out life-insurances under NLG 200000 (appr. $120000) without having been tested for HIV. If

death is the result of HIV/AIDS, the insurance company pays out, but is compensated out of the guarantee fund.

13   The proposed legislation became law on January 1st 1998.

References

AIDS COORDINATIE TEAM (1986) 'Voorlichting en preventie in het kader van Aids (beleidsnota)', Amsterdam: AIDS Coordinatie Team.

COHEN, H. (1996) 'Over verhitting gesproken', *Medisch Contact*, **51**, pp. 843–6.

COPPOOLSE, P.A. (1988) *AIDS, Preventie en Besluitvorming*, Rotterdam: Vereniging Humanitas Afdeling Rotterdam (Publikatie nr. 4).

COUTINHO, R. (1989) *Van Pokken, Syfilis en Aids. Geschiedenis van de Infectieziektenbestrijding door de Eeuwen heen*, Amsterdam: private edition.

GROENEVELD, F. (1989) 'Het ontwaken van politiek Den Haag', in H. VUIJSJE and R. COUTINHO (Eds), *Dilemma's rondom AIDS*, Amsterdam: Swets & Zeitlinger.

KAMERSTUKKEN 19218 nrs. 8–9 (1987) 'Het verworven immuun deficiëntiesyndroom (AIDS). Brief en Nota inzake Aids-beleid', Den Haag: SDU.

KAMERSTUKKEN 19218 nr. 10 (1988) 'Het verworven immuun deficientiesyndroom (AIDS). Notitie over de juridische aspecten van verzekering in geval van aids-risico', Den Haag: SDU.

KAMERSTUKKEN 19218 nrs 11–12 (1988) 'Schriftelijke vragen en antwoorden n.a.v. de nota inzake het Aids-beleid', Den Haag: SDU.

KAMERSTUKKEN 19218 nr. 39 (1990) 'Regeringsstandpunt inzake onderzoek naar de verspreiding van HIV-infectie in Nederland', Den Haag: SDU.

KAMERSTUKKEN 19218 nr. 40 (1990) 'Kabinetsstandpunt met betrekking tot de medische keuring bij instelling: het verworven immuun deficientiesyndroom (AIDS)', Den Haag: SDU.

KAMERSTUKKEN 19218 nr. 41 (1990) 'Het verworven immuun deficientiesyndroom (AIDS). Notitie AIDS/seropositiviteit, erfelijkheidsonderzoek en verzekeringen', Den Haag: SDU.

KAMERSTUKKEN 19218 nr. 51 (1992) 'Het verworven immuun deficientiesyndroom (AIDS). Brief van de Minister van Justitie', Den Haag: SDU.

NATIONALE OMBUDSMAN (1995) 'Openbaar rapport naar aanleiding van een verzoekschrift van de Nederlandse Vereniging van Hemofilie-Patiënten met een klacht over een gedraging van het ministerie van Welzijn, Volksgezondheid en Cultuur', Den Haag: Bureau Nationale Ombudsman, Rapportnr. 95/271.

NCAB (1987) 'Werkplan voorlichting en preventie 1987 (advies aan de Staatssecretaris van Welzijn, Volksgezondheid en Cultuur)', Amsterdam: NCAB.

NCAB (1995) *AIDS policy updated. The final recommendation by the National Committee on AIDS Control*, Amsterdam: Stichting AIDS Fonds.

REINKING, D. (1993) *Aids-beleid in Nederland. Een Reconstructie en een Aanzet tot Evaluatie*, Utrecht: NcGv.

ROZENDAAL, S. (1996) *Blus de Brand, Gesprekken over de Nederlandse AIDS Bestrijding*, Amsterdam: Stichting Aids Fonds/Mets.

SPIJKERMAN, S. (1986) *AIDS Voorlichting; de Voorbereiding van een Campagne*, Master Thesis, Utrecht: Universiteit Utrecht.

STG; STEERING COMMITTEE ON FUTURE HEALTH SCENARIOS (1992) *AIDS up to the Year 2000; Epidemiological, Sociocultural and Economic Scenario Analysis for the Netherlands*, Dordrecht: Kluwer Academic Publishers.

TILLEMANS, G. (1988) *AIDS, Beleid en Organisaties. Beschrijving en Analyse van de Beleidsvorming rondom AIDS en het Ontstaan van een Organisatienetwerk daarbij*, Master Thesis, Nijmegen: Katholieke Universiteit Nijmegen.

VAN WIJNGAARDEN, J. (1987) 'Epidemiologie als basis van voorlichting en preventie van Aids', in J. Blans (Ed.), *Aids Voorlichting en Gedragsverandering*, Amsterdam: Boom.

VAN WIJNGAARDEN, J. (1989) 'Aids-beleid in Nederland', in H. VUISJE, and R. COUTINHO (Eds), *Dilemma's rondom AIDS*, Amsterdam: Swets & Zeitlinger.

Chapter 8

No Anal Sex Please: We're Dutch. A Dilemma in HIV Prevention Directed at Gay Men

Onno de Zwart, Theo Sandfort and Marty van Kerkhof

While gay men in the United States and all other European countries were advised to use condoms when they were having anal sex, Dutch gay men at the beginning of the epidemic were recommended to refrain from anal sex altogether. Only if they were not able to give up anal sex, should they use a condom. This message became known as the 'double message' and was part of official Dutch AIDS policy from 1984 to 1992. It has subsequently been changed to advice that is more focused on the use of condoms.

The aim of this chapter is to analyze how such exceptional advice could be given. In order to understand this it is necessary to look beyond the superficialities of HIV prevention. In this chapter we will, with the luxury of more than a decade's hindsight, not only describe the history of the double message, but also look at the different actors involved in the process and their considerations in choosing it. We will discuss how the double message has been perceived by gay men, the effects it might have had, and the way HIV prevention has been changed. Furthermore we will analyze the way HIV prevention has been organized in the Netherlands and the history of how the Dutch gay movement has dealt with sexuality in general.

The Double Message and Its Presentation

The double message was first formulated during a local radio programme in Amsterdam in 1984 (Van Kerkhof, Sandfort and Geensen, 1991). Hans Moerkerk, then director of the Amsterdam Centre for Health Promotion, active in the Amsterdam gay health group and member of the National AIDS Policy Coordination team, declared that in order to prevent AIDS, gay men should stop having anal sex and that if gay men wanted to have anal sex they should use a condom. After being broadcast the text of this programme was published as a brochure by the Amsterdam Centre for Health Promotion and the Dutch Gay and Lesbian Association (NVIH COC).

There were several reasons why the AIDS Coordination Team, in which both health authorities and the gay organizations were represented, decided to choose a message that emphasized the avoidance of anal sex. First, realizing the significance of anal sex in the transmission of AIDS, they felt that the only logical, medical option at that moment was to advise gay men to stop having anal sex.[1] Based on earlier experiences with health promotion campaigns, the AIDS Coordination Team concluded that a clear and simple message was needed to introduce the norm of safe sex into the gay community – a message which was urgently needed to prevent large numbers of gay men becoming infected. The message therefore encouraged men to avoid anal sex. It was hoped that such a message would lead to a change in the sexual culture of gay men. No longer should the partner who did not want to engage in anal sex be the one who needed to negotiate; it should become the other way around (interview Van Wijngaarden, 1995; Van Kerkhof, 1991).

Condoms were not considered a reliable solution because at that time there existed no condoms designed for anal sex and the reported failure rate of vaginal condoms was too high, up to 20 per cent (Wigersma and Oud, 1987). Their acceptance within the gay community, too, was thought to be questionable. Coutinho, head of the Department of Public Health and Environment at the Amsterdam Municipal Health Service and member of the AIDS Coordination Team, expressed his doubts thus: 'The condom has proved its value as a prophylactic against STDs among heterosexuals, but whether this device will be accepted by homosexual men, remains to be seen' (Coutinho, 1984, p. 74).

It was assumed that anal sex was a significant, irreplaceable sexual technique for only a minority of gay men and thus the message was thought to be realistic. 'By calling for this behavioural change, and by "allowing" virtually all other forms of sexual contact, it was hoped that there would be only a minimal disruption of the culture of the gay community' (Van Wijngaarden, 1992, p. 261).

At that time, however, little was known about the significance of anal sex – only how often it was practised among a select group of gay men involved in a study on Hepatitis B carried out in Amsterdam between 1980 and 1984. Of the participants of this study, 74 per cent practised anal sex (Coutinho, 1984). This study showed, moreover, that Amsterdam had an exuberant sexual subculture, in which some gay men had many sexual partners with whom they had anal sex. To prevent the members of this subculture from becoming infected, a drastic change of behaviour was needed, which, according to the AIDS Coordination Team, could only come about through a radical message: the double message.

As the participants of this study, however, had been selected in such ways as to represent the group of gay men at highest risk of Hepatitis B infection, these figures were considered not to be representative for the Dutch gay community in general. Gay organizations stressed that the Dutch gay community was different from the American gay community. 'Gay organizations have frequently pointed out that the group of gay men was composed differently in the Netherlands and that there was a different subculture. While this was true, with regard to the ways the disease was transmitted there was no difference at all. I had concluded this from the figures on syphilis and Hepatitis-B' (interview with Coutinho in Coppoolse, 1988, p. 28).

The double message was considered necessary because of the particularly exuberant sexual subculture in Amsterdam. Despite the difference between this subculture and that of the larger gay community in the Netherlands, however, the use of this message was not limited to this group of gay men; it became the central message for all the national prevention campaigns. In contrast to other countries, it was hoped that avoiding anal sex would disrupt the gay community less than the introduction of condoms would.

While the key prevention message was to refrain from anal sex, the AIDS Coordination Team realized that there were gay men who would not be able do so. These men were advised to use condoms. Bearing in mind the high failure rate of regular condoms, the AIDS Coordination Team assumed that for anal sex only extra strong condoms would be sufficient. Such condoms, however, were not available and had to be developed. The Coordination Team supported manufacturers in developing these condoms. This official support for the development of extra strong condoms was unique in Europe.

The double message was presented to gay men in several ways. Famous, or perhaps notorious, was one of the first Dutch AIDS posters in 1986. Featuring a Robert Mapplethorpe photograph of a man's ass and the slogan 'Exit only', it formed the perfect icon of the double message. The poster not only found its way into many homes of gay men, it also infuriated some. For the latter, this poster and the double message were seen as stigmatizing anal sex (Van Kerkhof, De Zwart and Sandfort, 1995).

Leaflets and brochures quickly brought the message to the attention of gay men. These early leaflets stressed that the only safe option was to stop having anal sex. In a leaflet from 1986 it was stated that 'using a condom is never 100 per cent safe', and in a leaflet from 1989 anal sex with a condom was categorized as dangerous.[2] A year later the National Committee on AIDS Control (NCAB) made its position quite clear.[3] They wrote, 'The answer is simple: condoms do not offer enough protection during anal sex. Promoting the use of condoms could encourage men to continue having anal sex or to put fucking on their sexual "menu"' (NCAB, 1990, p. 4).

The first part of the double message, to avoid anal sex, was presented in many forms. The second part, to use a condom if one cannot refrain from anal sex, received far less attention. The AIDS Coordination Team had supported the development of stronger condoms. When in 1986 these condoms became available, however, they made clear that this should not lead to an increase in anal sex (Eijrond, 1986). No campaigns were organized to promote condoms or to teach gay men how to use them, and only the manufacturers advertised their products. Even in these advertisements it was made clear that using a condom was the second best option, 'Fucking is dangerous . . . if you want to fuck though use a condom' or 'Don't fuck or do it with DUO.'[4]

The failure rate of these stronger condoms was indeed lower, but not enough to cause a change in the main prevention message. 'No condom appears to be 100 per cent safe, even when used correctly. The primary prevention advice for homosexual men is therefore to refrain from anogenital intercourse. If this is not feasible a qualified anal condom should be used' (Van Griensven *et al.*, 1988, p. 346).

Cooperation and Pragmatism

Cooperation and pragmatism have always been the main features of the Dutch AIDS policy. A closer analysis of these characteristics will provide more insight into the background for the choice of the double message and for its retention.

The gay movement, working in close cooperation with the Amsterdam Centre for Health Promotion and the Amsterdam Municipal Health Service, developed the first AIDS prevention leaflet directed at gay men, which was distributed at Dutch Gay Pride in 1983.[5] Intersectoral cooperation was thought to be worthwhile by the gay movement as well as the health officials. Health officials considered cooperation useful since they were convinced this would make prevention efforts more effective. Based on his earlier experiences in developing STD campaigns, Coutinho wrote, 'It is extremely important that these educational programs [on STDs] for homosexual men, should be organized and directed by homosexual organizations themselves to avoid the moralizing issue' (1984, p. 73).

When the Dutch gay movement became aware of AIDS in 1982 there had already been forms of cooperation with health and other officials for more than a decade, and this was considered an effective way of promoting gay interests (Tielman, 1982). That cooperation on AIDS between health officials and the gay movement was possible can be illustrated by the so-called 'blood debate' (Coppoolse, 1988). When during late 1982 it became clear that HIV could be transmitted through blood and its products, the blood banks suggested that all gay men should be excluded as donors. Coutinho and Moerkerk organized a meeting with the blood banks, haemophilia organizations and the gay movement to discuss the issue. Despite differences, the groups reached an agreement: gay men would not be excluded from donating blood but the gay movement would call upon gay men to withdraw themselves voluntarily as donors. As a result of this agreement the gay movement gained credibility with health officials; it had also been made clear that AIDS was not only a medical problem and that a good knowledge of the gay community was a requisite for the development of effective AIDS policy.

By working together with health officials and calling upon the gay community to withdraw as donors, the gay movement had prevented what it considered to be discrimination and stigmatization and had assured itself of political influence. It has been suggested that as compensation for its political influence and the high priority to prevent discrimination, the gay movement and community had to behave responsibly (Mooij, 1993). While the primary reason for choosing the double message was to prevent gay men from becoming HIV-infected, one cannot exclude the possibility that choosing this option was also a way to show that gay men could behave responsibly by stopping having anal sex.

Cooperation between the gay movement and health officials was facilitated by the gay health groups as they were part of both the health system and the gay community. They played a major part in the development of an AIDS policy, more so than in other European countries (Van Wijngaarden, 1989). With their medical background they were convinced that a prevention message should discourage fucking as this posed the greatest risk. At the same time, being part of the gay movement, they were trusted and could therefore promote such a strict message without being considered unduly moralistic or homophobic (Van Wijngaarden, 1989; Veenker, 1989).

Informal cooperation became official in the form of AIDS Coordination Team which developed to coordinate Dutch AIDS policy. Both the gay movement and health officials were represented in this team. The aim was to develop a policy based on consensus, which included an active media strategy whereby the AIDS Coordination Team decided what could be told to the media. The consensus model gave rise to a group of insiders who took decisions behind closed doors, like those on the double message and on the question whether gay bath houses should be closed or not (Coppoolse, 1988; Van Wijngaarden, 1992). This approach has subsequently been criticized because the 'insiders' (sometimes called the AIDS élite) thereby prevented an open discussion taking place, created the impression everything was under control, caused rigidity and depoliticized AIDS (Duyvendak, 1995; De Graaf, 1995; Van Kerkhof, 1991; Van Wijngaarden, 1992; Moerkerk, 1990).

Cooperation has not been the only characteristic feature of Dutch AIDS policy; pragmatism is another one. In Dutch policy, pragmatism stands for finding a workable solution for a current problem without getting too involved in the ideological background of the problem or the actors involved. For AIDS policy this meant that AIDS prevention had to base itself on the actual lifestyles of those most at risk. The state did not want to moralize because it did not want to interfere in the private affairs of its citizens (Reinking, 1993). Decisions about prevention policies should be based upon medical facts about the risk of transmission and the results of epidemiological data (Reinking, 1993). Pragmatism prevented debates about whether the state by its HIV prevention strategy promoted homosexuality or not, or whether the state should promote monogamy.

The emphasis placed on epidemiological data and research findings, characteristic of a pragmatic approach, meant that only these arguments were considered valid in taking decisions about the double message. The results of the large-scale Amsterdam Cohort Study, which had been set up by the Amsterdam Municipal Health Service, pointed to an early decrease in anal sex.[6] These results, as well as the sharp decline in the incidence of rectal gonorrhoea and Hepatitis B, were interpreted as a sign that the message was successful (Van Griensven et al., 1989a and 1989b). Explaining these results to the gay press, the researcher Van Griensven concluded, 'It would be better to terminate fucking as a sexual technique among men all together' (Blans, 1987, p. 4).

Epidemiological research data, however, were more than data as such; they were considered the only valid arguments to judge whether the message was successful or not and should be altered or not. Kok, a professor in health promotion and in HIV prevention, declared, 'The most important argument for this [to change the message] is, that anal sex for all kinds of reasons (although quite serious ones) has such a significance for a large group of gay men, that to abandon it as an aim is not feasible at all. This is in my opinion, however, not a proper argument' (Kok, 1990, p. 134).[7]

By focusing on only epidemiological data in discussions about prevention, the debate became dominated by those actors who had access to such data: primarily researchers and health professionals. Arguments put forward by individual gay men or prevention workers were considered ideological – because they stressed the significance anal sex had for gay men and their identity – and not valid.[8] Such arguments were also considered methodologically unsound, since they were 'only' based either on men's own experience or the anecdotal evidence of prevention workshops. No research was done, however, into the meanings anal sex might have for gay men, which could have qualified or disqualified these arguments.

Being pragmatic meant that health professionals and researchers should accept as valid only the results of quantitative, scientific studies. As they were the only ones who had access to such data they limited, maybe unintentionally, discussion about the double message to themselves.

The Dutch Gay Movement and Anal Sex

The double message was certainly not invented by homophobic health officials: the Dutch gay movement considered it necessary and feasible advice and supported it wholeheartedly. To understand why the Dutch gay movement endorsed such a strict message it is necessary to examine its strategy through the years. In particular, an analysis of how the gay movement in the Netherlands has dealt historically with sexuality and anal sex reveals some of the origins of the double message.

The organized Dutch gay movement started in the 1910s. Since then, and in trying to achieve equality for gay men and lesbians, an important element in the strategy of the gay and lesbian movement until the 1970s has been to present itself as respectable (Tielman, 1982). This was done by soliciting the support of researchers and writers. These supporters took up the issue of sexuality, often presenting gay men and lesbians as chaste (Stokvis, 1939), as illustrated in the following quotation: 'It is not a rarity for two uranians to have a love-affair for years, without sexual contact taking place between them' (Aletrino, 1908, p. 69). In the 1950s the Dutch Gay and Lesbian Association introduced the word 'homophile' to replace the word 'homosexual', thereby taking the focus away from sexuality in an effort to promote a more human image of homosexuals. Efforts to become a respectable organization were not limited to questions of terminology; the Dutch Gay and Lesbian Association also distanced itself from paedophiles, sado-masochism and overtly effeminate or butch behaviour (Sandfort, 1987).

When anal sex was mentioned in general publications on homosexuality in the 1960s and the early 1970s, reference was limited to figures about the number of men practising anal sex. These varied between 8 per cent (based on Hirschfeld's findings) and 33 per cent (Straver, 1973; Tolsma, 1963; Overing *et al.*, 1961). These estimates were usually based on research done abroad, since in most research on gay men in the late 1960s and 1970s in the Netherlands, no attention was paid to sexual behaviour at all (Straver, Van der Heiden and Robert, 1980; Nelemans, 1977; Sengers, 1969). Instead, these studies focused on the nature of gay or lesbian identity or on the social situation of gay men and lesbians.

An examination of educational publications directed at young gay men, or focused on sex in particular, indicates the marginal position anal sex had in Dutch discourse on gay men's sexuality. In *Boy-Boy/Girl-Girl*, an educational book for young gay men and lesbians published in 1972, more than four pages were devoted to gay male sex, including anal sex. Apart from giving technical instructions, it stressed that there was no reason to consider anal sex dirty (AJAH, 1972). A decade later the Dutch gay movement published a new educational book directed at young gay men and lesbians (Bol *et al.*, 1981). Sex was of course one of the topics of this publication, but it was limited to one page and anal sex was discussed in two sentences, 'You can fuck each other from behind. Whenever you do it you have to be careful with each other and use a lubricant' (Bol *et al.*, 1981, p. 41).

In the early 1980s two books were published which dealt exclusively with gay male sexual practices. It is remarkable that both these books were translations. One might wonder whether sex was considered too private for the Dutch to write about or whether the Dutch gay movement and gay studies needed AIDS as a stimulus before being able to write about sexuality.

In 1980 the Dutch edition of *The Joy of Gay Sex* was published. In the introduction the Dutch editor made quite clear what he thought about anal sex, 'This book pays too much attention to anal sex. The American writers even suggest, although maybe unintentionally, that a homosexual relationship is not complete without anal contact. I think we, in Western Europe, have different opinions about that' (Silverstein and White, 1980, p. 11). The editor apparently assumed that Europeans, including the Dutch, practised less anal sex, without giving evidence for this. He had also chosen another title for the book: *Homosexuality among men*, 'as it is not only pleasure in the gay world' (p. 9).

Two years later *Mannenkoorts*, 'Male fever' was published.[9] This book was the translation from the German *Sumpf-fieber*, which was written by gay doctors (Coester, Feldman and Scholtyssek, 1984). The book described in detail how men could prepare themselves for having anal sex.[10] It was an exception in the Dutch tradition of down-playing the significance of anal sex.

The notion that anal sex had no great significance for gay men was not limited to the gay movement. On the contrary, the gay movement had succeeded in convincing others of this. This becomes clear in a publication of the Dutch Society of General Practitioners on sexual problems which described anal sex as a rare practice among gay men. By portraying homosexuality, or the less confronting 'homofilia' as it was referred to in the publication, in this way, this publication offers an example of how homosexuality had become integrated into Dutch society. 'Only very few queers are ass fuckers' was one of the summaries characterizing gay men's sexuality in the margins of the text to make the publication more readable (Nederlands Huisartsen Genootschap, 1977, p. 68).

From the 1910s onwards the Dutch gay movement had concentrated on promoting the political interests of gay men and lesbians. It had been far less interested in the desires of gay men and their community (Duyvendak, 1994). Sexuality and sexual techniques such as anal sex were not considered relevant in promoting such political interests. When in 1983 it became clear that anal sex was the most important risk factor for AIDS, it was – hardly surprisingly – decided to emphasize the importance of giving up anal sex. The choice for the 'double message' can be seen as the culmination of a long tradition of down-playing the role of anal sex in the lives of gay men.

Perceptions and Effects

After the double message was introduced in 1983 it remained undebated. In the monthly magazine *AIDS Info*, for example, this topic was not discussed until 1989.[11] Gay men seemed to support the prevention strategy. Findings from a national cohort of gay men, recruited through the gay press, from the years 1986 to 1989 show that few gay men considered the AIDS prevention messages directed at them to be patronizing (De Vroome, 1994). Most gay men also recognized the double message as the official prevention message (De Vroome, 1994; Sandfort, 1992).[12]

Results of a large-scale evaluation of the Dutch HIV prevention campaigns carried out in 1990 among 559 gay men showed that most men found the double message clear as well as wise, 94 per cent and 77 per cent respectively (for all these figures see Sandfort, 1992). Only 5 per cent of the men found the message patronizing, although this percentage was slightly higher for men who used condoms compared with men who had stopped having anal sex. When asked to compare the Dutch prevention message with those from abroad, the majority of the respondents, 52 per cent, considered the Dutch message the best. At the same time, however, 69 per cent would have liked to see more attention devoted to condoms in prevention efforts.[13] This wish to pay more attention to condoms can be related to the fact that many gay men considered the use of a condom rather safer than the policy makers did (De Kooning, 1992; Sandfort, 1992). Interestingly, 80 per cent of the men who used condoms felt supported in their behaviour by the double message. They presumably saw their needs being met by the second part of the message.

Although most men seemed to support the double message, some men considered it patronizing and unrealistic. For them it meant that anal sex was stigmatized (Van Kerkhof, De Zwart and Sandfort, 1995; Maasen, 1991). These differences in perception are related to the significance that anal sex has for the men involved and to differences in preferred styles of protection (Sandfort, 1992; Van Kerkhof, De Zwart and Sandfort, 1995). Some men for whom anal sex had great significance did not recognize themselves in the double message and felt their feelings were denied. The fact that anal sex was 'forbidden' led some men who already valued anal sex highly to become even more interested in it (Hospers, Molenaar and Kok, 1994).

The double message therefore seems to have been perceived fairly positively by most gay men, but what were the effects on their sexual behaviour? A definitive answer to this question is difficult to give. It is too simple to relate observed changes in sexual behaviour to official prevention messages only. The decision to engage in anal sex or not is the result of many factors, of which the risk of HIV infection is only one (Van Kerkhof, De Zwart and Sandfort, 1995).

This also means that it is impossible to determine what the effect of the double message has been on the number of HIV infections among gay men in the Netherlands, as some authors have tried to do (Duyvendak, 1995; Duyvendak and Koopmans, 1991). Official prevention messages are only one element on which gay men base their various prevention strategies. Besides, the number of gay men who have become infected with HIV is also related to factors such as the way different gay subcultures are organized and the time HIV was introduced into them. By over-emphasizing the importance of the official message, these authors fail to acknowledge the complexity of sexual behaviour and gravely overestimate the influence of prevention campaigns.

Despite difficulty in answering these questions, it is worthwhile looking at the results of studies used to support or oppose the double message. During the 1980s, several findings suggested that the double message was indeed successful, more than any other health promotion campaign carried out previously and more than originally expected. The incidence of STDs among gay men, a traditional marker of sexual activity, decreased dramatically (Van Griensven *et al.*, 1989a). Gay men in the Amsterdam Cohort Study also reported engaging in anal sex with fewer partners. The percentage of gay men who had not practised anal sex during the preceding six months increased from 13.5 per cent in 1984 to 46 per cent in 1988 (Van Kerkhof, De Zwart and Sandfort, 1995; Van Griensven *et al.*, 1989b). The limited number of special condoms being sold was also interpreted as a sign that gay men had decreased the number of sexual encounters in which anal sex took place (*AIDS Info*, 1988).

A closer analysis of the research findings of the Amsterdam Cohort Study, however, reveals more than only a decrease in anal sex. Although gay men practised less anal sex, this was mostly related to a decrease in the number of partners, with whom anal sex took place. In particular, with steady partners men continued to have anal sex, which was frequently unprotected. 'By comparing the decrease in the number of partners per sexual technique while taking into account the total number of partners of an individual, it was shown that the men in this study were more likely to reduce their number of partners than they were to change their specific sexual habits. Probably the reduction of partners was a more achievable goal than refraining from anogenital intercourse' (Van Griensven, 1989, pp. 83–4). De Vroome noticed the same phenomenon in a cohort study conducted among readers of *De Gay Krant*: 'It is remarkable that the relative popularity of specific sexual techniques during the period of study [1986–89] remained constant' (De Vroome, 1994, p. 45).

Compared with other European countries, however, and based on national figures for 1991, there was indeed a lower percentage of gay men in the Netherlands who engaged in anal sex.[14] Whereas in most countries 40 per cent of men did not engage in anal sex with casual partners, 70 per cent of Dutch men refrained from anal sex in such situations. In steady relationships, 50 per cent of Dutch gay men did not practise anal intercourse, whereas in other countries only 20 per cent did not do so (Bochow *et al.*, 1994). When Dutch gay men did have anal sex, however, they used a condom neither more nor less often (Bochow *et al.*, 1994).

Assumptions Being Questioned

When the double message was introduced it was assumed that for only a minority of Dutch gay men was anal sex significant, and that the message was realistic. Since then, research and the experiences of prevention workers have questioned these assumptions. Several studies, and not only Dutch ones, have made clear that for some men AIDS provided a reason to stop having anal sex (Van Kerkhof, De Zwart and Sandfort, 1995; Davies *et al.*, 1993). The fact that men needed this indicates that anal sex had become the norm in large parts of the gay community and thus anal sex had some significance for many men.

The significance given to anal sex also becomes clear in interviews with men who stopped fucking in the mid 1980s, but since then have started again (Van Kerkhof, De Zwart and Sandfort, 1995)[15]. For them anal sex was important, but the fear of AIDS, the double message and the unreliability of condoms made them stop having it. Improvements in the quality of condoms and the change of the Dutch policy made it possible for many of these men to start fucking again.

The other major assumption was that the message was realistic. From 1989 onwards it became clear, however, that the number of men engaging in anal sex increased again. In the Amsterdam Cohort Study the percentage increased from 51.4 per cent in 1988 to 59.5 per cent in 1992 (De Vroome, personal communication). In a study carried out in 1992, 60 per cent of young gay men reported engaging in receptive anal sex with a steady partner (Keet *et al.*, 1993).

Debates and Changes

The double message was already criticized for denying the significance and the symbolical value of anal sex for gay men, before data became known, indicating the significance that anal sex had for some men (*AIDS Info*, 1991; Maasen, 1991). The difficulties some gay men had in stopping having anal sex were first noticed by prevention workers. These prevention workers not only criticized the message for being unrealistic but they also tried, within the limits of the double message, to emphasize more the use of condoms for those men who could not stop having anal sex (Blom, 1990). In 1990, for example, the first 'condom workshops' were organized during which men were instructed how to use condoms. In these workshops, however, condom use was still presented as a second best option; condoms could make anal sex less unsafe, but avoiding anal sex remained the best option (Hoekzema and Dingelstad, 1991).

With the critique increasing and research findings indicating that gay men were having more anal sex again, the NCAB decided to reconsider the message. It had become clear to them that it was no longer feasible to focus predominantly on abstinence from anal sex, since as they reported 40 to 60 per cent of the men having sex with men were engaging in anal sex (NCAB, 1992). To reach its decision, the NCAB had asked the National Institute of Public Health and Environment (RIVM) to review the relevant literature. Two arguments played a major role in the final decision to change the message: the failure rate of condoms and the fact that the hierarchical double message made condom education more difficult.

New research indicated that the failure rate had become lower and that the main factor in condom failure was acceptance and incorrect use, not technical shortcomings of condoms themselves (Houweling, 1992; see also De Wit *et al.*, 1993). Gay men should thus be taught how to use a condom correctly and this could only be done through condom promotion.

The second argument was related to the fact that in order to educate men about condom use, it was not possible to focus on a particular group of gay men. Although many men had changed their sexual behaviour either by stopping having anal sex or by using condoms, their intentions with new partners could differ from their behavioural change (NCAB, 1992; Sandfort, 1992). Men who had stopped having anal sex did not exclude the option that with a new partner they would once again engage in anal sex. This meant there were no strictly separated groups of 'men who had stopped having anal sex' or 'men who used condoms' to whom condom promotion could have been directed. It was necessary therefore to inform all gay men about all aspects of condom use.

The arguments used to change the double message were valid and scientific. It was, however, not only because of these arguments that the policy was changed. While in the early 1980s only a small group of people, mostly from a medical background, concerned themselves with AIDS, by the early 1990s AIDS had become a central part of the life and work of many gay men. HIV prevention workers, with no medical background, had criticized the double message and a public debate had arisen. The former AIDS élite had expanded and, confronted with the critique and with what they considered valid arguments, the message was changed. In 1992, therefore, the NCAB decided the message would become: 'use a condom or do not fuck'.

Conclusions

In the 1980s the message addressed at gay men to refrain from anal sex, the so-called double message, raised many eyebrows internationally. This chapter has analyzed the origins of this message and how it came subsequently to be changed in 1992. As we have seen, this radical message was a response to events in the early 1980s within the sexual subculture in Amsterdam. Despite an awareness that this subculture was not representative of the gay population in the Netherlands, the message was used nationally. The double message was in line with the image of gay sex as it was put forward by the gay movement in the 1970s, and which had become common 'knowledge' among health professionals. Central within this image was the view that anal sex was practised infrequently by gay men. Additionally, at the time the gay movement focused predominantly on societal rather than on personal issues. Living with AIDS for over a decade has, however, made clear that anal sex is a central element in the sexual lifestyles of many Dutch gay men.

Against the background of the tradition of the Dutch gay movement in which the importance of anal sex had been played down, the double message was an understandable choice. It was, however, based on untested assumptions about the significance of anal sex for gay men and the feasibility of the message. Its widespread promulgation seems, nevertheless, to have resulted in a decrease of anal sexual activity. It is not clear what would have happened if a different message had been chosen. The lack of information and interest in the meaning that specific sexual practices have for gay men has undoubtedly hindered Dutch AIDS policy, as some men have felt that due to AIDS prevention a central element of their identity was stigmatized.

The important role the gay movement, and in particular the gay health groups, have played in the Dutch AIDS policy of the early 1980s, made the double message acceptable to the gay community. It was perceived as a 'gay' message and thus adopted by many gay men. The cooperation and pragmatism which enabled a quick, united and adequate response to AIDS, however, also resulted in the creation of a self-appointed élite. The initial general acceptance of the double message makes one wonder why later it became the topic of such heated debate. It seems that within the gay community the double message became a symbol of the way Dutch AIDS prevention had been organized. Opposing this message probably meant not opposing the message itself, but also the AIDS élite.

This chapter has made clear that to understand the double message it is necessary to place it in its historical and societal context. It has also pointed to the fact that prevention messages can be more than messages as such: they can be significant symbols of prevention policy or ways of decision making. In developing new, and more successful prevention messages this has to be taken into account.

Acknowledgements

The authors would like to thank Erik Brus and André Steffens for their useful comments on earlier versions of this chapter.

Notes

1   Interview with Jan van Wijngaarden, former AIDS Coordinator, 20 September 1995.
2   The leaflet from 1986 was called *Stop. Vrij veilig* and was produced by the Werkgroep Voorlichting AIDS Amsterdam. In 1989 Buro GVO produced the brochure called *Homoseks en AIDS*.
3   The NCAB had replaced the National AIDS Policy Coordination Team as the national organization responsible for AIDS control and prevention in 1987.
4   Advertisements of Gay Safe condoms and Duo condoms in *Homologie*, 1987, nr. 1, p. 52 and nr. 2, pp. 20, 21 respectively.
5   The history of the Dutch AIDS policy and prevention is discussed in Coppoolse (1988), Duyvendak (1995), Reinking (1993), Van Kerkhof, Sandfort and Geesen (1991) and Van Wijngaarden (1992).
6   Van Griensven (1989).
7   In an interview in *AIDS Info* in November 1992 Kok (looking back on the discussions on the double message) expressed his satisfaction with the fact that decisions had been based on epidemiological figures. He said, 'I'm glad ideology has no role to play in the decision making.' *AIDS Info* was a free magazine about AIDS directed at gay men, published by the Dutch Gay and Lesbian Association and *De Gay Krant* and funded by the government. *De Gay Krant* is the largest gay magazine in the Netherlands.

8   Looking back on more than a decade of AIDS prevention in the Netherlands, Van Wijngaarden said, 'I have great difficulty with reasonings that anal sex is an attainment of the gay subculture, the gay pride. I cannot stand that when a deadly illness is concerned' (Rozendaal, 1996, p. 58).

9   This book was translated by the members of the gay health groups. Members of these groups would play an important role in the development of the Dutch AIDS policy in the years to come. In 1984 the book was reprinted with a new section on AIDS.

10 It is remarkable that almost all information on anal sex in this book is written from the 'passive' perspective. This confirms the notion that there is still a special relationship between homosexuality and the 'passive' experience (Van Kerkhof, De Zwart and Sandfort, 1995). This topic deserves more attention.

11 It is significant that in an interview with Jan van Wijngaarden in *AIDS Info* in August 1988 when he was leaving as National AIDS Coordinator, no attention was paid to the double message. This suggests that the double message was of little concern at that time.

12 One might wonder, however, how far this is related to the fact that these were both quantitative studies in which the respondents had to select the correct answer from a range of descriptions of possible official prevention messages. In qualitative studies, using open questions, most men were not able to formulate the official message so precisely (De Zwart and Sandfort, 1993; Van Kerkhof, De Zwart and Sandfort, 1995).

13 See also De Kooning (1992).

14 This study made clear that the Netherlands had the lowest percentage of gay men who had engaged in anal sex. The study does not discuss, however, whether this percentage had always been lower or whether it had been the effect of the double message.

15 This is not only a Dutch phenomenon. Bochow (1994) has pointed out the same development in Germany.

References

Aids Info (1988) 'Verkoop condoms valt fors tegen', *Aids Info*, March, p. 4.

Aids Info (1991) 'Voorlichtingsdeskundige Peter Dankmeijer: "Symbolische waarde anaal kontakt door beleidsmakers ontkend"', *Aids Info*, September, p. 3.

Aletrino, A. (1908) *Hermaphrodisie en Uranisme*, Amsterdam: F. van Rossen.

AJAH; Amsterdamse Jongeren Aktie-groepen Homoseksualiteit (1972) *Jongen–Jongen/Meisje–Meisje*, Den Haag: Stichting Uitgeverij NVSH.

Blans, J. (1987) 'Amsterdamse steekproef: minder geneukt, meer condooms gebruikt', *Aids Info*, April, p. 4.

BLOM, C. (1990) 'SAD doorbreekt taboe rond neuken. Bij goed gebruik van condoom verminder je kans op infectie", *Aids Info*, September, p. 3.

BOCHOW, M. (1994) *Schwuler Sex und die Bedrohung durch Aids – Reaktionen Homosexueller Männer in Ost- und West-Deutschland*, Berlin: Deutsche AIDS-Hilfe.

BOCHOW, M., CHIAROTTI, F., DAVIES, P., DUBOIS-ARBER, F., DÜR, W., FOUCHARD, J., GRUET, F., MCMANUS, T., MARKERT, S., SANDFORT, T., SASSE, H., SCHILTZ, M.-A., TIELMAN, R. and WASSERFALLEN, F. (1994) 'Sexual behaviour of gay and bisexual men in eight European countries', *AIDS Care*, **6**, pp. 533–42.

BOL, B. *et al.* (Eds) (1981) *Ook zo?! Informatie voor Jongeren over Homoseksualiteit*, Amsterdam: NVIH – COC, Jhr. Mr. J.A. Schorerstichting.

BURO GVO (1989) *Homoseks en AIDS*, Amsterdam: Buro GVO.

COESTER, C.H., FELDMAN, J.H.R.S. and SCHOLTYSSEK, E. (1984) *Mannenkoorts*, Amsterdam: De Woelrat.

COPPOOLSE, P.A. (1988) *AIDS, Preventie en Besluitvorming*, Rotterdam: Humanitas.

COUTINHO, R.A. (1984) *Sexually Transmitted Diseases among Homosexual Men. Studies on Epidemiology and Prevention*, Doctoral Thesis, Amsterdam: Rodopi.

DAVIES, P.M., HICKSON, F.C.I., HUNT, J. and WEATHERBURN, P. (1993) *Sex, Gay Men and AIDS*, London: The Falmer Press.

DUYVENDAK, J.W. (1995) 'De Hollandse aanpak van een epidemie: Of waarom Act Up! in Nederland niet kon doorbreken', *Acta Politica*, **30**, pp. 189–214.

DUYVENDAK, J.W. (Ed.) (1994) *De Verzuiling van de Homobeweging*, Amsterdam: SUA.

DUYVENDAK, J.W. and KOOPMANS, R. (1991) 'Weerstand bieden aan aids: de invloed van de homobeweging op aids-preventie', *Mens en Maatschappij*, **43**, pp. 237–45.

EIJROND, B. (1986) 'Aan allen die betrokken zijn bij de voorlichting over AIDS aan mannen met homosexuele contacten' (letter).

DE GRAAF, R. (1995) 'Tien jaar beleid', *Tijdschrift voor Gezondheid en Politiek*, **13**, December, pp. 5–7.

VAN GRIENSVEN, G.J.P. (1989) *Epidemiology and Prevention of HIV Infection among Homosexual Men*, Doctoral Thesis, Amsterdam: Universiteit van Amsterdam.

VAN GRIENSVEN, G.J.P., DE VROOME, E.M.M., TIELMAN, R.A.P. and COUTINHO, R.A. (1988) 'Failure rate of condoms during anogenital intercourse in homosexual men', *Genitourinary Medicine*, **64**, pp. 344–6.

VAN GRIENSVEN, G.J.P., VAN DEN HOEK, J.A.R., LEENTVAAR, A. and COUTINHO, R.A. (1989a) 'Surrogate markers for HIV incidence among homosexual men', in G.J.P. VAN GRIENSVEN, *Epidemiology and Prevention of HIV Infection among Homosexual Men*, Amsterdam.

VAN GRIENSVEN, G.J.P., DE VROOME, E.M.M., GOUDSMIT, J. and COUTINHO, R.A. (1989b) 'Changes in sexual behaviour and the fall of incidence of HIV infection among homosexual men', *British Medical Journal*, **298**, pp. 218–22.

HOEKZEMA, C. and DINGELSTAD, A. (1991) *De Condoomworkshop. Evaluatie-rapport naar Aanleiding van een Preventie-activiteit van de SAD over Condoomgebruik bij Mannen met Homoseksuele Contacten*, Master Thesis, Utrecht: Universiteit Utrecht.

HOSPERS, H.J., MOLENAAR, S. and KOK, G. (1994) 'Focus groups with risk-taking gay men: appraisal of AIDS prevention activities, explanations for sexual risk-taking and needs for support', *Patient Education and Counseling*, **24**, pp. 299–306.

HOUWELING, H. (1992) 'Condom-failure. Notitie ten bate van het debat over HIV-voorlichting onder homoseksuele mannen', unpublished memoran-dum, Centrum voor Epidemiologie, Rijksinstituut voor Volksgezondheid en Mileuhygiëne.

KEET, I., VAN DEN BERGH, H., VAN GRIENSVEN, G., COUTINHO, R., SANDFORT, TH. and VAN DEN HOEK, J. (1993) 'HIV infectie en riskant seksueel gedrag onder jonge homoseksuele mannen te Amsterdam, 1992', *Nederlands Tijdschrift voor Geneeskunde*, **137**, p. 52.

VAN KERKHOF, M.P.N. (1991) 'Vastberaden of wankelmoedig. Over seks, zorg en moraal', in I. MEIJER, J.W. DUYVENDAK and M.P.N. VAN KERKHOF (Eds), *Over Normaal Gesproken. Over Hedendaagse Homopolitiek*, Am-sterdam: Schorer.

VAN KERKHOF, M., SANDFORT, TH. and GEENSEN, R. (1991) *Als Je Het Nou van Hard Werken Kreeg! Tien Jaar AIDS en Homocultuur*, Utrecht: Veen.

VAN KERKHOF, M.P.N., DE ZWART, O. and SANDFORT, TH. (1995) *Van Achteren Bezien. Anale Seks in het Aidstijdperk*, Amsterdam: Schorer.

KOK, G. (1990) 'Een dilemma in de Aidspreventie. De dubbele boodschap over anale seks', *Gedrag en Gezondheid*, **18**, pp. 134–9.

DE KOONING, D. (1992) *Evaluatieonderzoek Aidsfolders 'Homoseks & AIDS' en 'Stand van Zaken'*, Utrecht: Universiteit Utrecht.

MAASEN, T. (1991) 'Wat is er eigenlijk mis met homoseks?', *Homologie*, **13**, p. 39.

MOERKERK, H. (1990) 'AIDS prevention strategies in European countries', in M. PAALMAN (Ed.), *Promoting Safer Sex. Prevention of Sexual Transmis-sion of AIDS and other STD*, Amsterdam: Swets & Zeitlinger.

MOOIJ, A. (1993) *Geslachtsziekten en Besmettingsangst. Een Historisch-sociologische Studie 1850–1990*, Amsterdam: Boom.

NCAB (1990) 'Condooms en homosex', *Aids Info*, January, p. 4.

NCAB (1992) Unpublished letter to the Minister of Welfare, Health and Culture about the prevention message on anal sex directed at gay men.

NEDERLANDS HUISARTSEN GENOOTSCHAP (1977) *Helpen bij Seksuele Moeilijkheden. Een Boek voor Hulpverleners*, Deventer: Van Loghum Slaterus.

NELEMANS, W. (1977) *Leeftijd, Duur en Wijze van Bewustwording van de Homofiele Gerichtheid*, Tilburg: IVA.

OVERING, A.F.C. *et al.* (1961) *Homosexualiteit. Pastorele Cahiers 3*, Hilversum: Paul Brand.

REINKING, D. (1993) *Aids-beleid in Nederland. Een Reconstructie en Aanzet tot Evaluatie*, Utrecht: NcGv.

ROZENDAAL, S. (1996) *Blus de brand. Gesprekken over de Nederlandse Aidsbestrijding*, Amsterdam: Stichting Aids Fonds/Mets.

SANDFORT, TH.G.M. (1987) 'Pedophilia and the gay movement', *Journal of Homosexuality*, **13**, pp. 89–110.

SANDFORT, TH.G.M. (1992) *Homoseksuele Mannen en het AIDS-preventiebeleid. Een Evaluatie op Basis van de Tweede Meeting van het Tweede Nationale Cohort Homoseksuele Mannen*, Utrecht: Interfacultaire Werkgroep Homostudies.

SENGERS, W.J. (1969) *Homoseksualiteit als Klacht. Een Psychiatrische Studie*, Bussum: Paul Brand.

SILVERSTEIN, CH. and WHITE, E. [WAFELBAKKER, F. (Ed.)] (1980) *Homoseksualiteit bij Mannen*, Haarlem: Rostrum.

STOKVIS, B.J. (1939) *De Homosexueelen. 35 Autobiographieën*, Lochem: De Tijdstroom.

STRAVER, C.J. (1973) 'Hoe leven homofielen?', in B. WITTE *et al.*, *Homofilie. Informatie, Onderzoek en Herwaardering*, 2nd Edn, Amersfoort: De Horstink.

STRAVER, C.J., VAN DER HEIDEN, A.M. and ROBERT, W.C.J. (1980) *Tweerelaties, Anders dan het Huwelijk?*, Alphen aan den Rijn: Samson.

TIELMAN, R. (1982) *Homoseksualiteit in Nederland. Studie van een Emancipatiebeweging*, Meppel: Boom.

TOLSMA, F.J. (1963) *Homosexualiteit en Homoërotiek*, Den Haag, Bert Bakker.

VEENKER, J., (1989) 'De positie van de homobeweging', in H. VUIJSJE and R. COUTINHO (Eds), *Dillema's rondom AIDS*, Lisse: Swets & Zeitlinger.

DE VROOME, E.M.M. (1994) *AIDS-voorlichting onder Homoseksuele Mannen. Diffusie van Veilig Vrijen in Nederland (1986–1989)*, Doctoral Thesis, Amsterdam: Thesis Publishers.

WIGERSMA, L. and OUD, R. (1987) 'Safety and acceptability of condoms for use by homosexual men as a phrophylactic against transmisson of HIV during anogenital intercourse', *British Medical Journal*, **295**, p. 94.

VAN WIJNGAARDEN, J. (1989) 'AIDS-beleid in Nederland', in H. VUIJSJE, and R. COUTINHO (Eds), *Dillema's rondom AIDS*, Lisse: Swets & Zeitlinger.

VAN WIJNGAARDEN, J.K. (1992) 'The Netherlands: AIDS in an consensual society', in D.L. KIRP and R. BAYER (Eds), *AIDS in the Industrialized Democracies. Passions, Politics and Policies*, New Brunswick, NJ: Rutgers University Press.

DE WIT, J.B.F., SANDFORT, TH.G.M., DE VROOME, E.M.M., VAN GRIENSVEN,

G.J.P. and Kok, G. (1993) 'The effectiveness of the use of condoms among homosexual men', *AIDS*, **7**, pp. 751–2.

De Zwart, O. and Sandfort, Th.G.M. (1993) *'Gebruik een Condoom of Neuk niet' Een Kwalitatief Onderzoek naar de Wijze waarop de Nevenschikkende Boodschap Kan Worden Vormgegeven*, Utrecht: Universiteit Utrecht.

Chapter 9

The Impact of AIDS on the Dutch Health Care System

Frans van den Boom and Paul Schnabel

The AIDS epidemic, like any other epidemic, is not only a medical but also a social phenomenon. Medically, AIDS is a fatal disease which predominantly affects relatively young people. Regardless of the quantitative size of the epidemic, for the individuals infected and affected, AIDS is qualitatively a big problem, since their lives are disrupted by it. But numbers only identify the first and most obvious impact of the HIV/AIDS epidemic: the population of infected, sick and dying persons. Behind the statistics lies the biographical disruption of each individual who is infected. But the diagnosis of HIV or AIDS affects not only the person who is infected or ill, it also changes the life of people in his or her immediate and intimate environment. And beyond the individual and his immediate environment are the variety of institutions and practices that may also have been affected by the epidemic. Last but not least, epidemics may induce uncertainty, fear, blame and flight in those who are not (as yet) infected, and those who think that those who are infected pose a risk to them (Camus, 1947; McNeill, 1976).

At this point in the history of the epidemic, we may conclude that AIDS is still a quantitatively small problem, at least in the Netherlands with a population of 15 million. However, when the first cases of AIDS occurred in 1982, no one had any idea of its prevalence and incidence. The implication of this was that in the early years of the epidemic, decision making took place in an extremely uncertain situation. Because the earliest predictions of future incidence and prevalence generated very high estimates with very large confidence intervals, they were of limited use. Should one plan for the worst case or for the best case scenario, or for somewhere in between? Later on these early calculations were proven to be far too pessimistic.

In this chapter we will describe how the health care system has responded to the threat of AIDS in such a highly uncertain decision making situation, and try to analyze what the impact of HIV and AIDS has been on health care policy and the health care system. In particular, we will focus on the impact of AIDS on formal and informal health care provision, and on public health policies and practices. The impact of AIDS on the health care system cannot be understood if the baseline situation is not taken into account. By the baseline situation we are referring to the configuration of health and social services before AIDS first appeared. Evaluating the impact of

AIDS requires an assessment of principles, policies and practices prior to its appearance.

Before AIDS, countries differed dramatically with respect to health care organization, public health policies, patient rights, human rights, sex education and health promotion, attitudes towards drug use, homosexuality, prostitution, and so on. Prevailing principles, policies and practices have to a great extent influenced both the kinds of initiatives societies have taken, and those they have refused to take in the fight against AIDS. For example, in most of the countries where needle and syringe programmes are in place today, these programmes were only introduced because of AIDS. In the long term, therefore, AIDS may have an important effect on drug treatment systems and approaches in these countries. However, in countries where such programmes were already in place, the advent of AIDS may have had only an incremental effect. And the refusal of countries to begin with such programmes, despite all evidence of their effectiveness, is related to the fact that a harm reduction approach is believed not to fit with the prevailing principles and policies in the war against drugs. The impact of AIDS can therefore only be understood if the baseline situation is taken into account.

Principles of Dutch Health Care

Important characteristics of Dutch health care, public health, and health education policies and practices are an expression of deeply rooted moral and cultural principles. These principles include the following:

- The duty of all to help others when they are sick (the 'Samaritan' principle as Wulff (1995) calls it). If someone is in need of help, the moral norm is that help has to be provided. Today help is provided through a collectively-paid-for health care system. The fact that it is collectively paid for, reflects the principle of solidarity and its concomitant, the principle of distributive justice.
- The principle of self determination, which finds its expression in different areas such as the acceptance of free choice in relation to sexuality, as well as in medical decision making about the end of life (policy on the use of euthanasia and physician-assisted suicide). The principle of self-determination is closely linked to the fact that we live in a democratic society. We want to live our lives according to our own values and wishes while taking into account the freedom of others. This principle is closely linked to the belief in the ability of citizens to make rational and responsible decisions with respect to their health. For example the Dutch vaccination programme is executed on a voluntary basis with almost 95 per cent of the population participating. It implies an appeal to personal responsibility, a faith in the persuasive power of education and dialogue, and belief in the

integrative capacity of a society where there is a strongly developed sense of solidarity and mutual trust (Schnabel, 1989; Hofstede, 1991; Fukuyama, 1995).

- The principles of liberal pragmatism and non-moralistic pragmatism. The Netherlands is a liberal country. Citizens have the right to live their lives according to their own norms and beliefs within a legally and morally defined context. However, if there is a tension between law and public health, or between law and the principle of self-determination, a pragmatic and non-legalistic approach is often adopted. One of the best-known examples of this can be found in the harm reduction approach in the area of drug use (prosecute the traders, not the users), and the public health approach to sex work. Neither drug use nor prostitution is legal, but both are tolerated (in Dutch a new word to describe such a policy of repressive tolerance has emerged: *gedoogbeleid*), because it is believed that forbidding these practices will make the problem uncontrollable. The result is that groups and individuals already at the margin of society will go underground. It is believed that this should be prevented as much as possible.
- The principle of integration and participation: It is felt essential that all citizens should be able, and be enabled, to participate in society as much and for as long as possible. The integration of people with different backgrounds – in terms of religion, race, political orientation, gender – is promoted. Segregation should be prevented as much as possible. This principle is especially important since it also applies to marginalized and vulnerable groups. It is felt important to stay in touch as much as possible with vulnerable groups of people and patient groups, by establishing clear lines of communication between policy and political levels and 'vulnerable' groups and their advocates. Control is believed to be less effective if it takes the form of supervision and repression. Control in the shape of social control and self-control is believed to be more effective.
- Culture of consensus and commitment: decision making in the Netherlands aims at reaching consensus and obtaining commitment from all relevant parties. All relevant parties are involved in the decision making process in order to realize partnerships. In the area of health care, the Sick Fund Council exists where providers, financiers, patients, unions, employers, government and appointed independent experts meet and decide about what kind of services have to be reimbursed.

Policies and Practices at Baseline

The above principles are put to practice through political decision making and policy formulation and execution. The result of the principles of solidarity and distributive justice is an elaborate health care system which is available, accessible and affordable to all citizens as a result of obligatory health care insurance for all. Health care insurance in turn is part of a well developed social security system, covering, among other things, unemployment, sickness leave and disability. From the conviction that services should be available to all followed a policy that promotes general institutions and discourages categorical health care services and organizations. This formal policy, however, has never completely excluded the possibility of financing categorical institutions, as can be illustrated by the existence of specific institutions in the areas of oncology, epilepsy and – in the early 1980s – haemophilia.[1] More relevant to the care of AIDS, categorical organizations existed in the areas of drug treatment and mental health care provision for homosexual men and women. An elaborate network of drug treatment services, such as methadone and other treatment programmes, and needle exchange programmes (started as a method of preventing hepatitis B transmission among drug users) was already in place before the first case of AIDS was detected. With respect to homosexual men and women, the Schorerstichting, a mental health service organization for gay men and women, was financed by government and health care insurance. In the area of primary health care and sexually transmitted diseases, the Ancillary Service Department (SAD) provided additional services for gay men.[2]

The Netherlands is often pictured as a liberal society, one concerned with an openness about sexuality and the acceptance of different sexual lifestyles. There is a high tolerance towards homosexuality among the Dutch population. Since the 1970s, we have had an open policy with respect to the prevention of unwanted pregnancy – condom use, contraceptives paid by health care insurance, and pregnancy termination (abortion). Again, there are multiple principles at play including the principle of self-determination and the belief that citizens are capable of making rational and responsible decisions for themselves and others, and the principle of non-moralistic pragmatism.

Early Planning for the Future: 1982–87

When the first case of AIDS was diagnosed in 1982, the initial response came from professionals of varying backgrounds (infectious diseases, public health, health education and health promotion, medicine, blood transfusion and blood products), and community organizations (especially gay advocacy groups and gay service delivery organizations, such as SAD and Schorerstichting, and haemophilia groups). These individuals and organizations came together because of their shared anxiety about a new disease, possibly caused by a virus that apparently could be transmitted sexually and through blood and blood products. Most of the people who met together were not strangers to each other. In the gay community, the rise of STDs in the 1970s had triggered the foundation of the SAD, and in 1979 a large study about the occurrence of sexually transmitted diseases among homosexual men in and around Amsterdam was conducted by the Amsterdam Municipal

Health Department (Coutinho, 1984). The advent of hepatitis B had earlier created problems with respect to the safety of the blood supply. As a result, the health inspectorate already had working contacts with groups of gay men (the Dutch Gay and Lesbian Association, NVIH COC), sex workers (Red Thread), drug users (Junkie Union), as well as with public health officials.

In many ways, therefore, the Netherlands had an advantage over many other countries because of existing arrangements, which included, among other things, an elaborate drug treatment system, gay specific services in Amsterdam – the epicentre of the epidemic – and open lines of communication with representatives of other risk groups. All of this facilitated a quick response.

Bloody Sunday

A crucial date in the Dutch history of AIDS is 30 January 1983, which became known as 'Bloody Sunday'. Present were representatives from the blood sector, the health inspectorate, public health, an association of people with haemophilia, physicians, health education and health promotion, and gay advocacy groups. Apart from the health inspectorate and a representative of the National Institute on Public Health, neither the Ministry of Health nor the government was present. This may be perceived as strange, but within the Dutch context it is quite normal. As long as the relevant actors in the field take responsibility, policy and politics keep a distance. And in the area of AIDS, the front-line organizations took their responsibility, as they had in the past.

Bloody Sunday was the date when AIDS was first acknowledged as a problem in the Netherlands. The meeting was concerned with the safety of the blood supply in general, and, more specifically, how to prevent people at risk of HIV infection from donating blood. The collective decision that gay men should refrain from donating blood voluntarily instead of mandatorily debarring them, is illustrative of Dutch policy. An appeal to personal responsibility fitted the belief in the ability of citizens to make rational decisions with respect to their own health and the health of others. Moreover, it fitted very well the culture of consensus and commitment:[3] the decision taken was a common decision. In order to fight AIDS, collaboration and consensus became the key words. It was not gay men against physicians, not gay men against people with haemophilia, not a public health approach against a health education approach, but all should work together instead.

Self-organizing Capacity of Front-line Organizations

Bloody Sunday also marks the establishment of the National AIDS Policy Coordination Team, which was given responsibility for initiating and coordinating the response to AIDS. Until 1987, the AIDS Coordination Team and the affiliated extended council (Breed Beraad), and the front-line organizations defined the desirable course of action.

The first ministerial memorandum on AIDS presented to Parliament by the Secretary of Health was made in September 1985. Apart from offering an overview on ways in which front-line organizations could be facilitated in doing their work, and apart from stressing the importance and effectiveness of the AIDS Coordination Team in terms of coordination and information provision, the memorandum laid the foundations for the features of AIDS policy as we know it in the Netherlands today. Since no treatment was available, since the virus apparently could not be transmitted through everyday contact, since contracting the virus supposedly caused AIDS only in a minority of cases (in 5 to 10 per cent of affected individuals, it was at that moment assumed), and since revealing one's serostatus might lead to stigmatization, it was decided that AIDS should not be a mandatory reportable disease. Instead, physicians were requested to report cases of AIDS on a voluntary and anonymous basis. Not being a reportable infectious disease, involuntary partner notification would not occur. Testing could only be performed with informed consent and if accompanied by pre- and post-test counselling. Emphasis was to be placed on information and education as the main means of prevention.

With respect to care and treatment, the general principle of Dutch health care policy, that wherever possible care should be provided by general service delivery organizations, became a cornerstone for AIDS policy. Categorical organizations were only financed if absolutely necessary. The application of this principle did not exclude AIDS specific approaches, but the challenge was to balance general principles and specific needs.

AIDS: From a Specific to a General Problem

A second landmark in the Dutch history of AIDS is a 1986 meeting at the National Institute of Public Health where it was decided official policy should not be limited to 'high risk groups' but to the population as a whole. An information campaign was to be started, and the AIDS Coordination Team was transformed into the National Committee on AIDS Control (NCAB), to be established by the Ministry of Health and having the status of an official advisory body to government. The decision that AIDS should no longer be treated as a specific problem of gay men and other risk groups, but as a general problem, was not taken overnight. But there was consensus over the final decision, probably because the reconceptualization was a win–win situation for all the parties involved. From the start, gay men had emphasized that behaviourally homosexual men happened simply to be the first to be affected, and that they could not be seen as responsible for spreading the virus. AIDS might be a big problem for gay men, but that did not make it a gay disease. AIDS could very easily become a general problem. The population as a whole therefore needed to be addressed. AIDS should be considered a threat to every individual's health and sexuality.

The Period between 1987 and 1991

In 1987, the first policy document on AIDS was presented to parliament. This document described an integrated policy on AIDS involving:

- the implementation of an effective education and prevention programme;
- the development of an optimal AIDS care infrastructure;
- the stimulation of AIDS research, covering the basic sciences, clinical sciences, epidemiology, and the social and behavioural sciences;
- the monitoring of legal and ethical issues; and
- the prevention of discrimination and stigmatization towards people with HIV and AIDS.

An important means of executing the proposed policy was the NCAB, the successor of the AIDS Coordination Team. In terms of composition and working methods, the NCAB looked like other advisory bodies to government. All the stakeholding parties met in closed session to reach consensus on policy issues. On a regional level, Regional AIDS Platforms played an analogous role with respect to the organizations responsible for the execution of AIDS policy. It is accepted that all stakeholders carry with them specific interests and objectives, but it is believed that in the end specific interests will be made subordinate to collective interests and one common mission: the fight against AIDS. But there were differences with other advisory bodies as well. First, the NCAB focused on one disease, and operated next to general advisory bodies such as the National Health Council. Second, compared to other advisory bodies, patient organizations and community groups played a more prominent role.

The Normalization of AIDS

With the acceptance of the 1987 Policy Document on AIDS, the normalization of AIDS became an explicit aim of Dutch AIDS policy.[4] This was not as an expression of resignation, but as a strategy for adaptation to and control of a potentially large problem. Moreover, it was felt that normalization would divert attention from vulnerable groups, and therefore decrease the chance of discrimination and stigmatization. In this way normalization may be seen as part of the tradition of liberal pragmatism. Trust in personal and mutual responsibility can only be maintained as a starting point for policy when citizens have a sense of personal responsibility and trust is valued by the citizens. Normalization also explains why it turned out to be relatively easy to make AIDS policy, AIDS prevention, AIDS care and the fight against AIDS, a joint effort involving the state, science, health care, social services, education, people with HIV and AIDS, their advocacy groups and their solicitors.

The down-side of the normalization, however, was that the influence of gay advocacy groups and gay service organizations decreased, while the influence of patient organizations and general service organizations increased.

The Planning of Health Care Provision

From 1987 onwards, there was systematic attention to the planning, organization, and content of care and treatment. The challenge was to plan for the future while the decision making situation still was uncertain. Theoretical calculations did not exclude the possibility of an epidemic of considerable size. The risk could not be limited to relatively small groups at high risk, but had to be considered and responded to as a potential problem to all. This presupposition had a dramatic impact on ideas about the planning of health care services. If AIDS was to become a general problem of considerable size, then it did not make sense to invest heavily in categorical organizations. From 1987 onwards the planning of health care therefore became embedded within the existing configuration and became subject to prevailing principles.

The starting point for the planning and organization of AIDS care was the belief that AIDS-related problems could and should be dealt with within the existing health and social services policy framework and organizational network. Only if general policies, rules, regulations, and treatment and care facilities turned out to be ineffective and inefficient, was the possibility of categorical AIDS treatment facilities to be considered. A second starting point was the conviction that every Dutch citizen that was or might become HIV-infected, in whatever part of the country, should receive high quality care. This decision was made on the basis of distributive justice, but also on the hypothesis that AIDS might become a problem that was more or less evenly distributed over the country.

Consequences of this policy choice included efforts to inform and train everyone working in the health care system, and the expectation that every hospital and all hospital staff would treat and care for people with HIV and AIDS. This expectation applied to nursing home care as well. In order to prepare for a significant number of patients needing nursing home care, additional financial resourses were allocated to 29 nursing homes across the country. Similarly, the financing of volunteer programmes was not so much guided by the number of people with AIDS in a region, but by the expected number of people with HIV. By 1990 more than 30 volunteer programmes were spread over the country. By 1990 a structure had been created that could have dealt with a larger number of, and more widely spread, AIDS cases than were actually to transpire.

In a later stage 11 hospitals across the country were designated core hospitals, with the Academic Medical Centre in Amsterdam as national reference hospital. Important tasks of the core hospitals were the execution of clinical trials, the dissemination of information, the formulation of protocols and standards of care in the biomedical field as well as in nursing and psychosocial care. The policy principle that all hospitals should be willing to provide care did not exclude the possibility of AIDS specific approaches, treatment units, AIDS reference hospitals, AIDS specialists, AIDS nurses and AIDS consultative nurses; it merely meant that specific *services* should be part of the more general structures.

With respect to categorical service *organizations*, discussions were more problematic. With respect to the drug treatment system, it was acknowledged that these organizations played an essential role in the prevention of HIV. They executed the needle exchange programmes, they were in contact with drug users, and they knew in what language drug users should be addressed. However, HIV/AIDS treatment and care were to be provided by the general system. With respect to gay men, an analogous set of issues arose. Policy makers, financiers, and a majority within the NCAB discouraged the creation of gay specific AIDS services. From 1987 onwards gay specific services and advocacy groups were given primarily the task of executing policies, while their influence on the design of policies decreased. Operational tasks were not given to them with the objective to keep gay specific services and activities intact. Instead such organizations were seen as an important reservoir of knowledge and expertise that could be disseminated throughout the general health care system and public health services.

Getting Realistic: 1991 to 1995

In the early 1990s, an increasing number of factors suggested that AIDS might become a more limited health care problem than had hitherto been supposed, in terms of both size as well as costs. The Dutch scenario study (STG, 1992) prepared the grounds for a revision of AIDS policy.[5] Important conclusions from the scenario study included:

- AIDS will create a substantial but by no means insurmountable problem for the health care system;
- HIV has not become widespread outside the known risk groups; and
- the chances of a widespread epidemic among the heterosexual population are slight.

It was not concluded, however, that continued efforts for prevention were not needed. On the contrary, there is a continued need for AIDS education and prevention. Indeed, explicit information and education programmes have contributed to a containment of the HIV epidemic. To not continue with educational efforts might be seen as a signal that AIDS is no longer a threat to public and individual health, and might therefore have a negative effect on sustaining safe behaviours. The scenario report warned policy makers not to fall into the 'paradox of prevention' trap: effective prevention contributes to a containment of problems. By taking away the means of containment, the problem may in fact increase.

The revision of official AIDS policy did not occur overnight, but happened only after confirmation and the downward adjustment of calculations and epidemiological extrapolations based on the scenario study. Data from the HIV surveillance system and the AIDS reporting system made clear that the spread of HIV had indeed been limited. New infections among the heterosexual population had stayed well below 1 per cent (as measured through the HIV monitoring system), and most of these infections occurred amongst women and men coming from endemic areas. The prevalence of HIV among injecting drug users outside Amsterdam had stayed well below the Amsterdam percentage (20–25 per cent). And the steepness of the curve with respect to new infections among younger gay and bisexual men had decreased. Infections were still occurring, as well as risk behaviour, but not at any rate characteristic of gay and bisexual men in older age groups. Moreover, it had become clear that AIDS was a geographically focused problem with Amsterdam as its core, and that the AIDS and HIV epidemic was increasingly linked with lower socio-economic status. Last but not least, despite the fact that the percentage of gay men on the total number of AIDS diagnoses had decreased from 89 per cent in the period 1982–85 to 72 per cent in 1996, AIDS continued to be a serious problem for gay men.

It was against this background that the NCAB published its final advice in September 1995. Core elements of this were:

- Planning of services should be made more dependent on epidemiological data. This resulted in the advice to reduce the number of core hospitals and nursing homes.
- Services should take into account the different needs of different groups. A more supportive attitude towards categorical services for gay and bisexual men and women, and drug users was expressed.
- Continuation of support of volunteer care, taking into account the differential burden on the formal and informal care systems, and the different needs in different groups. At the same time, the planning of buddy projects should be made more dependent on epidemiological data. In a substantial number of regions, the number of volunteers exceeded the number of people with AIDS. Some volunteer programmes had stopped because there was a lack of patients in their catchment areas, and others had merged in order to improve efficiency. By 1996 the number of volunteer programmes had decreased from over 30 to 23.
- Continued provision of adequate psycho-social support, as provided by care givers with a double expertise, and by community mental health services.
- Continued attention to the social participation of people with HIV/AIDS.

This was considered all the more necessary, because of recent social policy changes. For example, the cost of the first 52 weeks of illness had become the responsibility of the employer, making selection on the basis of health more important. The conditions of the Disability Act had also become stricter and financially less favourable.

- Reaffirmation of patient organizations as key stakeholding parties and as an accumulated source of experience and expertise. Assigned tasks to patient organizations included 1) consolidation of advances in treatment and care, 2) ensuring that services and treatments – especially new therapies – stay or become available, accessible and affordable to all, 3) ensuring that proposed policy changes do not result in a curtailment of human and patient rights, 4) being an advocate for the optimal participation of PWHIV and PWAIDS in society and ensuring that selection on the basis of health status, access to the labour market and insurance becomes difficult or impossible, and 5) ensuring that preventive programmes and the resources they need remain available and accessible.

The bottom line of the advice was to preserve what is good, and invest in quality, efficiency and effectiveness. The policy recommendations have to be seen in the context of the then existing treatment possibilities, which were considered to be rather limited. AIDS was still very much seen as a fatal disease, and by implication much attention was paid to the quality of death.

New Drugs, New Hope, New Questions

Less than one year after the final NCAB report, the seemingly stable environment had changed dramatically. The XIth International Conference on AIDS (1996) in Vancouver was the first conference at which promising results were presented about new drugs, new combination therapies and new methods to determine viral load. The advent of protease inhibitors, it was felt, would have a compelling effect on AIDS care and prospects for people living with AIDS. These results gave rise to new hope. However, with the new drugs came new questions, not only for basic science and clinical science, but also for social science and behavioural research.

Compliance

New therapeutic regimens require considerable discipline on the part of the patient. He or she may have to take many different drugs, and he or she needs to take them regularly. From the literature we know that compliance is a major issue in patient treatment, and this is even more so in the case of AIDS. The drugs have quite serious side effects, and it is unknown what the side effects on the mid or longer term will be. Different drugs require different intake schedules (some on a full stomach, some on an empty stomach) – as a result life itself becomes medicalized. A substantial number of people with AIDS belong to groups that have a poor record in terms of compliance (drug users, sex workers, psychiatric patients, homeless people). Since non-compliance is an important factor in drug resistance, the question has to be addressed how these people can be assisted effectively.

Quality of Life

Not much information is available on the impact of the new drugs and drug regimens on the quality of life. Although the few data that we have are not too disquieting, several questions have to be addressed. First of all it is unclear what are the size and seriousness of the problems that arise due to the intake of toxic drugs, especially if they need to be taken lifelong. Furthermore, combination therapies make the simultaneous use of some other drugs impossible; how will starting these therapies and stopping others affect morbidity and mortality due to other diseases? We know little about the mid-and long-term efficacy if people already have developed symptoms of AIDS – is it a one-time chance? What will the individual psychological effect be if the drugs do not work? Finally, many people to a certain extent had adapted to the idea that they were going to die in the reasonably near future. Their perspective has suddenly changed. One cannot assume automatically that people will perceive this change as positive. What is a life without all the lost friends and a diminished social network, without a job, and having to live on a small income?

What Kind of Care?

The availability of new combination therapies will also have an impact on where treatment is going to be provided. Given the numerous combinations of therapy possible, and the complexity of viral load determinations, the role of physicians working in the core hospitals will most probably increase, and the role of GPs and home care will be limited to the final stages of disease. However, from the point of view of monitoring and compliance, the GP's office might be the better place, especially in Amsterdam where about 10 offices provide for 80 per cent of the total caseload. The work of volunteers will change as well, although it cannot be said what directions these changes will take. Is it possible, for example, to envisage volunteering for a period of 8 or 10 years? Will those who are infected but well, appreciate that kind of effort?

Who is going to pay?

At a more general policy level, the availability of new treatments requires decisions about the accessibility and affordability of these drugs. This will occur in the context of more general policies with respect to the reimbursement of drug treatments and increasing pressure on the health care budget. Thus far, the swiftness of decision making has been remarkable. By July 1996, finances for the new therapies were made available. This was the result of the network that has been established for the last 10 to 15 years, though the decision was taken under and after an influential alliance between the AIDS Fund and Patients Organization (HIV Society).

In summary, what seemed to be a rather predictable policy environment in 1995 had become more turbulent by 1996, especially in relation to health care. New combination therapies have already led to new questions and changing problems and needs. Their advent will require new responses from all parts of the health care system: hospitals, home care services, mental health care agencies, volunteer organizations, public health agencies and health education agencies.

So what is New?

The question arises, is there anything new in AIDS health care policy? After all, almost every kind of service is embedded in the already existing structures, and similar initiatives to these in the area of AIDS can be found in other areas (cancer, epilepsy). In an early interim evaluation, Schnabel (1989) characterized Dutch AIDS policy first and foremost as typically Dutch, and second as a specific AIDS policy. General principles and policies were applied and turned out to be applicable to the problems that AIDS created. We believe that this conclusion still stands at the level of principles and strategic health care planning. However, if we look at tactical and operational planning and practices, AIDS has had an influence that goes even beyond AIDS care. We will illustrate this by looking at practices and policies in community involvement, the influence of patient organizations, patient involvement in medical decision making, the health promotion approach to STDs and HIV testing policy, and psycho-social care.

Volunteer Care

AIDS affected the gay population first and hardest. Even now, more than 70 per cent of people with AIDS in the Netherlands are behaviourally homosexual men. Throughout the 1980s, gay men, gay organizations and gay advocacy groups were a powerful driving force behind the creation of AIDS policy, and had a decisive influence on the content of that policy. Simultaneously, they executed prevention campaigns and provided services, of which the so-called Buddy Programmes are one of the most striking examples. In the Netherlands, volunteer care and community involvement are most visible, innovative and effective in the gay population. The first Buddy Programme was introduced in

1985 by the Schorerstichting; it was inspired by the San Francisco Shanti Project and the New York Gay Men's Health Crisis' mutual support programmes (De Rijk and Van den Boom, 1989). It was striking, because there are no cities in the Netherlands where the same kind of gay neighbourhoods can be found as in San Francisco or New York. Gay men form part of a rather loose network. Nevertheless, AIDS triggered a community or more precisely a latent network response. Volunteer help served two purposes: first, by providing social, emotional and practical support to fellow homosexual men; second, it helped gay men come to terms with the epidemic. It is illustrative of collective behaviour in a period of social change, where gay men from a mixture of solidarity and personal involvement gave shape to an innovative form of psycho-social support. The programmes turned out to be so successful in terms of providing support that there was a wish to expand the concept to other groups, notably drug users, ethnic minorities and heterosexual men and women.[6]

Although specific programmes have been organized, it remains a question if volunteer care will have the same benefits to, and basis in, other populations. Driessen *et al.* (1991) have pointed to the problems that volunteer care in a drug using population can face. One of the main problems is the absence of a common social denominator other than drug use. A somewhat similar problem is described for the very heterogeneous group of women with HIV (Te Vaarwerk and Gaal, 1995).

The impact of the Buddy Programmes goes beyond AIDS care. In the early 1990s, at a policy level it was acknowledged that an extension of this model might also be applicable to other diseases. In practice, however, the application of the model has progressed slowly, and much will depend on the efforts of large volunteer organizations, such as the Netherlands Red Cross.

The Influence of Patient Organizations

From the 1970s onward, there has been increasing attention on the disequilibrium between patient and health service provider, at both individual and institutional levels. Laws and regulations to strengthen the position of patient organizations and empower patients have been enacted.[7] From this perspective, AIDS activists jumped on an already running train. But, although attention on the patient as a stakeholder within the health care system had been increasing, patient organizations did not meet on equal terms with other stakeholders (providers, financiers, government) in the mid 1980s. People with HIV and AIDS are prototypical for what De Swaan, Van Gelderen and Kense (1979) call 'proto-professionalized' patients, who wanted to be involved in decision making, including medical decision making, and had the knowledge and 'courage' to demand this right. PWAs challenged politicians, policy makers, public health officials, care givers and researchers since, generally speaking, they were well informed about the disease and its progression, the available drugs and the drugs under investigation, and their rights and obligations. Moreover, they organized a global information network, so that information was transferred very quickly from one part of the world to the other. There was and there still is a fast and intensive exchange of information, expertise, and experience. AIDS reinforced and accelerated changes already latent within the institutions and within policy making. AIDS patient organizations were among the first to negotiate about, and participate in, decision making with respect to research policy and execution, service quality, the financing of treatments and organizing new modalities of care.

It is salient that physicians and other care givers, researchers, policy makers and other health care professionals have perceived themselves more as partners of patients and patient groups than as opponents. There was a real willingness to enter discussion and dialogue. This dialogue was initially organized within the context of the NCAB, the regional AIDS Platforms and National AIDS Trial Evaluation Centre (NATEC). The role of the Ministry of Health in the positioning of the patient organizations should not, however, be underestimated. Progressive policy makers utilized the momentum created by AIDS activism to increase the role of the patient in the triad: patient, provider and financier. In the 1990s, the influence of patient organizations has increased on almost every aspect of health care policy.

Patient Involvement in Medical Decision Making

In line with principles of self-determination and personal autonomy, patients perceived their role as stakeholders and partners in decision making as one that was not limited to general decision making in the areas of care and treatment, education and prevention. They also wanted to be involved in decision making with respect to starting treatments, refusing treatments and the active termination of life. Increasingly, PWAs became involved in medical decision making. Informed consent procedures with respect to starting new treatments are now the rule rather than the exception, and many hospitals have formulated policy with respect to the drawing up of living wills. But the most salient expression of their involvement in medical decision making is the fact that almost 50 per cent of PWAs discuss the possibility of euthanasia and approximately 25 per cent now die after the administration of euthanasia and physician-assisted suicide (Van den Boom, 1995; Laane, 1995; Bindels *et al.*, 1996).[8]

The above does not imply that doctors simply do what patients demand. For example, treatments outside regular Western medicine have not been integrated into the health care system; and euthanasia is only performed if the necessary requirements are met. Self-determination has not become the only leading principle. Care givers in the area of AIDS and patients alike have been trying to find a balance between the Samaritan principle (implying the duty to help) and the principle of self-determination (Wulff, 1995).

A Health Promotion Approach to STDs

The HIV test, which became widely available in 1985, opened unknown possibilities for containment of the epidemic. By testing, people could be identified; by notifying them, transmission to others might be prevented. The darker side of identification, however, is the possibility of marginalization, exclusion, and isolation. This in itself is not unique to AIDS, but AIDS became special as an early test case of the relation between constitutionally given rights on the integrity of the human body and the right to the protection of personal privacy on the one hand, and the constitutionally given responsibility of the state to protect and promote public health on the other. The wish to protect the population against further HIV transmission had to be balanced against principles such as informed consent and autonomous choice, the protection of personal privacy, the integrity of the human body, and the confidentiality of medical information.

Whereas in other countries, especially the United States, initial resistance towards HIV testing and screening was very much linked to the fear that testing and screening might jeopardize the still unstable emancipation of gay men, this argument has never played a significant role in the Netherlands. Gay advocacy groups in alliance with leading Dutch experts on health law and health ethics, successfully defended the position that testing and screening were acceptable only after the informed consent of every individual was obtained: the result was that mandatory testing at an individual, let alone population level, was made impossible (with the exception of the screening and informing of blood and plasmapheresis donors). Other methods of containment that relied on community education and voluntary anonymous testing were advanced and accepted.

Although health education and promotion by means of mass media campaigns and school programmes were already used as a health policy strategy in the areas of smoking, drinking, and nutrition, health education and promotion did not occupy a central place in STD prevention. AIDS accelerated the adoption of such approaches and invited their intensive application to infectious diseases. Increasingly, AIDS prevention became the domain of representatives of health education and promotion, and became characterized by an approach and vision that had not played a significant role in the traditional, medical approaches to STD prevention thus far. Knowledge of the modes of transmission and the promotion of safe behaviours (sex, injecting drug use, universal precautions for health care personnel) became the byword in a prevention policy that was new both in the sense of approach and content.

Psycho-social Care

An integrated approach to health care, that is to say a policy that acknowledged that well-being and quality of life are the result of physical, psychological and social variables, was formulated and advocated in the mid 1980s, independent of HIV and AIDS. It was in the area of AIDS, however, where an integrated approach was not only formulated as one of the cornerstones of policy, but implemented as well. Attention to the psycho-social aspects thereby became an indissoluble and necessary component of quality care. It was in the area of AIDS that the gap between the conceptualization of disease as a bio-psycho-social problem and the practical implementation of this new approach to understanding disease was first bridged.

Conclusion

In assessing the impact of AIDS on the health care system, it is our conclusion that AIDS has not altered the *structure* of the institutions that we have discussed, but has had a significant impact on the *contents* of care and prevention. Organizational structure has not changed, partly because HIV remains a small epidemic in the Netherlands. Relatively few people are infected with HIV, and elaborate health care services were already available, accessible and afford- able as a result of obligatory health care insurance. No structural budgetary problems have arisen, and the denial of treatment due to being uninsured has *de facto* been neither an issue, nor a problem. In economic terms, AIDS has never seriously challenged the health care system as a system (STG, 1992). Since most of the effects could be dealt with in the already existing system, there was no compelling force for fundamental change in the structure of health care provision. And in order to change social institutions as complex as the health care and public health systems, a truly compelling force is essential. Moreover, early in the epidemic it was stated that AIDS care in all its facets should be or become an integral part of the existing health care system. This did not exclude the possibility of AIDS specific approaches, treatment units, and so on; it merely meant that specific services should be part of the more general structures.

In addition to being a quantitatively small problem, AIDS is a socially and geographically concentrated problem. Many geographical areas and strata of the population remain virtually untouched by the epidemic and hopefully and probably never will be. With respect to those specific groups affected by the epidemic, in the majority of cases specialist services were already in existence.

Given the size and character of the epidemic, it is the more surprising that AIDS has had a significant impact on health policy and practices. Although organizational structures have largely stayed intact, the often indirect and subtle influences of AIDS on health care and health care providers should not be underestimated. AIDS has made a difference in the area of STD prevention practices, volunteer care, patient involvement, and appreciation of the psycho-social aspects of somatic disease. AIDS reinforced and accelerated changes already latent both institutionally and in relation to health policy: attention for psycho-social problems and care, self-help and mutual support, support for patient organizations, and an emphasis on patient rights. The possibilities that were constitutionally and legally available, for example in the area of patient rights, were and are optimally used. An illustration of this is the financial compensation granted to HIV infected people with haemophilia. In 1995 the National Ombudsman decided that the demands of the National Haemophilic Patient Association were justified, and urged the government to arrange for compensation. By utilizing every possible legal instrument, the patient movement had finally realized what they had fought for for more than ten years. Some responses have acted as catalysts for similar responses in other areas of medicine. In many ways, therefore, AIDS policy became an experimental garden for health policy.

The many things that have been realized in the area of AIDS in a relatively short period of time cannot be ascribed to one single actor. The successes seem to be more the result of a complex interplay between many different forces entering into alliances. AIDS policy as we know it today, is the result of what one might describe as a pioneering network organization. The motor behind this organization in many cases have been people with AIDS themselves, their organizations and their advocates. This is not to say that there has not been an absence of conflict of interest, and sometimes heated discussions, but they have rarely resulted in schisms. Within this internal arena people were gathered who knew the ins and outs of the traditional policy cycle as well as policy making in the area of health care and public health. Their actions were aided by good links with key professionals, policy makers, and politicians.

Innovation and the Principle of Parsimony

Flexibility is needed now that with the introduction of combination therapies the environment has become dynamic once again. A dynamic environment requires new ideas and room for innovation as well as openness on the part of professional and institutional groups to discuss their own roles, futures and *raisons d'être*. The present and the future demand room for experimentation and innovation. But will there be room for innovation and experiments in the years to come?

The space for innovation is not automatically available. Due mainly to the small size of the epidemic, negotiations about financial recources will take place within stricter budgetary constraints. This will make less room for manoeuvre, as well as force innovation outside of the regular health care system. Advocacy groups, researchers, and care givers alike will be confronted increasingly with the third principle distinguished by Wulff: the principle of acknowledging that the health care budget is limited and henceforth requires parsimony.[9] The fight over a limited health care budget may become more fierce, since earlier configurations of 'consensus and commitment' have changed. Since late 1995, an NCAB has not existed. Its former tasks were transferred to the Dutch AIDS Fund, the National Institute on Alcohol and Drugs (NIAD), and the Foundation for STD Control. The AIDS policy unit at the Ministry of Health has virtually disappeared. The PccAo has become embedded within the Dutch Foundation for Scientific Research (NWO) with a link to the AIDS Fund. Dispersion of influence may make it more difficult to develop consensus on future policy and practice with respect to AIDS care.

Last but not least, there is an internal issue to confront. Peter Drucker (1973) once described the difficult transition from pioneering to established organizations. It is true that at as an organization grows, it cannot survive without adequate control and coordination. However, as soon as such mechanisms are implemented, the danger of dysfunctional bureaucratization arises. Instead of focusing on developments around themselves, organizations start focusing on internal processes and procedures and on self-preservation. Preventing this happening will be one of the most important challenges to all organizations involved in the fight against AIDS.

Notes

1 A general institution is accessible for every citizen who is in need of one of the services provided. A categorical institution is only accessible for people with a specific characteristic, for example a mental handicap, epilepsy, or belonging to a specific group (for example homosexual men and women, religious denomination). The Netherlands has a network of community mental health centers, which are financed through health care insurance. If a community mental health centre is founded that operates on a Christian basis, the rule is that this centre will not be financed out of public means, since such services are already provided.

2 The Schorerstichting is a mental health service organization for gay men and women; it was founded in 1967 and supported financially by government and health care insurance. The Ancillary Service Department (SAD) was founded in the early 1980s – before HIV and AIDS became a problem for the gay community – in order to deal more efficiently with the prevalence and incidence of sexually transmitted diseases in the gay population. Both foundations are located in Amsterdam. Recently the two foundations have merged into the SAD-Schorerstichting.

3 When the HIV test came available in 1985, the policy of voluntary non-donation stayed intact; but it was made clear to every donor that they would be informed about the test results. This policy of testing and informing everyone without the possibility of an individual opting not to receive the test result has been limited to the blood bank system.

4 On the premise that AIDS posed a threat to public health, and that the possible size of the epidemic might become substantial, AIDS was reconceptualized from a problem affecting small and distinguishable groups to a more general problem. General problems had to be dealt with

within the existing – normal – arrangements, even if the problem itself might have extraordinary characteristics. The adage was: deal with the extraordinary in as normal a way as possible.

5   In 1988, the Steering Committee on Future Health Scenarios (STG) asked the National Institute on Mental Health (NcGv) and the National Institute of Public Health and Environment (RIVM) to execute a scenario study in the area of AIDS. Prior to this study, scenario studies had been executed on cardiovascular disease, the elderly, cancer, chronic diseases, and on mental health. Scenario analysis first and foremost tries to incorporate representative data from different sources and process them into comprehensive and often new conceptual models. For an introduction in scenario analysis, the reader is referred to STG (1992); Jager and Van den Boom (1994); Van Genugten *et al.* (1996).

6   The National Haemophilic Patient Association has organized a mutual support programme for people with haemophilia.

7   For example, the 1983 change of the Constitution, adding to it the right of personal privacy and integrity of the human body. Several related laws have been passed including a law regulating the use of personal data; a law regulating the treatment contract between care giver and patient; and a law regulating the influence of patients or mentors on institutional functioning.

8   Again, it should be remembered that the issue of euthanasia has been discussed since the 1970s. In 1987, the Royal Academy of Medicine (KNMG) after a year-long discussion formulated criteria and general guidelines that had to be fulfilled in order to end the life of a patient by means of euthanasia and physician-assisted suicide.

9   The other two principles are: the Samaritan principle and the principle of self-determination.

References

AIDS FONDS (1996) *Behandelingsmogelijkheden bij HIV/AIDS. Inventarisatie van Consequenties en Aanbevelingen*, Amsterdam: Stichting AIDS Fonds.

BINDELS, P.J.E., KROL, A., VAN AMEIJDEN, E., MULDER-FOLKERTS, D.K.F., VAN DEN HOEK, A.R., VAN GRIENSVEN, G.P.J. and COUTINHO, R.A. (1996) 'Euthanasia and physician assisted suicide in homosexual men with AIDS', *Lancet*, **437**, pp. 499–504.

VAN DEN BOOM, F. (1995) 'AIDS, euthanasia and grief', *AIDS Care*, **7**, Supplement 2, 19, S. pp. 175–86.

VAN DEN BOOM, F., GREMMEN, T. and ROOZENBURG, H. (1991) *AIDS: Leven rond de Dood. Nabestaanden over Ziekte, Dood en Rouw*, Utrecht: NcGv.

VAN DEN BOOM, F., JAGER, J.C., LUMEY, L.H. and RUITENBERG, E.J. (1990) 'Het wetenschappelijk AIDS-onderzoek: randvoorwaarden van de onderzoeksprogrammering', in I. RAVENSLAG, M.A.M. DE WACHTER and

H.A.E. ZWART (Eds), *Aids. Instellingen, individu, samenleving*, Baarn: Ambo.

CAMUS, A. (1947) *La Peste*, Paris: Editions Gallimard.

COUTINHO, R.A. (1984) *Sexually Transmitted Diseases among Homosexual Men. Studies on Epidemiology and Prevention*, Doctoral Thesis, Amsterdam: Rodopi.

DRIESSEN, A., VAN DE VELDEN, L., VAN DEN BOOM, F. and DERKS, J. (1991) *Steun van de Regenboog. Vrijwillige Hulpverlening aan Verslaafden met AIDS*, Utrecht: NcGv.

DRUCKER, P. (1973) *Management: Tasks, Responsibilities and Practices*, New York: Harper & Row.

FUKUYAMA, F. (1995) *Trust*, London: Hamish Hamilton.

VAN GENUGTEN, M.L.L., RUTTEN, F.F.H. and JAGER, J.C. (1996) *Scenario Development and Costing in Health Care. Methodological Accomplishments and Practical Guidelines*, Utrecht: International Press.

HOFSTEDE, G. (1991) *Cultures and Organizations, Software of the Mind*, London: McGraw-Hill.

JAGER, J.C. and VAN DEN BOOM, F. (1994) 'Scenario analysis, health policy and decision making', in E.H. KAPLAN and M.L. BRANDEAU (Eds) *Modelling the Epidemic. Planning, Policy and Prediction*, New York: Raven Press.

KNMG (1987) 'Richtlijnen inzake euthanasie voor verpleegkundigen', *Medisch Contact*, **42**, 15, pp. 476–9.

LAANE, H.M. (1995) 'AIDS and euthanasia', in L. SHERR and F. VAN DEN BOOM (guest editors), *AIDS and Suicide. AIDS Care*, **7**, Supplement 2, 19, S. pp. 163–8.

MCNEILL, W.H. (1976) *Plagues and Peoples*, Garden City: Anchor/ Doubleday.

MINISTERIE VAN WVC (1986) *Gezondheid als Uitgangspunt. Nota 2000 in het Kort*, Den Haag: Ministerie van WVC.

MINISTERIE VAN WVC (1987) *Nota inzake het AIDS-beleid*, Den Haag: Ministerie van WVC.

NATIONALE OMBUDSMAN (1995) *Openbaar Rapport. Verzoekschrift van de NVHP met een Klacht over een Gedraging van het Ministerie van WVC*, Den Haag: Nationale Ombudsman.

NCAB (1995) *Het AIDS-beleid Geactualiseerd. Eindadvies van de Nationale Commissie AIDS Bestrijding*, Amsterdam: NCAB.

NCCZ (1995) *Werk op Maat. Advies Arbeidsmarktpositie van Mensen met Chronische Gezondheidsproblemen*, Zoetermeer: NCCZ.

NETHERLANDS MINISTRY OF WELFARE, HEALTH AND CULTURAL AFFAIRS (1992) *AIDS-policy in the Netherlands. Progress Report*, Den Haag: Netherlands Ministry of Welfare, Health and Cultural Affairs.

POSTMA, M., JAGER, J.C. and DIJKGRAAF, M. (1995) 'AIDS scenarios for the Netherlands: the economic impact on hospitals', *Health Policy*, **31**, pp. 127–50.

DE RIJK, K. and VAN DEN BOOM, F. (1989) *Psychosociale Hulpverlening AIDS. Vijf Jaar Hulpverlening door de Schorerstichting*, Utrecht: NcGv.

SCHNABEL, P. (1987) 'Het eigene en het aardige van de geestelijke gezondheidszorg', Rede uitgesproken bij de aanvaarding van het ambt van hoogleraar aan de Universiteit van Utrecht, 13 October.

SCHNABEL, P. (1989) 'De diepten van een epidemie. Over de maatschappelijke gevolgen van AIDS', in A. NOORDHOFF-DE VRIES (Ed.), *AIDS. Een Nieuwe Verantwoordelijkheid voor Gezondheidszorg en Onderwijs*, Amsterdam: Swets & Zeitlinger.

SOCIAAL EN CULTUREEL PLANBUREAU (1988) *Sociaal en Cultureel Rapport 1988*, Rijswijk: SCP.

STG; STEERING COMMITTEE ON FUTURE HEALTH SCENARIOS (1992) *AIDS up to the Year 2000; Epidemiological, Sociocultural and Economic Scenario Analysis for the Netherlands*, Dordrecht: Kluwer Academic Publishers.

DE SWAAN, A., VAN GELDEREN, R. and KENSE, V. (1979) *Sociologie van de Psychotherapie 2. Het Spreekuur als Opgave*, Utrecht/Antwerpen: Het Spectrum.

TE VAARWERK, M. TE and GAAL, E. (1995) *Vrouwen met AIDS. Een Onderzoek naar Aard en Omvang van Psychosociale Problematiek*, Utrecht: NcGv.

WULFF, H. (1995) *Medische ethiek en klinische praktijk. Op zoek naar het juiste evenwicht*, Amsterdam: De Volkskrant.

Chapter 10

AIDS: A Priority Issue in Foreign Assistance by the Netherlands

Hans Moerkerk

HIV/AIDS is considered a serious developmental issue by the Dutch government.[1] In consequence, support for HIV/AIDS-related activities has been included in Dutch foreign assistance since 1989. This includes multilateral support to UN Agencies and bilateral support to many countries (governments and non-governmental organizations, NGOs) in Asia, Africa, Central and South America and the Caribbean, both by the Dutch government (Ministry of Foreign Affairs) and through internationally operating Dutch NGOs. In addition, the Dutch Ministry of Health supports an extensive HIV/AIDS Programme of the World Health Organization (WHO) for the countries of East and Central Europe. In 1997, approximately 60 million Dutch Guilders (US$30 million) were spent on HIV/AIDS-specific activities in Central America, Latin America, Africa, Asia and Central and Eastern Europe.

At this moment, the Dutch government ranks as the third largest donor of international HIV/AIDS assistance in absolute US dollars, after the USA and the UK. Contrary to many governments in the industrialized world, the Netherlands has increased its contribution and will keep at least the same level for the remainder of the decade. Being a strong supporter of the establishment of the Joint United Nations Programme on HIV/AIDS (UNAIDS), the Dutch government increased its core contribution for this co-sponsored UN Programme in 1996 to 10 million Dutch guilders a year (US$5.3 million; Pronk, 1995). In 1997 and 1998 the Netherlands increased its contribution to 12 million Dutch guilders each year (US$6 million).

In this chapter, I will first discuss how HIV/AIDS affects the developing world and why HIV/AIDS is an important development issue for the Dutch government. Subsequently, I will describe the way in which HIV/AIDS is included in the Dutch international development policy.

The Pandemic at the Beginning of 1996

Since the early 1980s, AIDS has changed the world. Since the start of the epidemic, an estimated 30.6 million people worldwide have been infected with HIV, 10 per cent of them children. Globally, the male–female ratio is almost 50–50 (Mann and Tarantola, 1996). In terms of numbers, sub-Saharan

Africa is still the most affected area (63 per cent of global total of cases), with South-east Asia a fast runner-up (23 per cent of global total number of cases).

The epidemic is, however, as much about meanings as specific numbers. HIV/AIDS is a relatively new epidemic which is still unstable and dynamic, with the major impact, especially in the less developed parts of the world, still to come. As we examine the global picture of AIDS today, we have to recognize that, despite a remarkable and unprecedented worldwide response, existing efforts in terms of available financial resources are not sufficient to deal with the challenges of HIV/AIDS in the 1990s.

Although in some parts of the industrialized world the epidemic seems to be 'controllable', there is no reason for a declining societal commitment to HIV/AIDS both in the industrialized world and less developed countries. The lack of effective treatment, the long period of infectivity and the fact that through perinatal transmission HIV affects future generations as well, will disrupt existing projections for societal development in demographic, economic, cultural and political terms (Worldbank, 1993). A recent publication by the Global AIDS Policy Coalition confirms this analysis (Mann and Tarantola, 1996).

Prior to the HIV/AIDS pandemic, it was expected that the development of 'poorer' nations could be influenced in a 'positive' way by better sanitation, better nutrition and higher income. As a part of that process, positive health effects resulting in higher production and more effective schooling were expected. Now, however, HIV/AIDS has started a reverse process which threatens to destroy most of the recent improvements (Worldbank, 1993).

AIDS: A Developmental Crisis

In many poor countries, health for many years has not been considered as an investment for future development. The HIV/AIDS epidemic makes this manifest, as does the sharp increase of infectious diseases such as TB, STDs, opportunistic infections of various kinds, and other epidemics. Combined with poorly developed health service infrastructure, the advent of AIDS makes an already existing crisis more visible. Moreover, many governments, especially in Africa, have failed to give priority to health issues, because their health care systems have relied mostly on donors and on material support from Western countries. It is still not uncommon for African countries to spend less than 1 per cent of their annual budget on health. Donor countries have for too long encouraged the developing world to focus on health only as an issue of 'consumption' rather than as an 'investment' (Worldbank, 1993). AIDS is now forcing a change in priorities and a shift of attention towards prevention, both for HIV and STDs (Over and Piot, 1991). In most sub-Saharan countries 50 per cent of the available capacity in hospitals is now consumed by HIV/AIDS and related diseases. The lesson to be learned is that an isolated approach towards health problems is no longer acceptable, and that the characteristics of the epidemic should be included in a broader concept of development cooperation.

Although AIDS is much more than a health issue, this is especially true for developing countries. Poverty, poor health care, malnutrition, lack of respect for human rights, illiteracy, inadequate housing, discrimination against women and unresponsive political systems, all exacerbate the impact of HIV on any given society. In many developing countries, the HIV/AIDS epidemic has had a negative impact on social, economic and political development. In a vicious circle, the epidemic undermines earlier progress and reinforces many of the worst facets of underdevelopment (Moerkerk, 1992). It is not an exaggeration to state that HIV/AIDS threatens decades of progress towards improved health and sustained economic development in the Third World. The special attention given to the fight against the epidemic is more than justified.

Focusing exclusively on the public health aspects of HIV/AIDS ignores the many social, economical and political factors that influence the consequences of the epidemic. While it is true that the global attention paid to HIV/AIDS sometimes overshadows the fact that every year more people die of malaria, tuberculosis, infantile diarrhoea and bronchial diseases, there are four reasons at least why extra attention to HIV/AIDS in the context of development assistance is justified.

First, in economic terms, the fact that the disease mainly affects people in the most productive age group (15–45) has a detrimental effect on the development prospects of the society as a whole. This is particularly true for women, who play a central role not only in reproduction and in the individual household, but also in the economic process and in the educational sectors where qualified persons cannot be replaced any longer. Also vital sectors like transport and agriculture and, not least, health care are heavily affected.

Second, the fact that AIDS is concentrated in the most productive age group has other negative consequences for development: children lose one or both parents, which creates an enormous group of young people without any chance of a future in terms of education and stability.

Third, the violation of basic human rights and discrimination towards many vulnerable groups also has to be mentioned as being typical of this epidemic. People living with HIV/AIDS, refugees and migrants, ethnic minorities, sex workers, injecting drug users and gay men are stigmatized and blamed for the transmission of the virus, and are used as alibi for a lack of political attention.

Finally, AIDS leads to an increased prevalence of other diseases, most usually tuberculosis. A clear connection has been established between HIV and the large increase in 'traditional' venereal diseases in recent years, exposing the inadequacy of more general provisions for prevention and treatment. Connected with this, is the fact that HIV/AIDS imposes a considerable added burden on the health care sector, which detracts from the attention and resources that can be devoted to other health problems.

HIV/AIDS: A Policy Issue in Dutch Foreign Assistance

To understand the Dutch response to HIV/AIDS in developing countries, it is important to know that foreign assistance is a strong political issue in the Netherlands. The extent to which assistance will be made available for developing countries depends on political decisions and circumstances, but the issue as such is, in the Netherlands, not under discussion.

Since the beginning of the 1970s, the Netherlands has accepted the principle that developed countries have the moral duty to support less developed ones. Charity is obviously not the main reason for this attitude, although this policy is also not guided by mere national interests. In this respect, the Netherlands differs from many other countries in the Western world, where national and economic interest are the principles guiding their policies. Comparable countries to the Netherlands are those of the Nordic Council (Finland, Sweden, Norway and Denmark), Germany, Canada, Australia and, to a lesser extent, the United Kingdom. A stronger focus on their own national interests is shown by the United States, France and Japan, all of whom have an extreme desire for national benefit in return for foreign assistance. Due to the pressure from the Republican party in the USA, the support that country is giving internationally to HIV/AIDS-related activities is becoming more and more threatened.

Awareness of the consequences of HIV/AIDS for developing countries has ensured that fighting the epidemic became a vital part of the Dutch development assistance. To enable the government to introduce HIV-related priorities into the general framework of its development policy, the problem had to be understood in the context of other major issues for development cooperation. These issues include:

• political and economic destabilization;
• ecological destruction and exploitation;
• population growth, especially where the economic and ecological basis is already exhausted; and
• archaic warfare and forced migration.

These four elements have been used as the basis for setting priority in a development policy into which HIV/AIDS could be integrated. In the first place, the specific needs resulting from HIV/AIDS in developing countries were identified, as well as the most likely way the epidemic could develop in those areas. Second, the comparison and relationship between HIV/AIDS and other problematic issues with a high salience for developing countries was made. On the basis of this analysis, it was possible to choose priorities and to decide how and why scarce resources from the foreign assistance budget of the Dutch government should be used (Moerkerk, 1996).

Six key priorities were identified by this process. Considerations of a political nature were included as well, because they are regarded as the backbone of Dutch development policy (Pronk, 1990). Moreover, these priorities were in accordance with recommendations made by the World Health Organization's Global Programme on AIDS (Mann and Tarantola, 1996). The selected priorities are:

1. Strengthening existing national programmes, and the inclusion of NGOs and Community Based Organizations (CBOs) in a national strategy.
2. The promotion of an integrated multisector response.
3. Strengthening interventions to improve effectiveness in the (closely related) fields of prevention and care.
4. Supporting biomedical research focused on vaccines and clinical trials, and a stronger focus on social and behavioural research.
5. Countering discrimination against people living with HIV/AIDS and promoting their full participation in our common actions.
6. Fighting complacency and denial.

An important characteristic of the Dutch policy is that HIV/AIDS activities should be integrated into existing projects which focus on the improvement of economic and social conditions, on greater access to health care and education, and on improvement of human rights. The main elements of Dutch policy with regards to HIV/AIDS can be found in the conclusions and recommendations of several important meetings held in recent years. These include the International Conference on Population and Development (Cairo, 1994), the AIDS Summit of Heads of Government (Paris, 1994), the Social Summit (Copenhagen, 1995) and the World Conference on Women (Beijing, 1995). Linking HIV/AIDS to the main topics of these conferences, facilitates an integrated approach in which the promotion of reproductive and sexual health, the empowerment of women, sexual minorities and ethnic minorities, and measures to counter discrimination and deprivation are all vital preconditions for bringing the rapid spread of infection under control.

A further aim of Dutch policy is to more actively involve NGOs and groups of people living with HIV/AIDS in the implementation of government policy, with a particular emphasis on strengthening identity and cooperation with other similar groups. To ensure optimal relationships with community-based activities and independence from government interference, the Dutch government channels a part of its financial means to and through NGOs (both local and international). Especially in the field of HIV/AIDS, NGOs and CBOs are sometimes a more effective mechanism to initiate and to maintain activities than are national governments and national AIDS programmes. In relation to support for vulnerable groups, experience has taught us that strengthening the position of such groups themselves, also in institutional terms, contributed to the effectiveness and sustainability of their work. For this reason, the Dutch government tries to channel many of its resources directly to national and local NGOs. Sometimes Dutch NGOs are used as an intermediary for communication with such groups.

Hans Moerkerk

The Role of Dutch NGOs

Dutch developmental policy regarding HIV/AIDS is implemented in collaboration with several Dutch NGOs. There is a long-standing tradition of NGOs in the Netherlands operating in an international context. The political structure of the Netherlands whereby all religious and societal groups require representation, has created a variety of NGOs and CBOs that support the development cooperation in the Third World.

At this moment five so-called Co-financing Organizations (NOVIB, HIVOS, ICCO, BILANCE and SNV) are directly financed by the Ministry of Foreign Affairs to facilitate their work on different issues in developing countries. These organizations are independent from the government and have, besides substantial government funding, their own funding activities. HIVOS, ICCO and BILANCE are participating in many HIV/AIDS projects in developing countries and sometimes (as in the case of HIVOS), receive extra funding from the government for this work. But other NGOs too, such as MEMISA, SIMAVI and the Netherlands Red Cross Society have given priority to HIV/AIDS. They have organized themselves into an AIDS Coordination Group in which nine different NGOs cooperate and exchange their experiences. Both the Ministry of Foreign Affairs and the Ministry of Health are observers on this group (AIDS Coordination Group, 1996).

The Royal Tropical Institute (which underwrites support for a number of projects like TANESA) has established the AIDS Coordination Bureau which has set up a documentation centre, and is able to participate in research and desk studies for many intended projects. The AIDS Coordination Bureau and Group is also partly financed by the Dutch government.

The large funding organization AIDS Fund also finances some international activities; sometimes directly (they are the main funder of the Global Network of People Living with HIV/AIDS), and sometimes via NGOs which operate in developing countries. HIVOS, for example, has a specific agreement with AIDS Fund to ensure the implementation of different projects. In 1997 the Dutch government took over part of the core funding of the Global Network of People Living with HIV/AIDS.

Experience and expertise acquired in the Netherlands since HIV/AIDS activities started in 1983, is in many cases 'exported' outside the country. Both in bio-medical and social and behavioural research, Dutch researchers and institutions have made valuable contributions to international activities undertaken by WHO, UNICEF, UNFPA, the EU, IPPF and many other organizations. WHO and the EU have on some occasions requested Dutch organizations to execute specific activities for them. These include the Municipal Health Organizations of Amsterdam and Rotterdam, and the AIDS and Mobility Project which is part of the National Institute for Health Education. This latter institute is also the European focal point for HIV/AIDS and youth. Some universities (Amsterdam, Nijmegen and Utrecht) are involved in HIV/

AIDS-related activities in developing countries, including East and Central Europe.

Some Core Activities

The above-mentioned priority issues were reflected in a number of specific activities undertaken by the Dutch government. As a follow-up to the VIIIth International Conference on AIDS, held in Amsterdam in 1992, Dutch researchers were requested to draw up a plan to enable specific kinds of research, on vaccines and in other fields, to take place in developing countries. This resulted in the establishment in 1994 of ENARP (Ethiopian–Netherlands AIDS Research Project) which focuses on the scope for vaccine-related research to be carried out in Africa. The project will give particular attention to a wide variety of educational issues and to social and medical provision for study participants. The financial resources for the project are guaranteed for a number of years.

A second example of activities funded by the Netherlands, is the Tanzania–Netherlands Supporting AIDS Control Project (TANESA), which is now in its second five-year period. This project, which began as a joint activity between the Royal Tropical Institute in Amsterdam and three institutions in Tanzania, has focused on the development of an effective strategy to prevent infection with HIV. The project has led not only to important epidemiological and clinical research, but has also provided a detailed picture of behaviour patterns of the population of one particular district, enabling the introduction of specific interventions to allow people to make a conscious choice to use condoms (Borgdorff, 1994).

In Central America an important NGO project was established in 1992. The project is based in the Instituto Latinamericano de Prevención y Educación en Salud (ILPES) in Costa Rica, but conducts a variety of activities aimed at HIV prevention in seven Central American countries. ILPES gives priority to support for local NGOs. Via a special Embassy fund for AIDS prevention, a large number of small-scale NGO projects were set up in five Central American countries in 1993 and 1994. A recent evaluation made clear that this approach was satisfactory because it enabled small and emerging groups to develop different kinds of prevention activities for specific groups, including gays and lesbians, transvestites, refugees, indigenous people, and so on (De Man and Toro, 1994).

Dutch financing for UNICEF programmes for ethnic minorities in the border area of Thailand, Laos and Myanmar (1992–95) resulted in the development of a number of effective interventions for this poor, exploited and vulnerable population. The Dutch government and the UNICEF Association of the Netherlands decided to grant UNICEF 10 million Dutch Guilders (US$7.2 million) for extensive HIV prevention activities among ethnic minorities and children in difficult circumstances in six countries of that region.

The Dutch government is much involved in the financing of projects for the social marketing of condoms. Not only as a part of a prevention strategy for HIV, but also in relation to reproductive health, social marketing has proved to be a successful method of intervention. Projects are financed via an international NGO in Cambodia, Ethiopia, Tanzania, Mozambique, Benin and Haiti. Since 1997 the Dutch government has financed an NGO network on AIDS and Mobility in Southeast Asia, covering seven countries.

Finally, the Dutch government has supported the AIDS unit of the European Region of WHO with US$1.5 million to execute HIV/AIDS programmes in Eastern and Central Europe in the period 1990–95. This money was designated for the support of NGOs and CBOs in six different countries in that region.

The Near Future

At this moment, about 90 per cent of all cases of HIV/AIDS are in the developing world, where the poor and the oppressed are the most vulnerable. However, 92 per cent of the estimated US$14.2 billion annual spending on HIV prevention and care, is spent in the industrialized world. Unfortunately, this unbalanced situation will only increase in the near future, as a consequence of diminishing budgets for development assistance and non-health-committed priority setting by the developing countries themselves. At the same time, the burden in terms of the social and economic impact for the developing world will increase.

National budgets for foreign assistance are now under serious pressure in many countries. Perhaps not yet in the Netherlands, but in most of the above-mentioned countries, this is definitely the case. Due to its specific characteristics as a sexually transmitted disease and its connection with specific, vulnerable groups, HIV/AIDS will be one of the first issues to be touched by budget cuts. The fight against AIDS has for that reason reached a critical stage. The growing complexity of the consequences, the fast expanding epidemic and the confusion caused by so many different approaches, calls for a genuinely new initiative. Hopefully the recently established UNAIDS Programme, which brings together different UN efforts, will offer us new visions and challenges. The Global AIDS Policy Coalition has identified one such challenge: 'If current epidemic trends persist through the end of the century, it is most likely that between 60–70 million adults will have been infected by the end of the year 2000. Of these adults about 50 per cent will be in South-East Asia' (Mann and Tarantola, 1996, p. 27).

In 1988, in an article about AIDS as a new threat to the Third World, Lori Heise, a researcher at the Worldwatch Institute, made the important observation that 'AIDS is one of the few diseases that does not belong just to the "First

World" or the "Third World". This convergence of interests provides fresh opportunities to forge new paths for collaboration, new models for international cooperation. The global challenge of AIDS is simply expressed: If one country has AIDS, the world has AIDS' (Heise, 1988, p. 19). In relation to what we know now, this statement is even more true today than she could foresee eight years ago.

Note

1   In April 1993, a Parliamentary Report on *AIDS & Development* was published by the government and discussed in the Second Chamber (Lower House) of the Dutch Parliament. In June 1995 and January 1998, this report was updated and included a detailed review of activities since 1990 (Pronk, 1993, 1995 and 1998).

References

AIDS COORDINATION GROUP (1996) *Annual Report 1995*, Amsterdam: Royal Tropical Institute.

BORGDORFF, M. (1994) *Epidemiology of HIV-1 Infection in the Mwanza Region*, Amsterdam: Royal Tropical Institute.

HEISE, L. (1988) 'AIDS: new threat to the Third World?', *World Watch*, January–February, pp. 16–20.

DE MAN, F. and TORO, J. (1994) *And their Eyes Opened Like Flowers*, Den Haag: Directorate-General for International Cooperation.

MANN, T. and TARANTOLA, D. (Eds) (1996) *AIDS in the World, Vol. II*, New York: Oxford University Press.

MOERKERK, H. (1992) 'AIDS and development', in J. MANN, D. TARANTOLA and T. NETTER (Eds), *AIDS in the World, Vol. I*, Cambridge: Harvard University Press.

MOERKERK, H. (1996) 'Une Géographie politique du sida', *RAMSES 1996*, Yearbook of the Institut Français des Relations Internationales, Paris.

OVER, M. and PIOT, P. (1991) *HIV Infection and Sexually Transmitted Diseases, Disease Control Priorities in Developing Countries*, New York: Oxford University Press.

PRONK, J. (1990) *A World of Difference*, Netherlands Government Policy Paper on Foreign Assistance, Den Haag: Staatsdrukkerij.

PRONK, J. (1993) *Memorandum on AIDS and Development Cooperation*, Den Haag: Parliamentary Papers No. 21836/2.

PRONK, J. (1995) *Progress Report on Policy in the Area of AIDS and Development Cooperation*, Den Haag: Parliamentary Papers No. 21836/3.

WORLDBANK (1993) *Investing in Health, the World Development Report*, Washington: The Worldbank.

Part 3

Original Studies

Chapter 11

Sexual Behaviour in the Netherlands

Gertjan van Zessen and Theo Sandfort

When AIDS first appeared, Dutch health policy makers had little in-depth knowledge about the sexual behaviour of the population. Baseline information for the planning of well-targeted and effective HIV prevention was missing. At what age do young people start having sex? How many people have sex with someone of the same gender? How many men and women are involved in sex work, either as sex workers or clients? How many people are at risk of HIV transmission, and who and where are they? And what, as a consequence of these sexual interactions, is the likelihood of HIV spreading throughout the population as a whole?

Some knowledge about sexuality was already available, since sex surveys had been carried out in 1968 and 1981 before the emergence of AIDS (Kooy *et al.*, 1969, 1983). In accordance with the main concerns at the time, these studies focused on sexual norms and knowledge, rather than on the specific behavioural information which is needed to understand the risk of HIV transmission. In 1968, in the midst of the sexual revolution, the main concern fuelling research was a moral, not an epidemiological one.

Because of AIDS, new population level studies were needed to provide detailed information on sexual conduct, and to identify the knowledge base that future prevention campaigns should target. The Dutch government was one of the first in Europe to fund such work. In 1988, funding not only became available for an adult survey (Van Zessen and Sandfort, 1991) but also for one among young people (Vogels and Van der Vliet, 1990; see Chapter 13 in this book).

Although AIDS and HIV triggered this work, the focus of the adult population survey was sexuality in general, and not just risk-related behaviours. In order to promote healthy sexual behaviour, it is not sufficient to focus exclusively on sexual risk behaviour. An in-depth understanding of how sexuality in general is structured is a prerequisite for effective interventions. As a consequence, questions were included on topics such as masturbation and erotic fantasies, positive and negative (emotional) aspects of current sexual relationships, and sexual problems. In this chapter, we will describe the study itself and some of the key outcomes. The findings presented here reflect the situation in 1989, when data collection for this study took place. It is possible that the situation has changed since, as a consequence of AIDS or other factors. In fact, there are indications that condom use increased among people with mutiple partners. No study with a comparable design to the one presented here has been carried out since 1989.

Methods, Data Collection and Subjects

Conducting a large number of face-to-face interviews using a national sample is a costly matter, even in a relatively small country like the Netherlands with its 15 million population. A geographically well spread pool of trained interviewers is needed, and contacting households, getting individuals to participate and doing the actual interviews are time consuming. Balancing the desired minimum level of precision and the available funding, it was decided to draw two samples. The first one, which will be the focus of this chapter, is a random household sample, covering household members from 18 to 50 years old. This sample would provide information on sexual behaviour in the general population. An additional sample of unmarried people in larger towns and cities was expected to provide in-depth information on those people with sexual life-styles which would make them more vulnerable to the risk of HIV infection and STDs. This latter group was chosen to shed light on cognitions and behaviours related to preventive action.

For the general sample, 1001 men and women were interviewed in autumn 1989. A lower age limit of 18 years was set because younger people (aged 12 to 18 years old) were studied separately (Vogels and Van der Vliet, 1990). An upper age limit of 50 years was chosen because of the relatively low incidence of STDs in people of 50 and older. In the Netherlands, there are approximately 7 million inhabitants in the 18 to 50 year age range.

Sampling

The sampling frame consisted of addresses listed in the continuously updated national file of postal addresses. In a representative sample of communities, samples with sizes corresponding to the numbers of inhabitants were drawn and distributed among interviewers. These interviewers, 34 women and 7 men, were all experienced and had worked for the fieldwork agency for years.

Interviewers had to visit addresses in person, and in a fixed order. At addresses where a household was assumed to exist, they were to contact a member in person and to explain that they were involved in a government funded research project into 'Health and Relationships'. Only one person per household was selected. Interviewers were instructed to speak to a household member who fell within the specified age range. If more than one person qualified, the one who most recently had his or her birthday was selected. Selection by birthday introduces a random effect that prevents oversampling persons with an elevated probability of being found at home. Only to this person were the aims and contents of the interview explained.

If the person with the most recent birthday could not be contacted during the fieldwork, or refused to participate, he or she was marked as non-responder. Sometimes other members of the household volunteered to be interviewed, and on other occasions parents refused on behalf of their children, or husbands on behalf of their wife. All these were included as non-responses. Other exclusion criteria were serious language problems, serious illnesses or complete deafness.

Response

The overall response rate was 58.3 per cent, and appears to be somewhat lower than in other contemporary European sex surveys (Spira *et al.*, 1994; Field, Wadsworth and Bradshaw, 1994). The response should, however, be considered as relatively high in the Dutch context. Recent Dutch surveys in the realm of sex and relationships have all had higher refusal rates. Besides, willingness to participate in research studies has been known to decrease in the past 10 years.

Although one might expect that female interviewers would have more success in recruiting since they might be perceived as less threatening in relation to the subject of the survey, there were no differences in response rates between male and female interviewers. Instead, level of urbanization of the assigned interviewing area and individual skills, such as a good 'doorstep appearance', were the main factors responsible for the response rates.

To have a better understanding of the selective nature of non-response, we compared the sample with national census data. This showed that with respect to sociodemographic characteristics, the sample was fairly representative. This procedure is, however, insufficient to assess the representativeness of the non-responders' sexual lives. To assess this, people who initially refused to participate and those who could not be reached were approached again until 100 of them were found willing to complete an interview. To prevent people refusing on grounds of long duration, a shorter version of the original questionnaire was used, covering only the essential demographic and sexual variables.

While the non-response study was hampered by non-response itself, its outcomes were useful. Among men, no differences were found on any of the relevant 'sexual' variables (attitudes, past and present sexual conduct, protective behaviour, knowledge, and so on). The same was true for women who refused the initial interview. The only differences were found between the women in the main sample and the women who were initially not at home. The latter group reported a markedly more diverse sex life: they were less often married or cohabiting, reported more sexual partners, masturbated more often and had more sexual fantasies. They had more lifetime bisexual experience, and a higher proportion of them reported potentially risky behaviour with respect to HIV and STDs. We could conclude that women who are unlikely to be found at home, are more likely to lead more diverse, and potentially more risky sexual lives.

These findings led us to conclude that the male part of the sample seemed representative for the male population, but that findings somewhat underestimated sexual diversity, sexual activity and sexual risks in the female population. It is commonly accepted that the people who explicitly refuse to participate and not the people who cannot be reached introduce bias in the outcomes. The finding in our study that bias resulted from the women who were hard to reach indicates that the effects of non-response may be different in sex surveys.

The Questionnaire

Most interviews were conducted in respondents' homes. No partners, parents or others were allowed to be present – respondents who initially wanted their partner to be present were usually glad that (s)he was not when the questions on past and present sexual partners were asked. The interviewer used several booklets, following a flow chart to guide respondents through the structured, but heavily branched questionnaire. Most of the 550 questions were read aloud by the interviewer. The respondent provided answers using a set of printed cards with the appropriate answer categories. Some, more sensitive, questions on, for instance, sexual fantasies and masturbation, were asked in short self-completion questionnaires, which were filled out and placed in an envelope that was sealed at the end of the interview. Another reason for using a variety of approaches was to prevent the respondent from becoming bored.

In order to enhance the validity of the data, interviewers were trained in advance for three days, not only on working with the questionnaire but also on discussing sexuality in general, including their own sexual attitudes. Interviewers had to understand the purpose of the study, and feel at ease with the task they had to perform and the responses that might be given by respondents. In the training, detailed information was provided about AIDS and STDs, homosexuality, prostitution, traumatic sexual experiences like incest and (childhood or adult) abuse, sexual variation and life-styles, and on how to react when 'difficult' topics arose during the interview. How to handle sexual remarks or sexual overtures by respondents, and the interviewers' own emotions during interviewing were also discussed. Interviewers were provided with referral guidelines for respondents in need of professional help. The interviewers could also rely on professional counselling for themselves, should the need for this arise. Test interviews, and close monitoring and group exchanges of experiences during fieldwork were part of the process of quality control.

Interviews were structured in the sense that the intrusiveness of the topics gradually increased. After questioning on less sensitive topics such as daily worries, impulsiveness and attitudes, early sexual experiences with both genders (first love, first petting, first intercourse) were discussed. Then, sexual behaviour in the past year was asked about in detail, starting with steady relationships, whether one had sex with others besides the steady partner, and/or 'less steady' or casual partners in the last twelve months. Care was taken to avoid giving the impression that heterosexuality, long-term relationships or marriage were the 'proper' sexual contexts. Use of the labels homo-, bi- or heterosexuality was avoided as much as possible, and in questioning different types of partners or behaviours, we consistently asked whether this was with a man or a woman.

To avoid too general and imprecise answers, sexual practices, emotions, contraceptives and the like were not asked about globally, but were addressed in the context of specific relations or contacts. When a respondent reported having had sex in the preceding year with a steady partner, with casual partners, with someone abroad, and sex for money, (s)he was presented with the maximum number of six separate lists of questions, and asked to discuss these partners specifically. This method was chosen for two reasons. First, in order to make sexual network analyses possible we needed data on recent, specific partners. These data-hungry analyses require information on the demographic characteristics of partners, such as age, gender, class, as well as on HIV risk factors connected to recent partners such as same-sex experiences and injecting drug use. In relation to recent sex partners, data on over 30 of these characteristics were obtained.The second reason has to do with data validity. We believe that risk perception and protective behaviour are context specific and dependent, which makes general answers on these topics misleading. When people are asked to summarize several situations into one answer, for instance on whether they used condoms consistently, they tend to overestimate their safe behaviour, as becomes clear in qualitative interviewing on this topic (Van Zessen, 1995).

Following the detailed description of recent partnerships, the sexual life span was explored in a more global way. We asked questions about where and how people tried to find potential sexual partners (also relevant from a sexual network perspective), about the emotional evaluation of sex and relationships, sexual problems and dysfunctions, masturbation and sexual fantasies, and the extent to which they searched for sexual stimuli (pornography, videos, sex lines and so on). Finally, there was a large set of questions on AIDS and STDs, covering knowledge and beliefs, attitudes, risk perceptions, past and current intentions and protective behaviours. AIDS-related topics were discussed at the end of the interview since we assumed that an awareness of AIDS might have promoted socially desirable answers about sexual (risk) behaviour. The interview concluded with a self-administered evaluation of the questions and the interviewer.

Special attention was paid to the wording of the questions about sexuality.

Vernacular phrases and medical jargon were avoided. All key variables, like sexual partner and intercourse, were explained in simple, direct language, for example 'vaginal intercourse, means penis in vagina'. In comparison with the problems that Wellings *et al.* (1989) reported encountering in finding unambiguous formulations for the British general population sexual behaviour survey (Johnson *et al.*, 1994), the Dutch language appears to offer a sexual vocabulary that makes it easy to interview about sex. Presumably, greater public openness on sexual matters will have been helpful here as well. Interviewers were instructed to stick to the original phrasing of the questions. Respondents were free to use their own language and terms.

A typical interview lasted 75 to 90 minutes. There was virtually no refusal to answer specific questions or parts of the interview, and practically all post-interview evaluations were (very) positive. Very often, respondents confided afterwards to the interviewer that they had never before been so frank about their sexuality, not even with their husbands or wives, and that they had enjoyed talking about it.

First Intercourse

Respondents aged 42–50, born between 1939 and 1947, had their first sexual intercourse at a mean age of 20.4 years. The youngest respondents, 18–25 years old, born between 1964 and 1971, report a mean age of 17.2. On average, first intercourse took place six years after they had fallen in love for the first time and three years after they had sex for the first time. By the age of 15, 15 per cent of the men and 9 per cent of the women had experienced their first sexual intercourse. These percentages rose to 71 and 80 per cent respectively at the age of 20, and to 90 and 95 per cent at the age of 25.

Younger age cohorts reported having had first sexual intercourse at significantly younger ages than older age cohorts. The age at first intercourse seems to go down systematically. This trend is shown in Figure 11.1, where a later year of birth clearly coincides with an earlier median age of sexual experience. The time interval between the first kiss and first intercourse does not seem to change over the years. Recent research among young people showed that the decrease in age at first intercourse as well as in that of other sexual techniques, can even be observed in as short as a five-year period (Brugman *et al.*, 1995; Chapter 13 in this book). There is no indication that the emergence of AIDS has stopped or reversed this decrease.

The decrease in age at first intercourse can be observed all over Europe (Bozon and Kontula, forthcoming) and is probably a result of two processes. Presumably as a result of improved nutrition, menarche and puberty are known to start at an increasingly younger age (Wyshak and Frisch, 1982; Van der Vliet, 1992). There also seems to be an increased societal tolerance towards young people having sex and also an ever increasing visibility of sex.

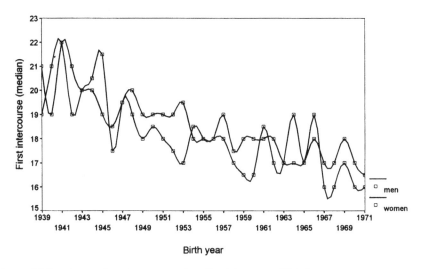

Figure 11.1 Age at first intercourse (median) by year of birth.

As young people start earlier in their sexual careers, this leads to an increase in sexual activity in the population.

Current Sexual Experience

One in eight adults reported having had no sexual partner in the 12 months preceding the interview (Table 11.1). In the study, a partner qualified as a 'sexual partner' when there had been intercourse, oral sex or manual stimulation of the genitals. Mutual masturbation was addressed because we did not want to miss those occasions when respondents purposely abstained from penetrative sex in order to prevent STDs, HIV or pregnancy.

The vast majority of respondents reported sexual partners of the opposite sex only. Of the men, 5.5 per cent reported having had sex with men or with both men and women in the past year. For women this was less than 1 per cent. When people were asked to indicate their sexual preference on a seven-point scale, the results match their actual behaviours: 4.0 per cent of the men and 0.9 per cent of the women described their erotic preference in the range between bisexual to exclusively homosexual. The comparatively low prevalence of same-sex behaviour among women is remarkable, and may partly be attributed to selective sampling. Other studies, however, did also find substantial gender differences in this respect (Kinsey *et al.*, 1953; Sandfort, forthcoming).

In a lifetime perspective, the various percentages are somewhat higher. Of all men and women, respectively 12.8 per cent and 10.2 per cent report having experienced sexual attraction to someone of the same gender at least

Table 11.1 *Sexual behaviour in past 12 months (%)*

	Men	Women
Heterosexual only	81.7	88.4
Homosexual only	3.6	0.3
Partners of both gender	1.9	0.5
No sexual partners	12.8	10.7
N	421	580

once; 11.9 per cent of the men and 4.3 per cent of the women reported having had sex (mutual masturbation or penetrative sex) with a same-sex partner. Data show that nearly all men who ever felt attracted to a boy or man had also experimented with sex, whereas for women experiencing same-sex attraction is in most instances not associated with actual experience. These latter percentages offer a striking contrast with earlier findings by Kinsey *et al.* (1948, 1953), who reported that 37 per cent of men and 19 per cent of women had ever had same-sex activity. If these proportions have indeed gone down, this might be a consequence of the stronger visibility of homosexuality. This stronger visibility of socially still unaccepted behaviour may also have increased awareness of its taboo character. When homosexual behaviour is seen as something practised by gays and lesbians, the barriers to 'straight' people engaging in sex with someone of the same gender may become higher (Sandfort, 1998).

At the time people were interviewed, three-quarters of the sample were involved in a steady relationship, 'steady' being defined as being involved with another person for at least a year. Twelve per cent had not had sex with someone else in the previous year; the majority of these people desired to be in a steady relationship. The remainder, approximately 13 per cent, reported having had more than one sexual partner or were involved in a relationship which had lasted shorter than 12 months (the 'non-steady relationships').

Somewhat to our surprise, 'one night stands' were quite rare, even among young adults. In our category of 'non-steady relationships', the mean frequency of sexual encounters with a partner was 25 times; only 12 per cent of these people reported partners with whom they had sex only once or twice. One 'protective' feature of these occasional contacts was that the risk of STD or HIV transmission was generally low, not because of condom use, but because penetrative intercourse often did not take place. It is important to note that this could not have been detected if the word 'intercourse' had been used as a criterion for sexual partnership. As sex happened more often with one partner, it was more likely that intercourse was practised and condom use became less likely.

From a risk perspective, long-term relationships are relevant only when third partners are involved. In sharp contrast to the alarming 'finding' that, for instance, 7 out of 10 married women have extramarital affairs (Hite, 1987), we found only small percentages of people who said that they (or their partners) also had sex with others. In the previous year, 6.4 per cent of men and 2.8 per cent of women reported one or more partners outside their steady, heterosexual relationship. Comparisons with earlier studies indicate that the prevalence of sex outside a steady relationship has decreased somewhat since 1981. In this study, men were three times as likely as women not to inform their partner about these contacts. More disturbing is the fact that in 75 per cent of the cases, the men had unprotected intercourse with both the third party and the, usually unaware, regular partner.

Of all heterosexual men, 2.8 per cent had paid for sex in the previous year. None of the women had done so. There was, however, one woman in the sample who reported exchanging sex for money. Lifetime data indicate that 13.5 per cent of all men have paid for sex at least once, and, again, none of the women. One per cent of both genders reported having been paid for sex; for men as well as for women, this was always by another man.

As in other Dutch studies on sex work, female sex workers were among the most regular condom users in the heterosexual population. In consequence, the potential contribution of female sex work to HIV transmission must be considered small (De Graaf *et al.*, 1992).

Number of Partners

Respondents were questioned in detail about the number of male and female partners they had had during their sexual career. The number of (new) partners in a given time period is an independent risk factor for HIV transmission. Given the relatively low prevalence of HIV in the Dutch population, this factor is probably more important than the frequency of sexual encounters per partner (Padian, Schiboski and Hitchcock, 1991).

Table 11.2 shows the mean number of partners in the preceding year, the preceding five years and lifetime. The categories in the rows are based on the sexual behaviour in the preceding year, as presented in Table 11.1. Two findings stand out: the reported numbers of partners vary strongly with gender and with sexual preference. Within each category, heterosexual men report (far) more partners than heterosexual women. The disparity between men and women is even greater for homosexual men. Women who had sex in the preceding year with both men and women, report a higher number of partners than women who had sex exclusively with either men or women. Since the distribution is very skewed and means are heavily influenced by a small percentage of respondents reporting very high numbers of partners, medians are a useful, though less spectacular way of presenting these data. Lifetime medians for heterosexual men and women are four and two respectively. It is important to stress that sample size for people with homosexual experience is small, especially in the case of women.

Table 11.2   *Number of sexual partners in three periods, by sexual behaviour in past 12 months (means)*

	12 months	5 years	Lifetime	N
Heterosexual				
Men	1.3	2.8	11.1	344
Women	1.1	1.4	3.9	512
Homosexual				
Men	9.1	48.6	270.3	15
Women	1.0	2.5	5.5	2
Bisexual				
Men	5.5	13.0	25.1	8
Women	2.3	3.3	14.0	3
No sex				
Men	0.0	0.5	1.7	54
Women	0.0	0.6	3.6	62

Table 11.3   *Number of sexual partners of those currently behaving or feeling heterosexual (%)*

	12 months		5 years		Lifetime	
	Men	Women	Men	Women	Men	Women
0	13	11	9	7	7	4
1	73	83	58	77	17	36
2–5	12	6	24	15	38	46
6–10	2	0.2	5	1	16	9
11+	–	–	4	0.4	22	5
N	398	584	398	584	398	584

Table 11.3 gives the distribution of partners for heterosexual men and women. The reporting difference between the genders is rather small in one year but substantial over life. Invariably in studies like these, men report far more partners than women. In this particular survey, part of the difference is due to sampling error: sexually active women are less well represented in this sample. Sampling error cannot, however, account for the gap completely: nearly 60 per cent of the total number of female partners reported by the males is unexplained. Various explanations for this gap have been formulated, including overreporting by men and underreporting by women, presumably related to the gender differences in meanings associated with sex and sexual reputations. It is also possible that men count every woman with whom

something slightly erotic happened as a sexual partner, whereas women seem to take their emotional evaluation of the situation more into account. Men also tend to have more homosexual experiences, usually during adolescence. Finally, there are strong indications in many European surveys that paid sex explains part of the gender gap (Leridon, Hubert and Van Zessen, forthcoming).

Since the number of partners has never been addressed in previous sex surveys in the Netherlands, it is impossible to identify any trends. Data on the sex life of senior citizens are completely lacking, but as people tend to get older in physically better shape, and as cultural norms condemning sex for older people diminish, it is likely that new cohorts of seniors will remain sexually active longer than their predecessors. A recent US survey including older people confirms this hypothesis (Janus and Janus, 1993).

When we combine these assumptions, it seems likely that overall levels of sexual activity in the population are slowly increasing. A consequence of this is that the infrastructure for STDs is slowly growing in density, giving STDs more chance to spread. At present, there is no indication that the emergence of AIDS has influenced this development.

Risks and Protection

Using a card sort test which covered 18 daily worries, we found that worries about HIV and STDs turned out to be the least prevalent, and worries about the environment most. This indicates that AIDS, at least in 1989, was not felt as an urgent problem, either by the person him- or herself, or by society at large. Data from other sources indicate that people's concern about AIDS has been relatively constant since 1988 (NSS Research and Consultancy, 1997).

Traditionally, pregnancy is the risk most closely related to sex, and we can see this priority reflected in the preventive actions that people take. Of the respondents with regular, heterosexual relationships, 84 per cent used some contraceptive method consistently – the majority of the remaining 16 per cent was presumably either pregnant or trying to become so. Of the people who used some kind of contraceptive, the pill and sterilization were most often mentioned, by 39 and 23 per cent respectively. Condoms were used by 18 per cent of people. Further questioning revealed that contraception was the foremost reason in 98.5 per cent of the cases where condoms were used. By those people who used condoms, 69 per cent used them inconsistently. Effective, consistent condom use was found in only 6 per cent of steady relationships.

Among respondents with short-term or casual relationships, consistent condom use was somewhat higher: 15 per cent used condoms every time they had vaginal or anal intercourse. Inconsistent condom use was reported by 31 per cent of people in short-term or casual relationships. Fifty-three per cent of these people had never used a condom in the previous year. In the whole sample, 28 per cent of the respondents said that they had never used a condom in their life. Of the whole sample, only 2 per cent claimed that they used condoms primarily to prevent HIV infection.

People did not seem to be particularly worried about HIV, and they also did not seem to use condoms very often. Since this might be caused by their current situation, we asked whether they would take protective action should they have sex with a new partner. Those who could imagine that this would happen were completely, or reasonably, sure that they would protect themselves against HIV. When asked how difficult this would be, 81 per cent foresaw no problems, 16 per cent expected minor problems and only 3 per cent feared it would be quite difficult to put the intention into practice.

A likely interpretation of these findings is that the general awareness of and basic knowledge about AIDS had been communicated effectively by the media campaigns that had been running for two years at the time of data collection. But at the same time, AIDS was not seen as a personal problem by the vast majority of this sample. Pregnancy was the risk that they felt should be avoided, and this was done effectively. HIV was a theoretical risk, and a theoretical reaction to a hypothetical situation was appropriate: use a condom or abstain from intercourse. Data on actual behaviour, however, show that the acknowledged necessity to use condoms and the high levels of personal efficacy associated with the intention to use them, only result in effective practice for a few people. This is even the case among people who frequently change partners and for whom AIDS and STDs are more than theoretical risks.

Data from another study show that for the period 1987 to 1993, the number of people who took preventive measures against HIV increased significantly among the young and the non-monogamous. Also, and especially in these groups, both actual and intended condom use had increased considerably (De Vroome *et al.*, 1994).

Potential Risk Behaviour

In order to estimate the levels of HIV-related risk, we considered respondents' sexual behaviour in the preceding year. Those who had had no sexual contacts, or those people involved in a regular, monogamous relationship were assigned a risk factor of zero. These people, constituting 84 per cent of the total sample, are very unlikely to be at risk of HIV. Some, but not many, of the people with casual and/or short-term relationships protected themselves consistently with condoms and/or by refraining from intercourse. These people, constituting 4 per cent of the total sample, also have low risk.

Twelve per cent of the total sample, according to their own reports, did run the potential risk of being infected in the preceding year, men more often then women (respectively 15 and 10 per cent), and younger people more often than older people. This risk was most often a consequence of the individual having had unprotected intercourse with one or more new partners. Some people, predominantly women, ran a risk because they had unprotected vaginal intercourse with a steady partner, who had had sexual contact with other people. This 12 per cent corresponds to approximately one million of the 18- to 50-year-old adults in the Dutch population. Because of the natural in- and outflow on the sexual partner market, the subpopulation at potential risk is constantly changing. Over a five-year period, the subpopulation at risk is estimated to be 25 per cent, a substantial part of the general population.

Some population subgroups were more likely to have run a risk than others. Risk behaviour occurs more frequently among people who do not consider themselves as exclusively heterosexual, people with higher levels of education, and people who live in urban areas. Risk is also more common among people who are not religiously involved and those who have politically a progressive instead of a conservative orientation.

Having been at risk and being aware of it, do not necessarily coincide. More than half of the people who have been at risk for HIV transmission declared that no risk was attached to their recent sex life. Most factors which were correlated with having been at risk also correlate with awareness of that risk. From those people who have been at risk, those who do not consider themselves to be exclusively heterosexual more often acknowledged their risk than those who do. Acknowledgement of risk was also more frequent among people with a higher level of education and those who were not religiously involved. Realistic acknowledgement of one's risk is also related to more accurate knowledge about AIDS and a higher awareness of AIDS. There was a negative relationship between playing down the overall risk of HIV and acknowledging that one actually had been at risk oneself (Sandfort and Van Zessen, 1992).

Sexual Networks

The data collected on sexual relationships enabled us to conduct sexual net- work analyses (Van Zessen and Jager, 1994). Because an anonymous, national survey does not permit the identification of real sexual networks, these have had to be modelled on the basis of the empirical information about the way sexual partners choose one another. Without going into the specifics of this method, the main conclusions are worth describing here.

Repeated analyses show that the chance of substantial sexual networks forming, wherein a large number of people are sexually closely connected, are extremely small. The main reason for this is the absence of frequent partner change; there is simply not enough sexual activity in the general population to form risky chains of sexual relations, as was already suggested by the findings shown in Table 11.2. Among gay men on the other hand, where there is a high frequency of partner change, such networks can come into being. These conditions are not found in the heterosexual population. The setting where heterosexual partner change is most frequent, sex for payment, is also, largely due to its professional structure, the setting where condom use is frequent and, usually, consistent.

Network analyses can help to focus prevention strategies. The aim of prevention should be to disrupt as many sexual chains between and within sexual networks as possible, in order to prevent HIV transmission. The most efficient way of doing this is to encourage the few people who have high numbers of partners to use condoms or refrain from intercourse. These people function as nodes connecting various chains of sexual relations with one another. Should the 1 per cent of people with the highest number of partners use condoms consistently, the sexual infrastructure of a population no longer consists of larger network structures but contains merely small fragments. A key recommendation from our network analyses has therefore been to give additional preventive attention to frequent partner changers.

On the basis of epidemiological findings and data on sexual conduct, it seems that HIV will not spread much beyond known risk populations in the future. This does not mean that heterosexual HIV transmission will not occur, but that such transmission will be rare and unpredictable – and therefore difficult to control. Educating the general population about the risks of HIV and AIDS will remain necessary, but as the contours of the epidemic become increasingly clearer, the task of promoting preventive behaviour will become more difficult.

The Netherlands in European Perspective

From a European perspective, the Netherlands has the image of being a sexually permissive society. To a certain extent our data lend support to this idea. Comparatively, values about sexuality and relationships are fairly permissive (Ester, Halman and de Moor, 1994), and the distance between masculine and feminine sex roles is small (Hofstede, 1992). One might wonder whether this higher level of permissiveness is also reflected in sexual behaviour. A comparison of the data presented here with findings of recent sex surveys carried out in other European countries, made possible by the EC Concerted Action on 'Sexual behaviour and risks of HIV infection' (Hubert, Bajos and Sandfort, forthcoming), shows that this is only partly the case.

Although there is a general trend across Europe towards sexual initiation at an earlier age, Dutch men and women start their sexual careers relatively late. This can be observed among older as well as younger age cohorts. Remarkable is the fact that the difference in median age between Dutch men and women in all age cohorts is relatively small. This is the same in Denmark, Switzerland and former West Germany, but different in France, Greece, Portugal and the United Kingdom, where men start earlier than women. In the latter countries, the difference between men and women has become smaller in younger age cohorts as well. As in other countries, early sexual initiation is an indicator of a more active sexual life in later life.

Compared to other countries, Dutch people in steady relationships have sex the least often, rather like in Belgium. The frequency of sexual interaction goes down with increasing age and with increasing length of relationships. Unlike in most other countries, where men report higher frequencies of sexual interaction than women, Dutch women report having sexual relations more frequently. Regarding specific sexual practices, oral sex seems to be practised more frequently, but with younger people doing so more frequently than older people. Anal sex seems to be practised by relatively few people in the Netherlands.

The number of people with lifetime homosexual experience is high compared to other countries. For men, this also applies to homosexual experience in the preceding year. This might be a consequence of a more open climate towards homosexuality, which makes it easier to report homosexual experiences, and which may also facilitate homosexual experiences (Sandfort, forthcoming). Demographic correlates of homosexual experiences are more or less the same in different European countries. As in other countries, Dutch people with lifetime homosexual experiences less often are, or have been, married. However, when one looks at Dutch men and women who report having had homosexual experience in the preceding year, the proportion who are or have been married is small compared to the same people in other countries. This may also be a reflection of a climate which is more accepting of homosexual behaviour.

The number of lifetime sexual partners is relatively high for Dutch people, compared to people in Finland, France, the United Kingdom, Norway and Switzerland. This may partly be caused by a wider definition of what counts as a sexual partner. With respect to number of sexual partners in the preceding year, Dutch men and women have an average score. As in other countries, people who live in urban areas report having had more partners.

In conclusion, Dutch society is a permissive but not a promiscuous society. Never before in history has there been so much opportunity to live a nonconformist sexual lifestyle openly, yet very few people choose to do so. The trend, among young people and presumably among adults as well, is an increase in the number of lifetime partners. Still, a steady, monogamous relationship is preferred by most people. An HIV epidemic in the general population, feared for in the mid-1980s when we started preparing this study, has never occured in the Netherlands – not so much because of effective protection, but because sexual pathways and sexual bridges are so scarce.

Acknowledgement

The 'Sexuality in the Netherlands' (1991) study was conducted by the Netherlands Institute for Social Sexological Research (NISSO) and the Department of Gay and Lesbian Studies of Utrecht University, under auspices of the Programme Coordinating Committee for AIDS Research (PccAo). It was funded by the Ministry of Welfare, Health and Culture and the Dutch Society for Preventive Medicine.

References

Bozon, M. and Kontula, O. (forthcoming) 'Sexual initiation and gender in Europe: a cross-cultural analysis of trends in the 20th century', in M.C. Hubert, N. Bajos and Th.G.M. Sandfort (Eds), *Sexual Behaviour and HIV/AIDS in Europe*, London: UCL Press.

Brugman, E., Goedhart, H., Vogels, T. and Van Zessen, G. (1995) *Jeugd en Seks 95. (Youth and Sex 95)*, Utrecht: SWP.

Ester, P., Halman, L. and de Moor, R. (Eds) (1994) *The Individualizing Society. Value Change in Europe and North America*, Tilburg: Tilburg University Press.

Field, J., Wadsworth, J. and Bradshaw, S. (1994) 'Survey methods and sample characteristics', in A.M. Johnson, J. Wadsworth, K. Wellings and J. Field (Eds), *Sexual Attitudes and Lifestyles*, Oxford: Blackwell.

De Graaf, R., Vanwesenbeeck, I., Straver, C.J., Visser, J.H. and Van Zessen, G. (1992). 'Condom use and sexual behaviour in heterosexual prostitution in the Netherlands', *AIDS*, **6**, pp. 1223–6.

Hite, S. (1987) *Women and Love: A Cultural Revolution in Progress*, New York: Knopf.

Hofstede, G. (1992) *Cultures and Organizations, Software of the Mind*, London: McGraw-Hill.

Hubert, M.C., Bajos, N. and Sandfort, Th.G.M. (Eds) (forthcoming) *Sexual Behaviour and HIV/AIDS in Europe*, London: UCL Press.

Janus, S.S. and Janus, C.L. (1993) *The Janus Report on Sexual Behavior*, New York: Wiley.

Johnson, A.M., Wadsworth, J., Wellings, K. and Field, J. (Eds) (1994) *Sexual Attitudes and Lifestyles*, Oxford: Blackwell.

Kinsey, A.C., Pomeroy, W.P. and Martin, C.E. (1948) *Sexual Behavior in the Human Male*, Philadelphia: W.B. Saunders.

Kinsey, A.C., Pomeroy, W.P., Martin, C.E. and Gebhard, P.H. (1953) *Sexual Behavior in the Human Female*, Philadelphia: W.B. Saunders.

Kooy, G.A. *et al.* (1969) *Sex in Nederland (Sex in the Netherlands)*, Utrecht: Spectrum.

Kooy, G.A. *et al.* (1983) *Sex in Nederland 2 (Sex in the Netherlands 2)*, Utrecht: Spectrum.

Leridon, H., Hubert, M. and Van Zessen, G. (forthcoming) 'Numbers of partners: variations across Europe', in M.C. Hubert, N. Bajos and Th.G.M. Sandfort (Eds), *Sexual Behaviour and HIV/AIDS in Europe*, London: UCL Press.

NSS Research & Consultancy (1997) *Multi dimensionele indicatoren voor betrokkenheid bij maatschappelijke problemen*, Den Haag.

PADIAN, N.S., SHIBOSKI, S.C. and HITCHCOCK, P.J. (1991) 'Risk factors for acquisition of sexually transmitted diseases and development of complications', in J.N. WASSERHEIT, S.O. ARAL, K.K. HOLMES and P.J. HITCHCOCK (Eds), *Research Issues in Human Behavior and Sexually Transmitted Diseases in the AIDS Era*, Washington DC: American Society for Microbiology.

SANDFORT, TH.G.M. (1998) 'Homosexual and bisexual behaviour in European countries', in M.C. HUBERT, N. BAJOS and TH.G.M. SANDFORT (Eds), *Sexual Behaviour and HIV/AIDS in Europe*, London: UCL Press.

SANDFORT, TH.G.M. and VAN ZESSEN, G. (1992) 'Denial as a barrier for HIV prevention within the general population', *Journal of Psychology and Human Sexuality*, **5**, pp. 69–87.

SPIRA, A., BAJOS, N. and the ASCF GROUP (1994) *Sexual Behaviour and AIDS*, Aldershot: Avebury.

VAN DER VLIET, R. (1992) 'Love without ties: a new phase in the sexual life course', in W. MEEUS, M. DE GOEDE and W. KOX (Eds), *Adolescence, Careers, and Cultures*, Berlin/New York: Walter de Gruyter.

VOGELS, T. and VAN DER VLIET, R. (1990) *Jeugd en Seks (Youth and Sex)*, Den Haag: SDU.

DE VROOME, E.M.M., PAALMAN, M.E.M., DINGELSTAD, A.A.M., KOLKER, L. and SANDFORT, TH.G.M. (1994) 'Increase in safe sex among the young and nonmonogamous: knowledge, attitudes and behavior regarding safe sex and condom use in the Netherlands from 1987 to 1993', *Patient Education and Counseling*, **24**, pp. 279–88.

WELLINGS, K., FIELD, J., JOHNSON, A., WADSWORTH, J. and BRADSHAW, S. (1989) *Notes on the Design and Construction of a National Survey of Sexual Attitudes and Lifestyles*, London, internal report.

WYSHAK, G. and FRISCH R.E. (1982) 'Evidence for a secular trend in age of menarche', *The New England Journal of Medicine*, **306**, pp. 1033–5.

VAN ZESSEN, G. (1995) *Wisselend Contact (Changing contact)*, Leiden: DSWO Press.

VAN ZESSEN, G. and J.C. JAGER (Eds) (1994) *Analyse van Seksuele Netwerken (Analysis of sexual networks)*, Bilthoven: RIVM, rapport 431502004.

VAN ZESSEN, G. and SANDFORT, TH.G.M. (1991) *Seksualiteit in Nederland. Seksueel Gedrag, Risico en Preventie van AIDS (Sexuality in the Netherlands. Sexual Conduct, Risk and the Prevention of AIDS)*, Lisse: Swets & Zeitlinger.

Chapter 12

Determinants of Safe Sex among Adult Heterosexuals: Towards Theory-Based Interventions

Arnold Bakker, Bram Buunk, Regina van den Eijnden and Frans Siero

Recent epidemiological studies from the United Kingdom and from the United States suggest that the heterosexual population may increasingly be at risk for infection with the human immunodeficiency virus (HIV) (Clumeck *et al.*, 1989; Karon *et al.*, 1992). A similar trend has been observed in the Netherlands, although the cumulative number of reported cases of AIDS involving heterosexuals is still small in both a relative and an absolute sense. As of April 1995, this number was 357, that is 10.2 per cent of the total number of 3488 people with AIDS. However, it must be noted that the estimated incidence of new infections with sexually transmitted diseases (STDs) other than AIDS is 110000 a year, and that the majority of these infections are due to unprotected sexual activities between people with a heterosexual orientation (Stichting SOA-BESTRIJDING, 1995). Despite the clear success of the public campaigns on AIDS in the Netherlands (De Vroome *et al.*, 1995; De Vroome *et al.*, 1994), it has been consistently shown that half of those who engage in a new heterosexual relationship never use a condom when they have sexual intercourse. Moreover, 5 per cent of those with a regular partner have engaged in sex outside their relationship in the previous year, and about half of these did not use a condom when having sexual intercourse with someone other than their steady partner (Bakker, 1995a; Van Zessen and Sandfort, 1991). Because most individuals do not inform their regular partner about their sexual activities outside their relationship, these individuals put not only themselves, but also their partner at risk for HIV infection (Buunk and Bakker, 1997; Buunk and Bakker, in press).

Because the virus that causes AIDS is transmitted primarily through unprotected sexual contact, using condoms, especially with new partners, is an effective way of preventing such transmission. Thus, in order to prevent the transmission of HIV and other STDs among heterosexuals, it is important to identify the determinants of condom use that are sensitive to intervention. This chapter offers an overview of Dutch research that has examined the social psychological determinants of safe sex among adult heterosexuals. It also describes several experiments in which theory-based interventions (formalized as persuasive communications in flyers and brochures) were used to change these determinants in order to promote safe sex.

Determinants of Safe Sex among Adult Heterosexuals

In research on the determinants of safe sex among adult heterosexuals, it is common to use social psychological models of health behaviour, such as the health belief model, protection motivation theory, the theory of reasoned action, and the theory of planned behaviour (see Stroebe and Stroebe, 1995, for an overview). Although these models emphasize different determinants of behaviour, when applied to safe sex, they focus particularly on factors such as beliefs about safe sex, attitudes towards this behaviour, barriers towards implementing safe sex, and perceived social norms towards engaging in this behaviour. The goal of research based on these approaches is to identify those factors that are independent and important predictors of the intention to practise safe sex. On the basis of such research, prevention programmes can be developed aimed at changing the most relevant variables related to safe sex intentions.

Despite the widespread use of social psychological models in research and prevention, some researchers have criticized these models as being too 'individualistic' and 'rationalistic' (Kippax and Crawford, 1993; Rademakers *et al.*, 1992; Van Zessen, 1995). These researchers claim that there is too much reliance on cognitive factors to explain behaviour and too little on emotional and social factors. In their view, quantitative models insufficiently reflect the social and emotional nature of sexuality and are not informative about the barriers (for example uncooperative partners, overwhelming sexual arousal) that may be encountered when people want to act on their intentions. Additionally, Gold (1993) has claimed that research on the predictors of safe sex has examined only those cognitions that are present in respondents' minds at the time they are answering the researcher's questions ('off-line cognitions'), rather than those that are present during actual sexual encounters ('on-line cognitions'). Gold argues that there may be considerable differences between on-line and off-line AIDS-related cognitions, and he provides some preliminary evidence for his proposition. He suggests, for example, that people may engage in unsafe sex instead of safe sex because they are emotionally blackmailed, too intoxicated to prevent it from happening, or because perceptible cues evoke self-justifications (for example 'This guy looks so healthy, he can't possibly be infected'). It is quite conceivable that these on-line cognitions are activated in actual sexual encounters, and that these cognitions will never be identified by survey or experimental research. Indeed, the prevalence of on-line cognitions during 'the act' may partly explain why intentions often do not account for very much of the variance in behaviour.

Although it is true that in a concrete sexual interaction, behaviour may be determined by factors other than those proposed in the common social psychological models, in a number of ways criticisms of these models do not seem very relevant. First, these models do not focus only on cognitive factors, and can easily incorporate emotional and social factors. For instance, Richard, Van der Pligt and De Vries (1995, in press) have shown that anticipated regret is an important predictor of actual condom use, and we have also included the perceived norm of future partners in our research (Bakker, 1995a). Other factors suggested by critics of existing models can also be taken into account in research designs. Second, it is difficult to study 'in vivo' what happens when individuals do not use condoms in a sexual interaction, and researchers generally have to rely on self-reports. Finally, and most importantly, in order to develop adequate interventions, researchers must study the most important determinants of safe sex, assuming that behaviour change can be achieved by changing such determinants (compare Fishbein and Middlestadt, 1989). Those criticizing current models usually offer no suggestions for interventions based on the determinants they find important, and have rarely developed and evaluated such interventions. We have focused on identifying determinants of unsafe sex, and on modifying this behaviour through persuasive communication. Such an approach does not ignore social and emotional factors, but assumes indeed that people at least take notice of safe sex messages, which implies that the 'cognitive route' has to be travelled in order to change behaviour.

In one of the first attempts to identify the modifiable social psychological factors that underlie condom use among adult heterosexuals that might be targeted in subsequent intervention research, we conducted two studies, the first involving 711 males and females (mean age 32) (Buunk *et al.*, in press), the second involving 218 young adults (mean age 21) (Bakker, 1995a). Our recruitment procedures (for example announcements on Dutch television and advertisements in *Playboy* magazine) ensured that both samples were likely to include a substantial number of individuals who had engaged in unprotected sex with new partners. For example, members of the sample in our first study reported an average of 6 opposite-sex partners in the previous five years. In many of these contacts unprotected vaginal intercourse had occurred. The fact that 16 per cent of this sample reported having had an STD at least once in their lives indicated that participants had put themselves at risk for HIV infection.

To employ variables and concomitant operationalizations that are optimally relevant for the population and behaviour under consideration, both studies used an eclectic approach, and drew from the health belief model, protection motivation theory, and the theory of anticipated regret. Moreover, various types of social norms were examined, and the role of self-efficacy was assessed. The results showed that in both studies about 50 per cent of the variance in the intention to use condoms with new sexual partners could be predicted on the basis of a limited number of predictors, namely perceived risk, self-efficacy, anticipated regret, and social norms. Moreover, a one-year follow-up among the young adults indicated that the intention to use condoms was positively related to actual condom use (for women: r = .38; and for men: r = .57; p's < .01).

Because support for each of the above-mentioned predictors of condom use has been found consistently in other Dutch research (Paulussen *et al.*, 1989; Richard, Van der Pligt and De Vries, 1995; Schaalma, Kok and Peters, 1993), we will first discuss the theoretical basis of each of these variables, and their empirical relation to HIV preventive behaviour. Next, we will present data on the 'false consensus' phenomenon, showing that individuals tend to project their unsafe sexual behaviour onto others. Finally, we will discuss a number of studies examining interventions aimed at changing behavioural intentions as related to unsafe sex by aiming at the various behavioural determinants.

Perceived Risk

In most theories of health behaviour, the perceived risk of a specific negative event is assumed to be the primary motivation for the avoidance of risky behaviour and for the initiation of preventive action (Weinstein, 1993). However, although there is fairly compelling evidence that risk perceptions motivate a wide variety of precautionary and preventive actions, including inoculation against influenza, blood-pressure screening and compliance with an insulin-dependent diabetic regimen (Harrison, Mullen and Green, 1992), there is little empirical support for the hypothesis that perceptions of the risk of acquiring HIV motivate precautionary sexual behaviour. In a review of the evidence for the correlation between perceived vulnerability to HIV infection and HIV preventive behaviour, Gerrard *et al.* (1993) concluded that in cross-sectional as well as prospective studies, sometimes negative, sometimes zero, and sometimes positive correlations are found between perceived risk of contracting HIV and HIV preventive behaviour.

How can HIV preventive behaviour be unrelated to risk perceptions? One of the reasons for the conflicting results in the literature may be that usually what we will refer to as *absolute risk* has been assesssed, that is the plain perceived risk of HIV infection. In these studies, respondents are typically asked how large they think their chances are of becoming infected with HIV. It seems obvious that individuals may estimate their risk as low if they have taken, or intend to take precautionary measures. Thus, perceived vulnerability operationalized in this way may not be a predictor, but rather an effect of the intention to use condoms. Therefore, a more appropriate way to operationalize vulnerability would be to assess to what extent individuals feel they would be at risk for HIV infection when they would not use condoms. This *conditional risk* would more likely predict condom use because it may indeed motivate individuals to take precautionary measures.

The conceptual distinction between absolute and conditional risk has consistently been supported in our research programme. For example, in line with many other studies (see Gerrard *et al.*, 1993), Buunk *et al.* (in press) showed that the perceived absolute risk of HIV infection was negatively related to the intention to use condoms (for men: $r = -.14$, $p < .05$; for women: $r = -.25$, $p < .01$), suggesting that those inclined to take precautions felt they had a relatively low chance of acquiring HIV. In contrast, conditional risk – the perception that one was at risk for HIV infection when not using condoms with new sexual partners – was not only positively correlated with condom use intentions (for men: $r = .29$; for women: $r = .21$; p's $< .01$), but still had a significant relation with this intention when controlling in regression analyses for all other relevant predictors (for example self-efficacy, various types of norms, and anticipated regret). These findings may offer an explanation for the contradictory results reviewed by Gerrard *et al.* (1993), and suggest that in future research the operationalization of conditional risk may be a more appropriate way of assessing perceived vulnerability than absolute risk.

Self-Efficacy

One of the reasons why the correlation between perceived vulnerability to HIV infection and HIV preventive behaviour may not be very high, is the complicated and socially complex nature of preventive sexual behaviour. Avoidance of the risk of HIV infection clearly requires a complex series of behaviours, for example negotiating with a sexual partner, and overcoming strongly ingrained habits or drives associated with sexual behaviour. For many people, the process of communicating with one's sexual partner, and negotiating cooperation in practising safe sex, may be quite difficult. It has indeed been shown that people sometimes do not engage in safe sex because they feel too embarrassed to talk about it, because they find it difficult to buy or to bring out a condom, and because they fear offending their partner by implying the partner has a disreputable past (Bakker, Buunk and Siero, 1993; Miller *et al.*, 1993).

Indeed, a health risk may only lead to behavioural change if individuals believe they are capable of performing the behaviours necessary to reduce that risk. According to Bandura's (1986) social cognitive theory, translating knowledge about HIV transmission into effective HIV preventive behaviour requires a sense of personal power to exercise control over the sexual situation, that is a sense of self-efficacy:

> People's beliefs about their capabilities affect what they choose to do, how much effort they mobilize, how long they will persevere in the face of difficulties, whether they engage in self-debilitating or self-encouraging thought patterns, and the amount of stress and depression they experience in taxing situations. When people lack a sense of self-efficacy, they do not manage situations effectively even

though they know what to do and possess the requisite skills. (Bandura, 1989, pp. 128–9).

There is considerable support for self-efficacy as a predictor of condom use and other safe sex behaviours among heterosexuals in the Netherlands (Bakker, 1995a; Bakker, Buunk and Siero, 1993; Paulussen *et al.*, 1989; Richard and Van der Pligt, 1991; Richard, Van der Pligt and De Vries, 1995; Van der Pligt and Richard, 1994; Van der Velde and Van der Pligt, 1991), as well as in other countries (Nucifora, Gallois and Kashima, 1993; Wulfert and Wan, 1993). Moreover, Buunk *et al.* (in press) proposed a conceptual and operational extension of self-efficacy to enhance the predictive value of their model. They reasoned that in general individuals prefer to feel they are better than others in relevant abilities (compare Hoorens, 1993), and that this feeling will motivate them to actually perform a behaviour in which that ability is used. Because using condoms with new sexual partners is likely to be viewed as an ability, *comparative* self-efficacy, that is the perception of being better able than other individuals to perform HIV preventive behaviour, may have an additional effect upon the willingness to use condoms with new partners. The results of this study showed that, when controlling for absolute self-efficacy, comparative self-efficacy was an independent predictor of the intention to use condoms: a feeling of having less difficulty than others in using condoms helped to support condom use intentions.

Two Dutch studies contribute to our knowledge about the factors underlying self-efficacy for HIV preventive behaviour. Rademakers *et al.* (1992) conducted a comprehensive qualitative study among adult heterosexuals. Their sample included 100 participants aged between 18 and 39 who had had heterosexual contact with two or more partners in the previous year. The results indicated that consistent condom users not only possessed better communication and negotiation skills than inconsistent users, but also reported less fear that the partner would reject them as a sexual partner. In sharp contrast, inconsistent condom users engaged in safe sex only when they thought the partner had a positive attitude towards safe sex.

In an unpublished empirical study among 200 young heterosexual adults, Bakker (1995b) also identified several factors related to self-efficacy. Self-efficacy regarding condom use among participants was higher the more they were convinced that one can talk about past sexual relationships before having sex, the more they thought that talking about condom use before having sex was useful, the less they thought that it was difficult to discuss using a condom with a new partner and to actually put a condom on the penis, and the less they expected that the sexual partner would be reluctant to use a condom.

Because research has consistently shown that self-efficacy is a crucial, independent predictor of safe sex, and because we have identified the most salient self-efficacy beliefs, self-efficacy would seem a relevant target for intervention. Even more so, it seems plausible that emphasizing in persuasive messages the risk of not using condoms with new sexual partners, may not be sufficient to promote safe sex, but will only encourage HIV preventive action if simultaneously the sense of self-efficacy is enhanced.

In order to test this hypothesis, Bakker, Buunk and Siero (in press) conducted an experiment among 85 adult heterosexuals (mean age = 33). In the previous five years, 34 per cent of this sample had had one, 48 per cent had had two to five, and 18 per cent had had more than five sexual partners. A majority of the sample (80 per cent) indicated having had sexual intercourse with a new partner without using a condom during this same period. While AIDS-risk perceptions were manipulated by providing participants with information about the prevalence of AIDS and about the risk of HIV infection (low versus high), self-efficacy was manipulated in two different ways. A first experimental group was exposed to concrete information, that is suggestions for safe sex strategies that bolstered their sense of personal power to exercise control over the sexual situation. A second group was asked to generate at least three personal arguments to engage in safe sex. The purpose of this manipulation was to explore whether people's self-efficacy perceptions could be changed in the absence of any direct persuasive message. These two groups were compared with a control group who performed an unrelated task. Persuasive messages were allegedly taken from a magazine. The final design in this experiment was a 2 (AIDS-risk: low, high) × 3 (Self-efficacy (SE): low (unrelated task), high (SE-message), high (self-generated SE-message)) between-subjects design with a pre- and post-test. Changes in attitudes towards condom use (that is the favourableness of a person's evaluation of the behaviour) and in behavioural expectations were the main dependent variables.

Both manipulations were succesful. First, the manipulation checks revealed that participants who received the high-risk message perceived a higher risk of becoming infected with HIV than those who received the low-risk message. In addition, both participants who were asked to generate safe sex strategies themselves, and those who received an SE-message reported a stronger sense of self-efficacy than subjects who completed the unrelated task. As can be seen in Figures 12.1 and 12.2, consistent with our view that translating knowledge about HIV transmission into effective HIV preventive behaviour requires a sense of self-efficacy, we found that most persuasion occurred when participants received a relatively high AIDS-risk message *and* were led to believe that they could protect themselves when needed (either by reading a message targeting at self-efficacy beliefs, or by self-generating a message). Similar results were found in a follow-up study (IJzer *et al.*, 1996) among female undergraduates from the University of Connecticut employing a 2 (AIDS-risk: low, high) × 2 (Self-efficacy: low, high) between-subjects design. Participants in this study received a message that was presented as a newspaper article. The motivation to engage in AIDS preventive behaviour was highest among those women who received the information that their risk of getting infected with HIV was high *and* who were led to believe that their self-efficacy was high. Interestingly, the results of this last experiment also indicated that participants in the high-risk/high self-efficacy condition were least likely to deny their AIDS-risk.

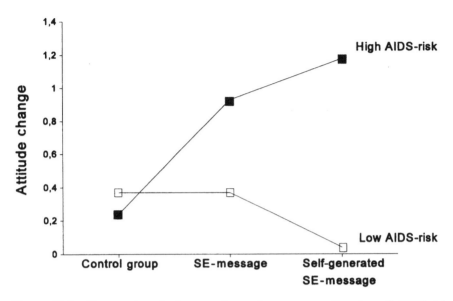

Figure 12.1 *Changes in attitude towards condom use as a function of AIDS-risk information and self-efficacy.*

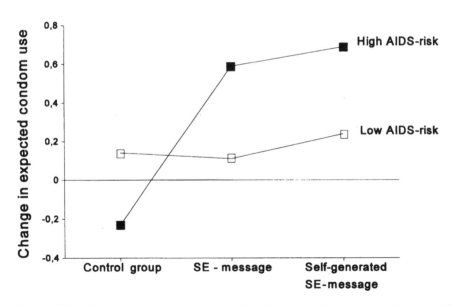

Figure 12.2 *Changes in expectation regarding future condom use as a function of AIDS-risk information and self-efficacy.*

211

In summary, consistent with Bandura's (1986) social cognitive theory, the findings by Bakker, Buunk and Siero (in press) and by IJzer *et al.* (in press) demonstrate that AIDS-risk information will especially have a positive impact on attitudes and behavioural intentions if recipients are encouraged to believe they can engage in safe sex if necessary. The results suggest that programmes to promote safe sex should not only offer strong arguments in favour of safe sex, but should also target self-efficacy beliefs and attempt to change them. This can be done by increasing positive and decreasing negative self-efficacy expectancies regarding safe sex with a new partner, for example by stressing that safe sex shows that one is a caring and responsible person, and by using a parallel of other, more routine, health behaviours. Furthermore, challenging people to generate concrete behavioural strategies that ensure safe sex might be especially effective, as it enhances a sense of self-efficacy which forms the basis for adaptive cognitions and behaviour.

Anticipated Regret

A difference between the risk of contracting HIV and many other health threats such as heart disease and cancer is that a single act (that is unprotected sex) may result in a deadly disease. When individuals realize this, they may anticipate a large amount of regret and self-blame if they have engaged in a behaviour that put them at risk and that could easily have been prevented. In line with other theoretical and empirical work on counter-factual thinking, anticipated regret theory (Janis and Mann, 1977; Richard, 1994) states that individuals who anticipate negative consequences before undertaking an action will be motivated to take protective measures. If, for instance, a person has had sexual intercourse with a new partner without using a condom, he or she might worry about the possibility of becoming infected with HIV, and therefore regret having taken the wrong course of action. Although this unpleasant affective state will perhaps motivate the person to use condoms in the future, it cannot undo a possible HIV infection. However, to the extent that people *anticipate* such negative feelings before undertaking action, they will be more cautious (Richard, 1994). Indeed, Richard and his colleagues (Richard, Van der Pligt and De Vries, 1995, in press) have convincingly shown that the anticipated consequences of unsafe sex can be a powerful antecedent of HIV preventive behaviour, which has explanatory power over and above other relevant predictors, such as perceived AIDS risk, attitudes, and self-efficacy (see also Buunk *et al.*, in press).

Anticipated regret is especially relevant because it is quite amenable to intervention by, for instance, inducing individuals to engage in imagining how they would feel if they had not used condoms with a new partner and then found out that this partner had a rather promiscuous past. Indeed, in two recent experimental studies among 439 young adult heterosexuals, Richard (1994) showed that individuals who were requested to focus on the feelings that they would experience after unsafe sexual practices expressed stronger expectations to use condoms in future 'casual' interactions (as compared to a control condition), and found that these persons were more consistent condom users in the five-month period following the experimental manipulation.

Social Norms

The previous factors all concern intra-individual cognitions and perceptions, and do not include the influence of the social environment on HIV preventive behaviour. However, as has been argued by Fisher and Misovich (1990), social context can play an important role in this regard. For example, individuals may not want to look more concerned and less risky than their friends, may fear sanctions when being cautious with new sexual partners, and may be afraid of rejection when they discuss condom use with a new partner. Indeed, in the theory of reasoned action (Fishbein and Ajzen, 1975) and the theory of planned behaviour (Ajzen, 1991) social context is given an important place in addition to attitudes and behavioural control by the inclusion of social norms, referring to what one perceives that others in the referent group think one should do.

Despite the potential importance of social norms for AIDS preventive behaviour, studies based upon the theory of planned behaviour have as yet found limited evidence for an independent role of subjective norms (Fishbein *et al.*, 1992; Paulussen *et al.*, 1989; Richard and Van der Pligt, 1991; however, see Ajzen, 1991, for more supportive evidence). One of the reasons for this may be the way in which the normative component is usually conceptualized, that is as the perceived approval of condom use in one's reference group (compare Ajzen, 1991; Fishbein and Ajzen, 1975). However, such perceived approval is only one possible type of social influence (Fisher, 1988), and may play a role only when it concerns relations with others upon whom one is more or less dependent (including parents, physicians or superiors). It is perfectly conceivable that in the case of condom use in new sexual relationships the norms of the new partner will play an important role.

Furthermore, to the extent that social influence from the reference group does indeed affect condom use with new sexual partners, it may not be as important what others are perceived to *approve*, but rather what others are perceived to *do* themselves. Indeed, in line with conformity studies and with research on the 'false consensus' phenomenon, that is the tendency to overestimate the prevalence of one's own characteristics in the population (Marks and Miller, 1987), one would expect that the perceived behaviour of comparable others is a central determinant of behaviour (Allen and Wilder, 1977). The perceived behaviour of one's friends refers to a *descriptive* norm about what is most common in a specific situation ('this is the way things are done'), whereas the subjective norm refers to an *injunctive* norm about what one ought to do in a given situation ('this is what you should do') (compare Cialdini, Reno and Kallgren, 1990).

Whereas to comply with injunctive social norms, one does not necessarily have to accept the opinion of others as valid, when it comes to descriptive social norms, the informational component may also play a role ('If everyone does this, then there must be a reason for it'). In other words, one may accept the fact that one's friends behave in a certain way as information about objective reality. Because there is much uncertainty about the way people should cope with AIDS, such social comparison processes may be important for AIDS preventive behaviour (Buunk, 1991; Fisher, 1988).

On the basis of these considerations, Buunk *et al.* (in press) examined the role of three types of normative influence: injunctive norms and descriptive norms as perceived in the reference group, as well as injunctive norms as perceived in potential new partners. The results supported the importance of the distinction between the various types of social norms. When controlling for both other measures of social norms, each social norm was an independent predictor of the intention to use condoms with new sexual partners. Moreover, in regression analysis including all relevant predictors, all types of social norms made independent contributions to condom use intentions, underlining the role of the social environment with respect to AIDS preventive behaviour that has been emphasized by Fisher and Misovich (1990).

An important implication of these results is that interventions highlighting that others in one's reference group value using condoms in new sexual contacts might be quite effective. However, earlier studies have shown that researchers have found it difficult to manipulate social norms through persuasive messages (O'Keefe, 1991). For this reason, and because the findings by Buunk *et al.* (in press) showed the apparent important role of the descriptive norm as a determinant of HIV preventive behaviour, we assumed that the descriptive norm would be a more promising focus for intervention. It is important to note that the mean scores on descriptive norms in the Buunk *et al.* (in press) study indicated that both women and men did not consider it very likely that their friends and acquaintances actually would use condoms in the case of sexual contact with a new partner. This finding and the positive correlation between descriptive norms and HIV preventive behaviour suggests that abstinence from HIV preventive behaviour in case of sexual contact with a new partner may be encouraged by the perception that most others one knows have unprotected sexual contacts.

False Consensus

Although the perception that others engage in unsafe sex may increase one's own tendency to engage in sexual risk behaviour, the opposite may also be true. Having unsafe sexual contacts oneself may increase the perceived prevalence of unsafe sex among others. A large body of evidence indeed shows that people tend to give relatively high prevalence estimates for their own behaviours (Leventhal, Glynn and Flemming, 1987). This phenomenon is often referred to as the false consensus effect (FCE; Ross, Green and House, 1977) and has been demonstrated for several attributes, such as attitudes, preferences, and characteristics. Recently, we have found that the FCE also applies to unsafe sexual behaviour (Van den Eijnden, Buunk and Bakker, 1993). Our study among 729 heterosexual Dutch adults showed that individuals who engaged in unsafe sex gave higher prevalence estimates of unsafe sex in the population than individuals who did not engage in such behaviour, and this finding was replicated in a follow-up study among a representative sample of adults who said they might engage in sex with new partners in the future (N = 384). A consistent and remarkable finding in these studies was that the FCE was much stronger for men than for women.

Although it is often suggested that cognitive processes account for the FCE, when it comes to behaviours which are commonly seen as undesirable this effect particularly seems to be the result of motivational mechanisms (Agostinelli *et al.*, 1992). By projecting one's undesirable behaviour on to others, this behaviour becomes less deviant, less inappropriate, or at least to some extent defensible (Suls, Wan and Sanders, 1988). The idea that many people engage in unsafe sex may normalize or justify one's own unsafe sexual behaviour. This may explain the gender difference in the false consensus effect with respect to unsafe sex. Because women have stronger intentions to use condoms than men (Bakker, Buunk and Siero, 1993; Van Zessen and Sandfort, 1991), they may justify their unsafe sex by emphasizing their intention to practise safe sex in the future, whereas men may feel the need to justify their behaviour by assuming that most others do the same.

Towards Theory-Based Interventions

Prevalence Information and Intention Change

In order to examine whether information about the prevalence of safe sexual behaviour could promote HIV preventive behaviour, we conducted several experiments. A first study included a sample of 120 undergraduate students from the universities of Groningen and Nijmegen with a heterosexual orientation (Van den Eijnden *et al.*, 1994). A high prevalence of safe sex was framed in two different ways. Participants either received a bogus newspaper article with the information that 88 per cent of their fellow students had safe sex, or with the information that 12 per cent of their fellow students had unsafe sex. These two experimental groups were compared with a control group who received no information. The results showed that the '88 per cent have safe sex' information increased the intention to use condoms of both male and female students, whereas the '12 per cent have unsafe sex' information elevated condom use intentions among male students alone. Moreover, in line with the assumption that prevalence information about safe sex can inhibit projection mechanisms, this increased intention to use condoms was accompanied by a lowered risk perception. Similar results were found in an intervention study among adult Dutch citizens (Van den Eijnden *et al.*, submitted).

A follow-up study among adult heterosexuals (Van den Eijnden *et al.*, in press) examined if the effects of prevalence information upon condom use intention and perceived risk were mediated by changes in the perception of the social norms among friends and among potential future partners. Unlike earlier studies, participants in this study received information about the safe sexual behaviour of either male students or female students. More specifically, one group of students received the information that 88 per cent of male students engage in safe sex, a second group obtained the information that 88 per cent of female students engage in safe sex, and a third group received no information. The results showed only effects of information about the prevalence of male students' safe sexual behaviour. Among male students, this information only led to a decrease in perceived vulnerability to HIV. Among female students, however, the information that most male students practised safe sex led to the perception that potential future partners would have a favourable norm towards safe sex. In turn, this perception enhanced the intention to use condoms in contacts with new partners. However, prevalence information did not affect the perceived social norm among friends. Thus, these studies suggest that information about a high prevalence of safe sex, particularly when the information refers to male students, may enhance the intention to use condoms with new sexual partners, particularly among women.

Message Discrepancy, Elaboration, and AIDS Prevention

In the foregoing, little attention has been paid to the specific ways through which various messages may lead to changes in risk perceptions, attitudes and behaviour. In a number of studies, we reasoned on the basis of social judgement theory (Sherif and Hovland, 1961) that messages aimed at persuading individuals to practise safe sex would have to be moderately discrepant from the recipient's own position. Messages that are relatively extreme, as well as messages that are not different from what recipients already think, would generate little change. Our studies were also based on the elaboration likelihood model developed by Petty and Cacioppo (1986), according to which attitude change due to a persuasive communication about AIDS prevention can occur through one of two relatively distinct 'routes' to persuasion. The *central route* involves effortful cognitive activity whereby the person carefully scrutinizes and evaluates the issue-relevant arguments presented in the communication. This route is followed when the message recipient possesses sufficient motivation and ability to think about the information provided, which will be the case when, for instance, the message is personally relevant (Petty,

Cacioppo and Schumann, 1983), and when individuals are high in need for cognition, that is have an intrinsic motivation to engage in and enjoy thinking (Cacioppo and Petty, 1982). In contrast, in the *peripheral route*, individuals use simple heuristics to evaluate the validity of the message (for example 'Experts are correct'). This route is followed when people are not motivated or able to engage in message- or issue-relevant thinking, which will, for instance, be the case when the message is not personally relevant, and when the recipient has a relatively low 'need for cognition' (Cacioppo and Petty, 1982).

Although peripheral processing of AIDS education – for example hearing that a well-known celebrity uses condoms (as in the Dutch 1987 public campaign) – can cause the same amount of attitude change as central processing, the consequences of these changes for preventive sexual behaviour are quite different. That is, individuals who have based their attitude change on a thoughtful consideration of the personal risks of unprotected sex – for example because they are motivated to do so – will be better able to persuade an unwilling partner to use a condom, because they possess more convincing arguments.

On the basis of social judgement theory and the elaboration likelihood model, we predicted that moderately discrepant messages advocating safe sex would generate most attitude change among individuals who engage in central processing, that is individuals highly involved with AIDS (Experiment 1) and individuals high in their need for cognition (Experiment 2) (Bakker, 1995a). Participants in these two experiments were 215 and 218 heterosexual adults, who were exposed to a message allegedly taken from a newspaper. The results showed, as predicted, that for individuals with a high involvement with AIDS and for those with a high need for cognition, moderately discrepant messages produced most attitude change (see Figures 12.3 and 12.4). In contrast, for those unmotivated to think, there was no reliable effect of discrepancy. These results support our view that as the motivation to think increases, the content of the information becomes a more important determinant of persuasion.

In another study, we evaluated two AIDS prevention communications which have been disseminated on a wide scale in the Netherlands (Bakker, Siero and Buunk, 1995). Young people were classified as being high or low in need for cognition and expressed their knowledge about AIDS, attitudes towards condom use and perceived social norms after being exposed to a cartoon or a written message. The main difference between both messages was the *format* in which the information was presented: The cartoon message 'Think about it, play safe' adopts an airy, humorous tone to present information about AIDS/STDs, and to communicate with pictures that condom use is needed. In sharp contrast, the written brochure 'Have safe sex or no sex' contains concise information, and presents the information formally without using pictures. The content of both brochures is not essentially different, although the cartoon message contains somewhat less detailed information. It was predicted that students with a high need for cognition would show more

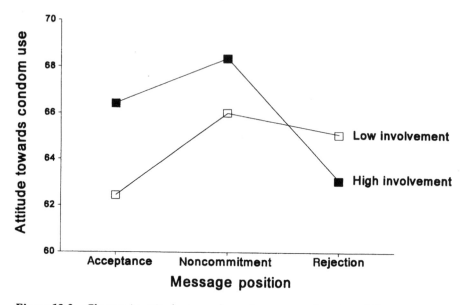

Figure 12.3 *Changes in attitudes towards condom use as a function of discrepancy and involvement with AIDS.*

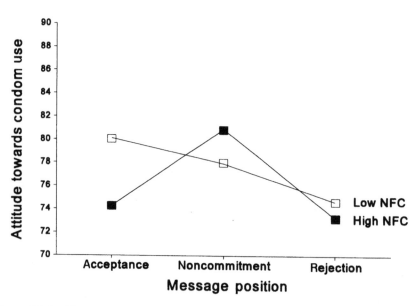

Figure 12.4 *Changes in attitudes towards condom use as a function of discrepancy and need for cognition (NFC).*

change (in terms of attitudes and subjective norms) in response to the written brochure than in response to the cartoon, and that the opposite would be the case for individuals with a low need for cognition. As can be seen in Figures 12.5 and 12.6, the results supported our hypothesis. An explanation for these findings is that individuals with a high need for cognition were indeed motivated to process the concise, written brochure, and were distracted – and maybe even annoyed – by the format of the cartoon message (for example 'How childish'). In contrast, individuals low in need for cognition were presumably not intrinsically motivated to engage in a thoughtful consideration of the written information, but were apparently only encouraged to process such information when it was visually presented in a cartoon format.

The studies described here suggest that it is important to consider the original attitudes of the audience as well as individual differences in the audience motivation to process information about safe sex when aiming to change attitudes towards safe sex. Our findings suggest that messages developed to foster such change may sometimes be too extreme, and sometimes not extreme enough. Moreover, whereas among some individuals attitude change can be attained by presenting messages evoking a thoughtful reasoning process, others will change their attitudes primarily on the basis of relatively simple cues. Because the goal of persuasive communications about AIDS is to produce long-lasting changes in attitudes with behavioural consequences, the central route to persuasion appears to be the preferred influence strategy. Because not all people have the ability and motivation to process the new

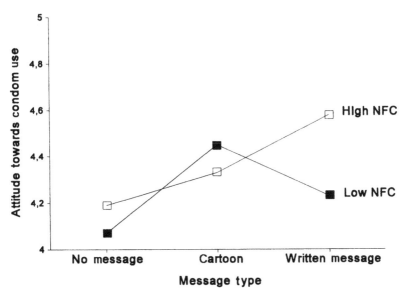

Figure 12.5 *Attitude towards condom use as a function of message type and need for cognition (NFC).*

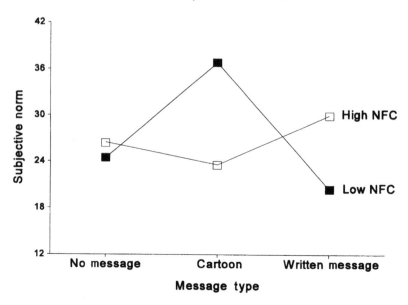

Figure 12.6 *Subjective norm as a function of message type and need for cognition (NFC).*

information, it is important to find ways to change the attitudes of those who are unmotivated to engage in a careful analysis of the AIDS prevention information. Our cartoon study (Bakker, Siero and Buunk, 1995) showed that using cartoons may offer one way to realize this.

Conclusions

Several studies in the Netherlands have documented the importance of perceived risk, self-efficacy, anticipated regret, social norms and false consensus in relation to the intention to use condoms with new sexual partners. Because these studies were mostly conducted in samples of adult heterosexuals, many of whom showed a considerable degree of risky sexual behaviour, the findings seem particularly relevant for designing intervention strategies. We have presented evidence from field and laboratory experiments that most factors related to unsafe sex are amenable to intervention. Moreover, we have shown that it is important to take into account the original attitudes of the audience as well as the motivation to process information when implementing strategies aimed at behavioural change. Although the effects in the various studies were often modest, and although we were often unable to assess long-term behavioural change, we hope that the research described here will contribute to developing more effective AIDS prevention strategies that are adapted better to the group for which they are intended.

Acknowledgements

We are grateful to Theo Sandfort and Peter Aggleton for their valuable comments on a previous version of this chapter. Preparation of this chapter was facilitated by grant 93026 from the Dutch AIDS Prevention Foundation.

References

AGOSTINELLI, G., SHERMAN, S.J., PRESSON, C.C. and CHASSIN, L. (1992) 'Self protection and self-enhancement biases in estimates of population prevalence', *Personality and Social Psychology Bulletin*, **18**, pp. 631–42.

AJZEN, I. (1991) 'The theory of planned behavior', *Organizational Behavior and Human Decision Processes*, **50**, pp. 179–211.

ALLEN, V.L. and WILDER, D.A. (1977) 'Social comparison, self-evaluation, and conformity to the group', in J.M. SULS and R.L. MILLER (Eds), *Social Comparison Processes: Theoretical and Empirical Perspectives*, Washington, DC: Hemisphere.

BAKKER, A.B. (1995a) *Denk Na, Vrij Veilig: Descriptief en Experimenteel Onderzoek naar Attitudes tegenover Condoomgebruik* (Think About It, Play Safe: descriptive and experimental research on attitudes towards condom use), Ridderkerk: Ridderprint.

BAKKER, A.B. (1995b) 'How self-efficacy and anticipated regret affect HIV preventive behaviour', unpublished raw data.

BAKKER, A.B., BUUNK, B.P. and SIERO, F.W. (1993) 'Condoomgebruik door heteroseksuelen: een vergelijking van de theorie van gepland gedrag, het health belief model en de protectie-motivatie theorie' (Condom use among heterosexuals: a comparison of the theory of planned behavior, the health belief model and protection motivation theory), *Gedrag & Gezondheid*, **21**, pp. 238–54.

BAKKER, A.B., BUUNK, B.P. and SIERO, F.W. (in press) 'Translating AIDS-threat information into safe sex motivation requires a sense of self-efficacy', *Basic and Applied Social Psychology*.

BAKKER, A.B., SIERO, F.W. and BUUNK, B.P. (1995) 'Ik vrij veilig of ik vrij niet: een evaluatie van AIDS-voorlichting aan jongeren' (Have safe sex or no sex: persuasive communication about AIDS among adolescents), *Gedrag & Gezondheid*, **23**, pp. 166–78.

BANDURA, A. (1986) *Social Foundations of Thought and Action: a Social Cognitive Theory*, Englewood Cliffs, NJ: Prentice-Hall.

BANDURA, A. (1989) 'Perceived self-efficacy in the exercise of control over AIDS infection', in V.M. MAYS, G.W. ALBEE and S.F. SCHNEIDER (Eds), *Primary Prevention of AIDS: Psychological Approaches*, London: Sage.

BUUNK, B.P. (1991) 'Sociale vergelijking en coping onder stress: implicaties voor AIDS' (Social comparison and coping under stress: implications for AIDS), *Nederlands Tijdschrift voor de Psychologie*, **46**, pp. 208–17.

BUUNK, B.P. and BAKKER, A.B. (1997) 'Commitment to the relationship, extradyadic sex, and AIDS-preventive behavior', *Journal of Applied Social Psychology*, **27**, pp. 1241–57.

BUUNK, B.P. and BAKKER, A.B. (in press) 'Responses to unprotected extradyadic sex by one's partner: testing predictions from interdependence and equity theory', *The Journal of Sex Research*.

BUUNK, B.P., BAKKER, A.B., SIERO, F.W. and VAN DEN EIJNDEN, R. (in press) 'Predictors of AIDS-preventive behavioral intentions among adult heterosexuals: extending current models and measures', *AIDS Education and Prevention*.

CACIOPPO, J.T. and PETTY, R.E. (1982) 'The need for cognition', *Journal of Personality and Social Psychology*, **42**, pp. 116–31.

CIALDINI, R.B., RENO, R.R. and KALLGREN, C.A. (1990) 'A focus theory of normative conduct: recycling the concept of norms to reduce littering in public places', *Journal of Personality and Social Psychology*, **58**, pp. 1015–26.

CLUMECK, N., TAELMAN, H., HERMANS, P., PIOT, P., SCHOUMACHER, M. and DE WIT, S. (1989) 'A cluster of HIV infection among heterosexual people with apparent risk factors', *New England Journal of Medicine*, **321**, pp. 1460–2.

VAN DEN EIJNDEN, R.J.J.M., BUUNK, B.P. and BAKKER, A.B. (1993) 'Vermeende consensus en onveilig seksueel gedrag' (False consensus and unsafe sexual behaviour), *Gedrag & Gezondheid*, **21**, pp. 184–93.

VAN DEN EIJNDEN, R.J.J.M., BUUNK, B.P., PLAGGENBORG, I.E. and HOORENS, V. (1994) 'Informatie over seksueel gedrag van anderen en de intentie tot veilig vrijen' (Information about sexual behaviour of others and the intention to have safe sex), in P.A.M. VAN LANGE, F.W. SIERO, B. VERPLANKEN and E.C.M. VAN SCHIE (Eds), *Sociale Psychologie en haar Toepassingen, Vol. 8*, Delft: Eburon.

VAN DEN EIJNDEN, R.J.J.M., BUUNK, B.P., BAKKER, A.B. and SIERO, F.W. (submitted) 'Gender differences in false consensus and risk perception with respect to unsafe sexual behavior'.

VAN DEN EIJNDEN, R.J.J.M., BUUNK, B.P., BAKKER, A.B. and SIERO, F.W. (in press) 'The impact of information about the prevalence of AIDS-preventive behavior among men and women: the mediating role of social norms', *Psychology and Health*.

FISHBEIN, M. and AJZEN, I. (1975) *Belief, Attitude, Intention and Behavior: an Introduction to Theory and Research*, Reading, MA: Addison-Wesley.

FISHBEIN, M. and MIDDLESTADT, S. (1989) 'Using the theory of reasoned action as a framework for understanding and changing AIDS-related behaviors', in V. MAYS, G. ALBEE and S. SCHNEIDER (Eds), *Primary prevention of AIDS: Psychological approaches*, Newbury Park, CA: Sage.

FISHBEIN, M., CHAN, D.K., O'REILLY, K., SCHNELL, D., WOOD, R., BEEKER, C. and COHN, D. (1992) 'Attitudinal and normative factors as determinants of gay men's intentions to perform AIDS-related sexual behaviors: a multisite analysis', *Journal of Applied Social Psychology*, **22**, pp. 999–1011.

FISHER, J.D. (1988) 'Possible effects of reference group-based social influence on AIDS-risk behavior and AIDS-prevention. Special Issue: Psychology and AIDS', *American Psychologist*, **43**, pp. 914–20.

FISHER, J.D. and MISOVICH, S. (1990) 'Social influence and AIDS-preventive behavior', in J. EDWARDS, R.S. TINDALE, L. HEATH and E.J. POSAVAC (Eds), *Applying Social Influence Processes in Preventing Social Problems*, New York: Plenum.

GERRARD, M., GIBBONS, F.X., WARNER, T.D. and SMITH, G.E. (1993) 'Perceived vulnerability to HIV infection and AIDS preventive behavior: a critical review of the evidence', in J.B. PRYOR and G.D. REEDER (Eds), *The Social Psychology of HIV Infection*, Hillsdale, NJ: Erlbaum.

GOLD, R.S. (1993) 'On the need to mind the gap: on-line versus off-line cognitions underlying sexual risk taking', in D.J. TERRY, C. GALLOIS and M. McCAMISH (Eds), *The Theory of Reasoned Action: its Application to AIDS-preventive Behaviour*, Oxford: Pergamon.

HARRISON, J.A., MULLEN, P.D. and GREEN, L.W. (1992) 'A meta-analysis of studies of the health belief model with adults', *Health Education Research*, **7**, pp. 107–16.

HOORENS, V. (1993) 'Self-enhancement and superiority biases in social comparison', in W. STROEBE and M. HEWSTONE (Eds), *European Review of Social Psychology, Vol. 4*, Chichester: John Wiley.

IJZER, M.C., FISHER, J.D., BAKKER, A.B., SIERO, F.W. and MISOVICH, S.J. (in press) 'The effects of perceived vulnerability and self-efficacy on intentions to engage in AIDS preventive behavior', *Journal of Applied Social Psychology*.

JANIS, I.L. and MANN, L. (1977) *Decision Making: a Psychological Analysis of Conflict, Choice, and Commitment*, New York: Free Press.

KARON, J.M., DONDERO, T.J., BERKELMANN, R., BUEHLER, J., CURRAN, J., FLEMING, P., GREEN, T., GREENSPAN, A., GWINN, M., HOLMBERG, S., MORGAN, M., BLATTNER, W., VERMUND, S. and BRUNDAGE, J. (1992) 'HIV prevalence estimates and AIDS case projections for the United States: report based upon a workshop', *AIDS-Forschung*, **6**, pp. 314–21.

KIPPAX, S. and CRAWFORD, J. (1993) 'Flaws in the theory of reasoned action', in D.J. TERRY, C. GALLOIS and M. McCAMISH (Eds), *The Theory of Reasoned Action: its Application to AIDS-preventive Behaviour*, Oxford: Pergamon.

LEVENTHAL, H., GLYNN, K. and FLEMMING, R. (1987) 'Is the smoking decision an informed choice?', *Psychological Bulletin*, **88**, pp. 370–405.

MARKS, G. and MILLER, N. (1987) 'Ten years of research on the false consensus effect: an empirical and theoretical review', *Psychological Bulletin*, **102**, pp. 72–90.

MILLER, L.C., BETTENCOURT, B.A., DeBro, S.C. and HOFFMAN, V. (1993) 'Negotiating safer sex: interpersonal dynamics', in J.B. PRYOR and G.D.

REEDER (Eds), *The Social Psychology of HIV Infection*, Hillsdale, NJ: Lawrence Erlbaum.

NUCIFORA, J., GALLOIS, C. and KASHIMA, Y. (1993) 'Influences on condom use among undergraduates: testing the theories of reasoned action and planned behaviour', in D.J. TERRY, C. GALLOIS and M. McCAMISH (Eds), *The Theory of Reasoned Action: its Application to AIDS-preventive Behaviour*, Oxford: Pergamon.

O'KEEFE, D.J. (1991) *Persuasion: Theory and Research*, Newbury Park, CA: Sage.

PAULUSSEN, T., KOK, G.J., KNIBBE, R. and KRAMER, T. (1989) 'AIDS en intraveneus druggebruik' (AIDS and injecting drug use), *Tijdschrift voor Sociale Gezondheidszorg*, **68**, pp. 129–36.

PETTY, R.E. and CACIOPPO, J.T. (1986) *Communication and Persuasion: Central and Peripheral Routes to Persuasion*, New York: Springer-Verlag.

PETTY, R.E., CACIOPPO, J.T. and SCHUMANN, D. (1983) 'Central and peripheral routes to advertising effectiveness: the moderating role of involvement', *Journal of Consumer Research*, **10**, pp. 135–46.

VAN DER PLIGT, J. and RICHARD, R. (1994) 'Changing adolescents' sexual behaviour: perceived risk, self-efficacy, and anticipated regret', *Patient Education and Counseling*, **23**, pp. 187–96.

RADEMAKERS, J., LUIJKX, J.B., VAN ZESSEN, G., ZIJLMANS, W., STRAVER, C. and VAN DER RIJT, G. (1992) *AIDS-preventie in Heteroseksuele Contacten: Risico-inschatting, Voornemen en Interactie* (AIDS prevention in Heterosexual Contacts: risk-appraisal, intention, and social interaction), Amsterdam: Swets & Zeitlinger.

RICHARD, R. (1994) *Regret is What You Get: the Impact of Anticipated Feelings and Emotions on Human Behavior*, Amsterdam: University of Amsterdam.

RICHARD, R. and VAN DER PLIGT, J. (1991) 'Factors affecting condom use among adolescents', *Journal of Community and Applied Social Psychology*, **1**, pp. 105–16.

RICHARD, R., VAN DER PLIGT, J. and DE VRIES, N. (1995) 'Anticipated affective reactions and prevention of AIDS', *British Journal of Social Psychology*, **34**, pp. 9–21.

RICHARD, R., VAN DER PLIGT, J. and DE VRIES, N. (in press) 'Anticipated regret and time perspective: changing sexual risk-taking behavior', *Journal of Behavioral Decision Making*.

ROSS, L., GREEN, D. and HOUSE, P. (1977) 'The "false consensus effect": An egocentric bias in social perception and attribution processes', *Journal of Experimental Social Psychology*, **13**, pp. 279–301.

SCHAALMA, H., KOK, G. and PETERS, L. (1993) 'Determinants of consistent condom use by adolescents: the impact of experience of sexual intercourse', *Health Education Research*, **8**, pp. 255–69.

SHERIF, M. and HOVLAND, C. (1961) *Social Judgment, Assimilation and Con-*

trast Effects in Communication and Attitude Change, New Haven: Yale University Press.

STICHTING SOA-BESTRIJDING (1995) *Fact Sheet SOA* (Fact Sheet STD), Utrecht: Stichting SOA-Bestrijding.

STROEBE, W. and STROEBE, M.S. (1995) *Social Psychology and Health*, Buckingham: Open University Press.

SULS, J., WAN, C.K. and SANDERS, S. (1988) 'False consensus and false uniqueness in estimating the prevalence of health-protective behaviors', *Journal of Applied Social Psychology*, **18**, pp. 66–79.

VAN DER VELDE, F.W. and VAN DER PLIGT, J. (1991) 'AIDS-related health behavior: coping, protection motivation, and previous behavior', *Journal of Behavioral Medicine*, **14**, pp. 429–51.

DE VROOME, E.M.M., PAALMAN, M.E.M., DINGELSTAD, A.A.M., KOLKER, L. and SANDFORT, T.G.M. (1994) 'Increase in safe sex among the young and non-monogamous: knowledge, attitudes and behavior regarding safe sex and condom use in the Netherlands from 1987 to 1993', *Patient Education and Counselling*, **24**, pp. 279–88.

DE VROOME, E.M.M., DINGELSTAD, A.A.M., KOLKER, L. and SANDFORT, T.G.M. (1995) 'Evaluatie van de algemene vrij veilig-campagne "Ik vrij veilig of ik vrij niet"' (Evaluation of the Dutch general public safe sex campaign 'Have safe sex or no sex'), *Tijdschrift voor Sociale Gezondheidszorg*, **73**, pp. 3–10.

WEINSTEIN, N.D. (1993) 'Testing four competing theories of health-protective behavior', *Health Psychology*, **12**, pp. 324–33.

WULFERT, E. and WAN, C.K. (1993) 'Condom use: A self-efficacy model', *Health Psychology*, **12**, pp. 346–53.

VAN ZESSEN, G. (1995) *Wisselend Contact: Seksuele Levensverhalen van Mensen met veel Partners* (Changeable Contact: sexual lifestories of people with many partners), Leiden: DSWO Press.

VAN ZESSEN, G. and SANDFORT, T. (Eds) (1991) *Seksualiteit in Nederland: Seksueel Gedrag, Risico en Preventie van AIDS* (Sexuality in the Netherlands: sexual behaviour, risk, and AIDS prevention), Amsterdam: Swets & Zeitlinger.

Chapter 13

Sex, Relationships and Risks among Young People: Trends between 1990 and 1995

Ton Vogels, Gertjan van Zessen and Emily Brugman

In reputation and practice, the Netherlands is considered to be a permissive country, with a predominantly liberal normative climate, sex education that recognizes sexual pleasure and services that are easily accessible, for young people as well as for others. Unwanted teenage pregnancies are comparatively rare and the number of abortions is reportedly among the lowest in industrialized countries (Jones *et al.*, 1986). To date, there are no signs of substantial HIV transmission among young people. By April 1995, only nine cases of AIDS had been diagnosed in the age group 13–19, out of a total of 3488 such cases (AIDS-Bestrijding, 1995). The prevalence of other sexually transmitted diseases is, however, much higher: about one out of 10 young people is likely to become infected with a sexually transmitted disease before the age of 25 (Stichting, 1995).

This chapter will describe the sexual conduct of young people (12–18 years of age) in the Netherlands, focusing on the following themes: sexual fantasies and orientation, norms, actual sexual experiences and relationships, and protection against pregnancy and sexually transmitted diseases, as assessed in a nationwide study carried out in 1995 (Brugman *et al.*, 1995). In order to identify relevant trends, findings from this study will be compared with those from an earlier study carried out in 1990, with an almost identical design (Vogels and Van der Vliet, 1990).

Both studies were possible because of the emergence of AIDS, which in turn led to an upsurge in studies into human sexual behaviour. In HIV prevention in the Netherlands, young people are considered to be a group that deserves special interest, for two reasons. First, more than older people, young people are thought to experiment with sexual behaviour and sexual relations, before developing more stable behavioural patterns and relations. This experimenting might lead to increased HIV risks. Second, as sexual behaviour in the formative stages is thought to be moulded more easily, preventive campaigns aimed at people beginning their sexually active lives may be more effective in the long run, thereby laying a solid foundation for safer sexual behaviour in adulthood.

In the late 1980s, when the first HIV prevention campaigns for the general public were started, most people were optimistic that safe sex education would lead to safer behaviour. The prevailing open and relaxed attitude towards teenage sexuality made it possible that by 1989, 85 per cent of all secondary schools had AIDS education voluntarily in their curriculum (Mellink, 1989). Much of this early work, however, had weaknesses, such as a predominance of verbal information and insufficient attention to training in skills. Such weaknesses were attributed, however, to the relative newness of the subject and the lack of proper teaching materials and training facilities for teachers involved in AIDS education. These deficiencies were expected to disappear as soon as better educational programmes and materials became available. The development of adequate interventions should be based on empirical, up to date knowledge about actual behaviour and its motivating factors.

Abstaining from or postponing intercourse has never been part of the general prevention message in the Netherlands. Dutch adolescent girls protect themselves quite effectively against pregnancy, in most cases by using the contraceptive pill (Rademakers, 1990). Since this is regarded as the main cause of the low rate of adolescent pregnancies, few were prepared to risk a decrease in pill use by campaigning for the use of less reliable condoms against pregnancy and infection with other sexually transmitted diseases (STDs). This led to a situation in which the 'Double Dutch' method was advocated: using both condoms and the contraceptive pill.

In 1994 a study (Mellink and Gijtenbeek, 1995) revealed that by then almost all schools (92 per cent) provided safe sex education for their pupils. No generation of school pupils has had such massive and intensive education on sexuality and safe sex as the generation participating in the 1995 study to be described here. We therefore expected to find substantial knowledge about AIDS, more positive attitudes towards condoms and greater reported condom use than in the previous study.

The Studies

Both the 1990 and the 1995 study should be seen as independent studies within the context of an ongoing research programme of the Dutch Sentinel Stations of Youth Health Care, aimed at monitoring general health and health behaviour of Dutch children and young people. Data were collected by means of paper and pencil questionnaires, administered in the classroom by school doctors and school nurses. The Dutch secondary school system is non-comprehensive and contains different types of schools ranging from technically oriented preoccupational education, to theoretically oriented pre-academic schools. Furthermore, many schools are not directly governed by central or local authorities but by autonomous boards, often based on religious affiliations. These affiliations are related to characteristics of the school population. Therefore, to obtain a representative sample of pupils, a stratified sample of schools was drawn with type of education and type of school government as key sampling criteria.

School doctors first approached the management of selected schools, and asked permission for data collection. Based on previous experiences, about one-third of the schools were expected not to participate in the study. These refusals are sometimes based on moral objections, educational principles and so on, but more often technical or organizational problems are the main reason for non-participation. In consequence, non-participating schools were replaced by randomly selected schools of the same type and denomination. This procedure does not entirely protect the sample against bias due to drop-out of more conservative schools, but does protect against bias due to other factors.

A few days before the administration of the questionnaires, parents were sent a letter announcing the study and stressing the fact that they could decide whether or not their child would participate. In class, pupils were also told that they were free to participate.

About two-thirds of the schools in the original 1995 sample were willing to participate. Only 7 per cent of the schools refused because of moral reasons or other reasons related to the subject of the study. Nearly all refusing schools could be replaced by a similar school. In both studies, the selected schools were almost completely identical to those specified in the original sample with respect to type of education and denomination of the school.

Response at an individual pupil level was high. In 1995, 91 per cent of all pupils completed the questionnaire. Non-response at this level is to be attributed mainly to absenteeism due to sickness and truancy. Less than 2 per cent of the pupils or their parents actually refused to participate. As a result, we consider the samples to be highly representative of all pupils in secondary education, with respect to type of education and type of management. The same applies to the grade, age, sex and religion of the pupils. Participation of schools, parents and pupils in the 1995 study was fully comparable to the participation in the 1990 study, which allows for meaningful comparisons (compare Vogels and Van der Vliet, 1990; Brugman *et al.*, 1995).

After data collection, the validity of the answers was checked thoroughly, using built-in checks in the questionnaires and unlikely answers or combinations of answers as a starting point. A rating procedure with three independent judges resulted for both studies in the removal of less than 1 per cent of the questionnaires because of answers judged to be unreliable or invalid.

In 1995, a total of 7299 completed and reliable questionnaires were received. The sample differs only slightly from the 1990 sample. The mean age in the sample was 14.8; 97 per cent were less than 19 years of age. Fifty-three per cent were girls.

In 1995, the proportion of pupils from ethnic minorities was 18 per cent, compared to 15 per cent in the 1990 sample. This rise reflects a real increase of ethnic groups in this age range in the population. Seven per cent were born to Turkish or Moroccan parents, the major minority ethnic groups in the Netherlands, and 7 per cent came from Surinam, the Netherlands Antilles and Indonesia. Four per cent came from other countries, a majority of them probably from Western European countries.

To ensure that differences between the samples are actual differences and are not due to differences in sample composition, the 1990 sample was weighted to bring it in line with the 1995 sample. The weighting procedure which was followed ensured that each combination of the categories ethnicity, type of education, age and sex occurs in the same proportion in both samples. To avoid too much technical detail, this chapter does not describe the details of all the statistical analyses. However, all differences reported as such were tested using appropriate statistical procedures, with $\alpha = .05$. Differences between 1990 and 1995 were tested on the unweighted samples, using multiple analysis of variance or logistic regression, with year of measurement and sample characteristics, such as age and sex, as test factors. This procedure assesses significant effects of year of measurement, which may not be explained by differences in sample composition.

The questionnaire was divided into sections addressing different aspects of young people's sexuality. The first section contained questions on the way young people think and feel about sexuality and sexual orientation. The second one asked for actual sexual experiences, including contraception and condom use. The questions on experiences were formulated in simple, direct language. Medical or street jargon was avoided. Key terms were explained (for example 'vaginal intercourse means: penis in vagina'). A third section addressed knowledge and attitudes regarding AIDS, other sexually transmitted diseases and safer sex.

When applicable, the questionnaire explored respondents' sexual relationships with their two most recent partners in detail. This was done for two reasons. The first one is the theoretically based aim of the study: asking about specific characteristics or social attributes of specific partners makes it possible to study the principles of partner selection. The choice of sexual partners bears a direct relationship to the formation of sexual networks and to the existence of sexual 'bridges' between networks and these concepts are essential when studying sexual disease transmission in a population (Laumann *et al.*, 1994; Kretzschmar *et al.*, 1994; Van Zessen and Junger, 1994).The second reason is methodological: we believe that even when using a very structured, and therefore rather global questionnaire, one should try to measure the key outcome behaviour (safe or unsafe sex) so far as is possible within its direct social and symbolic context: the relationship between two individuals. More general questions tend to illicit less focused answers, which may bear little relationship to actual conduct, and hence do not lead to useful intervention guidelines.

Sexual Norms

Using a Dutch adaptation of the Reiss scale (Reiss, 1960; Kooy, 1976), we asked respondents to indicate when they felt a boy and a girl were permitted to have intercourse: when planning to get married, when having a stable relationship, when liking each other a lot, and without liking each other much.

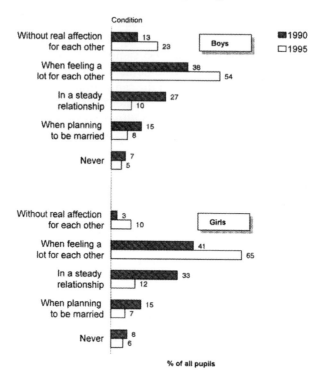

Figure 13.1 *Minimal conditions in which premarital intercourse is not disapproved of (changes between 1990 and 1995, by sex).*

The Reiss scale is a Guttman scale, which means that respondents who do not object to sex under a less strict condition (for example when liking each other), in general, also do not object to sex in stricter conditions. Figure 13.1 presents the distribution of the pupils over the most lenient condition in which they do not object to intercourse between a boy and a girl.

The answers in 1995 show marked differences with those given in 1990. In both years only a few pupils objected to sex in all these premarital situations. Also, only small proportions felt that intercourse is allowable only when partners plan to get married. However, in 1990 a minority of the pupils (48 per cent) believed that intercourse was permitted in an affective relationship or in the absence of such a relationship. In five years, this percentage increased markedly to 76 per cent.

Figure 13.1 shows some differences between boys and girls, the latter being somewhat more restrictive in their views. These differences, however, are rather small and, compared to older studies, seem to have grown smaller in the last decades (Deggeler *et al.*, 1969; Kooy *et al.*, 1983).

With increasing age – and increasing sexual experience – attitudes towards sex grow more liberal and permissive. At the age of 12 to 13, for example, 33 per cent of respondents disapproved of sex outside a formal relationship. At the age of 18 and older this is only 15 per cent.

Young people from minority ethnic groups are not as liberal as those of Dutch origin. Pupils with a minority ethnic background disapprove much more often of any form of premarital sex, regardless of the nature of the relationship, than their Dutch counterparts (14 versus 3 per cent). And whereas the norms of Dutch girls closely resemble those of Dutch boys, there are large differences between boys and girls from ethnic minorities, the latter being far more restrictive. The largest differences between boys and girls are to be found among adolescents from Turkish and Moroccan families (Brugman, Van Zessen and Vogels, 1997).

The original Reiss scale only covers norms about heterosexual intercourse. We added identically phrased questions on the attitudes towards two boys or two girls having sex (in this situation the phrase 'having sex' rather than 'having intercourse' was used). Thirty-four per cent of the sample disapproved of sex between two boys who like each other a lot. A similar rate of disapproval (33 per cent) was found regarding two girls wanting to have sex. These percentages compare to 25 per cent disapproval of intercourse between a boy and a girl in an affective relationship. Among boys, however, the percentages approving of male and female homosexual contacts is significantly less (52 and 58 per cent respectively) than for heterosexual contacts (75 per cent). Girls are more tolerant towards (or perhaps feel less threatened by) the idea of homosexual behaviour, and the rate of approval for homosexual contacts is similar to that for heterosexual contacts (76 per cent for both male and female homosexual contacts, and 74 per cent for heterosexual contacts).

Sexual Fantasies and Orientation

Both boys and girls were asked about sexual fantasies concerning boys and girls. Almost all pupils (91 per cent) report having sexual fantasies. This holds for both boys (94 per cent) and girls (89 per cent). Sexual fantasies are already quite common (84 per cent) among members of the youngest age group (11–13) and this percentage increases only slightly with age. Usually these fantasies concern the other sex (91 per cent), but 4 per cent of the boys and 6 per cent of the girls admit fantasizing sexually about members of the same sex. This percentage increases with age, from 4 per cent of the age group 11–13, to 8 per cent among those aged 18 or older. Most young people (94 per cent) with homosexual fantasies have fantasies about the other sex, too.

We asked pupils whether they saw themselves as being gay or lesbian. Only a few labelled themselves as such (0.5 per cent boys and 0.2 per cent girls). Another 0.6 per cent are uncertain and answer 'Yes, perhaps'. Four per cent (boys 3 per cent, girls 6 per cent) answered that they were uncertain in the past, but that they saw themselves not being gay or lesbian now. The percentage of respondents labelling themselves homosexual does not increase significantly with age.

Seven per cent of pupils said they sometimes thought they were able to fall in love with both boys and girls. This percentage is not related to age.

Combining the three different sorts of information, some indication of a potential homosexual orientation was found among 12 per cent of all young people surveyed. However, the different data do not present a consistent picture at all. For 9 per cent of respondents, only one of the three indicators pointed towards potential homosexuality, and 35 per cent of those who saw themselves as (possibly) being homosexual, said they did not fantasize sexually about the same sex. Most young people with such indications of homosexual thoughts or fantasies also report heterosexual thoughts and fantasies.

The relation between the indicators of homosexual orientation and actual homosexual experiences is inconsistent, too. Two per cent of all respondents indicated – somewhere in the questionnaire – that they had participated in French kissing, petting or more with someone of the same sex. This percentage increases with age from 1 per cent in the youngest age group to 4 per cent in the oldest one. For young people without any indication of a homosexual orientation, this percentage is less than 1 per cent; for those with some indication it is 11 per cent. However, heterosexual experiences are much more common in the latter group. Fifty-three per cent reported having had such experiences, a percentage which is comparable to that found among young people without any indication of a homosexual orientation (51 per cent).

In summary, sexual fantasies are quite common among Dutch adolescents, even in the youngest age group. Mostly such fantasies concern members of the opposite sex, but among 5 per cent they also concern members of the same sex. Twelve per cent of respondents gave some indication of homosexual fantasies, desires or self-labelling. Such indications, however, do not concur and are only weakly related to actual homosexual experiences. Clearly, a final homosexual identity, let alone a homosexual life-style, has only rarely been formed in this age group.

Actual Sexual Experiences

Experience of sexual contacts in the youngest age group is rather limited. From 12 years onwards actual contacts start to develop. This development is characterized by a mostly gradual transition from less to more intensive sexual experiences (Van der Vliet, 1990). The following 'first experiences' were distinguished: deep kissing, fondling under the clothes, naked sex without (vaginal/anal) intercourse and, finally, intercourse. The order in which these different experiences occur among young people seems to be quite fixed and is the same for boys and girls, and also for pupils from different ethnic groups.

Deep kissing is an experience reported by the majority of the sample: 64 per cent of all young people did so at least once. The median age for deep kissing – that is the age by which half of the sample had had this experience – is 13.9. On average, it takes more than one year before making the next step, 'feeling under the clothes' or petting, which 48 per cent had done at least once. Thirty per cent of all pupils had had sex with someone fully undressed, but without having intercourse. Doing this seems to be quite a big step, as the median age for naked sex lies just before the seventeenth birthday, more than two years after the median age for petting. By age 17.7, a few months before the eighteenth birthday, half of the respondents had had their first intercourse. Of the total sample, 23 per cent had experience of (vaginal) intercourse.

Despite increasingly liberal norms with regard to the question of when intercourse is permitted, the percentage of young people reporting coital experience has *not* increased in the last five years. Still, there are strong indications that the historical trend towards sexual experience commencing at a younger age has not yet reached its lowest point. The median age for deep kissing has decreased by six months. The median age for first intercourse has decreased too, by 3.5 months. Although this difference does not reach statistical significance, we assume that there may well be an indication of a historical trend here.

The development of sexual experience follows the same pattern for boys and girls. Yet there are marked gender differences in speed. In general, boys tend to start earlier. In the younger age groups, greater proportions of boys report having had some sexual experiences, mostly deep kissing and petting. Girls tend to start later, but progress faster towards more intimate forms of sex. By age 16, the boys have been overtaken, and the girls have more sexual experience. In the oldest age group (18 and up), 60 per cent of all girls have had their first intercourse, whereas for boys in the same age group only 49 per cent report having done so.

Apart from gender, two other demographic variables clearly have an important role to play with respect to sexual experience. The first is type of education. Pupils from vocational education schools start much earlier than those from higher general or pre-academic education schools. Among the lower age groups, pupils from vocational education therefore have a much higher degree of experience than pupils from other schools. So, by age 14 or 15 one out of five pupils from vocational schools has had intercourse at least once. For pupils from higher general and pre-academic schools, this figure is one out of 10.

Ethnicity is the other major factor. About two-thirds of pupils from minority ethnic groups are from Turkish or Moroccan origin and have an Islamic background. The Koran contains severe restrictions on premarital sex. In practice, for boys these restrictions are applied far less strictly. Girls from Islamic backgrounds, however, are confronted by strong restrictions with regard to social and sexual contact with boys. These cultural characteristics are reflected in the sexual experiences of young people from minority ethnic groups. The proportion of boys of Dutch origin reporting experience of intercourse is almost half of that of boys of non-Dutch origin (18 versus 38 per cent). The figures for girls are reversed, with 27 per cent of Dutch girls and 17 per cent of non-Dutch girls reporting experience of intercourse. Moreover, most of the non-Dutch girls reporting coital experience come from countries other than Turkey and Morocco. These differences cannot be explained by differences in age or type of education.

Cultural restrictions on the sexual contacts of Turkish and Moroccan girls also have far-reaching consequences for boys of these same groups. Whereas, in general, intercourse partners tend to have the same ethnic background, Turkish and Moroccan boys often have intercourse with girls from an ethnic background other than their own (84 per cent). In their eyes, girls from other backgrounds are more 'available' and they are willing to develop sexual relationships with these girls, so as to be able to acquire the experiences and skills deemed necessary for first intercourse in marriage (Danz, Vogels and Gründemann, 1993). For marriage, mostly Turkish or Moroccan girls are preferred.

These cultural restrictions, real as they are, do not mean that Turkish and Moroccan girls refrain fully from any form of sexual contact. A qualitative study of Danz, Vogels and Gründemann (1993) showed that a significant proportion of Turkish and Moroccan girls, although accepting restrictions on premarital intercourse, strongly resent these restrictions. With the support of friends and sometimes of brothers, they are prepared to go a long way to circumvent such constraints, such as, in one case reported in this study, drugging their parents with sleeping pills! Yet most of them want to remain a virgin until marriage and the percentage of Turkish and Moroccan girls reporting having had intercourse is, indeed, very small, as our quantitative study shows (6 per cent).

No Experience of Intercourse Yet

Thirty-four per cent of all the pupils in 1995 had not yet had any experience of French kissing, petting, or having sex with or without intercourse. Twenty-three per cent had had intercourse, at least once. And nearly half of the respondents had at least once experienced French kissing or petting with someone, or even naked sex, but had not yet had intercourse. We labelled this last group as 'sexual starters'. Often these starters had already had sex – but had not yet had intercourse – with several partners, with boys reporting an average of 4.9 partners and girls 5.5. It is clearly rare in the Netherlands today for young people to have intercourse with their first sexual partner.

Sexual starters differ in several aspects from their more fully experienced peers. Of course, they are younger; the mean age is 14.8 for the starters and 16.4 for those with experience of intercourse. Somewhat more often they report having a religious background (48 versus 43 per cent). They report other leisure-time activities. More often, sexual starters have not (yet) started to use alcohol (13 versus 25 per cent of the coitally experienced group) or visit bars or discotheques regularly (6 versus 17 per cent). The latter differences are related to differences in age, of course, but remain significant when age is controlled for. Visiting bars and drinking alcohol, however, do seem more important than religious background when it comes to explaining patterns of sexual activity.

We asked sexual starters to describe the partner with whom they had had most intimate sexual experience (usually the most recent partner). We asked if had they considered intercourse with this partner, would they have liked to have intercourse? Sixty-one per cent of the boys and 50 per cent of the girls replied that neither they nor their partners had wanted intercourse. A small proportion of the boys (6 per cent) and a large proportion of the girls (34 per cent) answered that their partners had actually wanted intercourse, but they themselves had not. Summing these percentages reveals that 67 per cent of the boys and 84 per cent of the girls abstained from intercourse on their own accord. Eleven per cent of starting boys actually wanted to have intercourse, but their partners did not. The remaining 23 per cent of the starting boys and 16 per cent of the starting girls, had also wanted to have intercourse, but had not succeeded due to circumstances, such as being disturbed by others or the location being not suitable.

When asked why they had not had intercourse, the most frequent answer, for both boys (55 per cent) and girls (71 per cent), was that they were not yet up to it. Twelve per cent of the girls answered that they had not wanted to have intercourse with this particular boy. Boys rarely gave this answer. They were more likely to have a partner who did not want to have intercourse (30 per cent) or no opportunities to have intercourse were available. Other motives, like having no condoms or wanting to remain a virgin, were hardly mentioned.

In summary, the majority of sexually active boys and girls have not yet had intercourse. Their sexual experience is quite extensive and already they have had several partners. Opportunities to have intercourse seem available in principle, but they decide to postpone on their own accord, until the time is right or until they have met the right partner. Accepting these self-reports as a reflection of the real motives, one cannot but conclude there are rather high levels of self-regulation and interactional competence ('no' means 'no') among sexual starters, both for boys and girls. This, however, should not be interpreted as meaning that sexual interaction is perfect. About one-third of all starters never actually talked about sex with their most recent partner. Forty-two per cent had ever felt the necessity to slow down an overly enthusiastic partner and 22 per cent of the boys and 16 per cent of the girls admitted ever having gone further than the partner wanted.

Intercourse Partners

As mentioned before, 23 per cent of the pupils in the 1995 sample had had intercourse at least once. This figure had not changed significantly since 1990. We asked respondents the number of partners with whom they had had (anal or vaginal) intercourse in the last 36 months, without specifying their partners' gender. For 91 per cent of the boys and 96 per cent of the girls the first intercourse was less than three years ago. The answers, therefore, present a fairly accurate picture of lifetime experiences. In the subsequent analysis we excluded 1.7 per cent of the respondents (mostly boys) who reported more than 20 partners, since we doubted the reliability of their answers and inclusion of their responses would have inflated the average picture unrealistically.

Boys with intercourse experience reported an average 3.0 partners. For girls the average number of reported intercourse partners was 1.7. Since the figures found in 1990 were 2.2 and 1.5 respectively, this reveals a substantial (and significant) change in sexual behaviour among young Dutch people. Figure 13.2 presents more detailed data. The percentage of boys with only one partner decreased from 48 per cent to 32 per cent. Among girls this percentage also decreased, albeit to a lesser degree. The percentages with more than two partners increased, especially among boys.

These figures point to a higher level of sexual activity, but do not necessarily mean that sexual relationships are on average less monogamous. The majority of all young people with experience of intercourse remained sexually

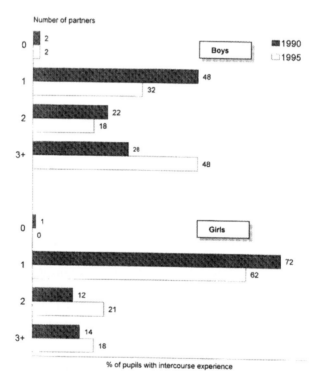

Figure 13.2 *Number of intercourse partners over the last three years (changes between 1990 and 1995, by sex).*

faithful towards their sexual partners – although 20 per cent of the boys and 5 per cent of the girls did not – and the percentage of intercourse relationships labelled as 'stable' remained unchanged in the last five years. The increased number of intercourse partners indicates a growing number of different, sequentially developing relationships, in which intercourse is one of the accepted forms of sexuality.

One could wonder whether AIDS and/or sex education played some role with regard to the increase in sexual activity. We did not try to assess the overall exposure to different forms of AIDS and/or sex education. However, we did ask the pupils whether they had received sex and/or AIDS education at school. Furthermore, we were able to link our data to data from a survey concerning school-based AIDS education among their teachers (Mellink and Gijtenbeek, 1995). Using logistic regression and controlling for other relevant variables (such as age and gender) we did not find any significant differences in the percentages of pupils with experience of intercourse or the number of intercourse partners between pupils who had received AIDS and/or sex education at school, and those who had not.

Contraception and Protection against Sexually Transmitted Diseases

Almost all pupils, including the younger ones, knew that AIDS exists and their knowledge of preventive measures is in general sufficient. Knowledge about sexually transmitted diseases in general, however, remained as unsatisfactory in 1995 as it was in 1990. Intentions to use condoms during intercourse increased. More than four out of five respondents said they would 'always' or 'nearly' always use condoms during intercourse. This increase was not associated with a decreasing use of the contraceptive pill. On the contrary, in 1995 63 per cent of all sexually experienced pupils reported always using the contraceptive pill during intercourse with their most recent partner. This is an increase compared to the situation found in 1990, when 54 per cent reported using the contraceptive pill. These percentages may even be an underestimate, since many boys did not know – or did not remember – whether the pill was used at that time. The advocates of 'Double Dutch' have gained some ground: 18 per cent of all experienced pupils reported using the contraceptive pill and condoms consistently during intercourse with their most recent partner, an increase of 5 per cent since 1990.

Although the intentions improved, other effects of the massive safe sex campaigns in schools and media appear to be limited. In 1990, knowledge of AIDS prevention was quite good already and did not improve overall. The percentage of respondents reporting condom use during first intercourse did increase from 58 to 70 per cent. With increasing age, however, more girls begin using the contraceptive pill and condom use decreases, as is shown in Figure 13.3.

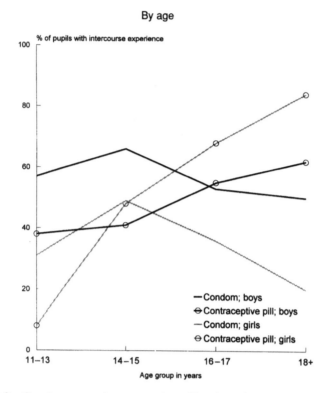

Figure 13.3 *Consistent use of contraceptive pill and condoms (by age).*

When having intercourse with their most recent partner, only 42 per cent of all boys and girls used condoms consistently, a percentage similar to that found in 1990. So, overall, despite a promising increase at the beginning of the sexual career, reported condom use among Dutch youngsters has *not* increased in the last five years.

This discarding of condoms in favour of the contraceptive pill suggests that the main motive for using condoms is not protection against STDs, but to protect against pregnancy. From this perspective it is only logical that condoms should be seen as something superfluous, both annoying and possibly distracting, once contraception is assured by the use of the easily available and reliable pill. This interpretation is corroborated by the answer most frequently given to the question why one had not used condoms: 'We used the contraceptive pill.'

Apart from the pill, another relevant factor in the decrease of condom use with age is type of the relationship. As mentioned before, a large majority reported intentions to use condoms (nearly) always during intercourse. However, these global answers to a global and superficial question hide important differentiations in intentions. When asked whether they where going to use

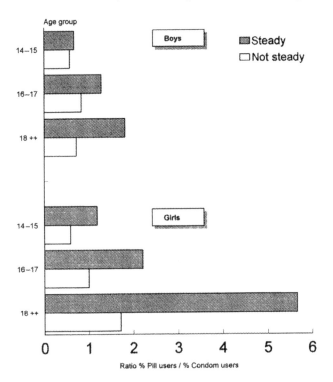

Figure 13.4 *Proportion of consistent users of the contraceptive pill (As a ratio of the proportion of consistent condom users by type of relationship and age group).*

condoms in specific situations, for example during intercourse in a steady relationship or with a partner who prefers not to use condoms, quite another picture emerges. A significant proportion of the boys said they would probably not use condoms when the girl would prefer not to, and a majority of boys and girls did not intend to use condoms during intercourse in a steady relationship.

These negative intentions towards condom use in steady relationships lead to a decrease in condom use at later age. At an early age, a relatively large proportion of relationships in which intercourse occurs are really not very stable. Partners may not have known each other for a long enough period of time. With increasing age, this changes. Older young people do know their partner better, have been acquainted for a longer period and label their relationships more often as steady. And, completely in accordance with their more differentiated intentions, they switch to the pill and leave condoms aside. This phenomenon increases with age. This is illustrated in Figure 13.4 which presents the proportion of consistent users of the contraceptive pill as a ratio of the proportion of consistent condom users.

The ratio was calculated by simply dividing the percentage of consistent users of the contraceptive pill by the percentage of consistent condom users. A value of 1 means that the proportion of consistent users of the contraceptive pill equals that of consistent condom users. A value of 5 means that the proportion of consistent pill users is 5 times that of the consistent condom users. Figure 13.4 shows clearly that in steady relationships and with increasing age, the pill is used more and more. This holds true for boys, but is much stronger for girls.

Due to the way the ratio was calculated, consistent users of both the contraceptive pill and condoms are included in the denominator as well as in the numerator. As using both the pill and condoms is found more often in non-steady relationships (24 per cent) than in steady relationships (16 per cent), the increased practice of Double Dutch cannot explain the trend.

In steady relationships the use of condoms is frequently discussed before having intercourse (in 80 per cent of the cases). This is more often than in not-steady relationships (52 per cent). In the latter case such discussions tend to be more directly related to more consistent condom use, but this is not the case in steady relationships. Young people who discuss condom use with a steady partner usually decide to abstain from condom use.

In summary, we found different attitudes towards condom use, dependent upon specific situations; systematic differences in condom use depending upon type of relationship; and differential outcomes from discussions about condom use, also depending upon type of relationship. All this suggests that, apart from contraception being the most important motive for condom use, a second explanation for the decreasing use of condoms lies in a differentiated risk assessment, or, better perhaps, a differentiated weighting of pros and cons of condom use. Pros are weighted more heavily in 'one-night stands' or in sexual contacts with relatively new partners, not in sexual contacts with steady partners. This is probably a phenomenon not unlike that which can be observed in the adult population. The main relevant difference is that younger people tend to have more partners per unit of time.

Risks of Infection with Sexually Transmitted Diseases

Despite high behavioural intentions, not more than 30 per cent of all coitally experienced adolescents used condoms consistently during intercourse. They took the most sensible precautions against infection with HIV and (most) other STDs, although they did so, probably, for the sake of contraception, not to protect themselves against STDs.

This does not mean, however, that the other 70 per cent have, consciously or unconsciously, run an actual risk of being infected with HIV or other sexually transmitted diseases. More than half of them (37 per cent of all coitally experienced boys and girls) reported having intercourse only with a partner who never had intercourse before and who never injected drugs. It is safe to assume that the vast majority of these inexperienced partners are not infected themselves and are therefore not incurring any health risk for their partners. A small proportion (6 per cent) of coitally experienced boys and girls may have taken some risk – consciously or unconsciously – as they had had unprotected intercourse with a partner without knowing anything about their sexual past and (possible) use of drugs. That leaves 27 per cent who certainly took the risk of being infected by having intercourse, knowing that their partners had had intercourse with other persons or had injected drugs. Therefore, one out of three young people with coital experience took avoidable risks or may have done so. In the whole sample, including those without coital experience, this is 6 per cent.

Three factors are clearly, and independently, related to being classified as belonging to the risk group defined above. Older age (and having more sexual experience) is the first. The second factor is gender. Not boys, with their higher levels of reported sexual activity, but girls are more prone to having taken avoidable sexual risks. Only 3 per cent of all boys belong to the risk group, compared to 9 per cent of the girls. The main explanation is that girls in most cases have intercourse in the context of a steady relationship, usually with an older male partner. Since most of these partners have had sexual contacts before, they form a greater health risk than the relatively young female partners of the boys. This gender difference in risk exposure increases strongly with age. While at the age of 18 and higher 15 per cent of *all* boys are classified as belonging to the risk group, the corresponding figure among girls is not less than 31 per cent. The third factor which should be mentioned, is a life-style of regularly going out, visiting bars and discotheques and using marijuana or Ecstasy. These life-style characteristics are strongly related to levels of sexual experience in general and sexual health risks in particular. For example, among boys and girls who never go out, hardly anybody belongs to the risk group (1 per cent). For those who regularly visit bars and discotheques the corresponding figure is 14 per cent. Comparable figures are found when distinguishing between young people who never drink alcohol and those who do so regularly. Among those who have ever used marijuana, Ecstasy or drugs such as heroin, 19 per cent belong to the risk group. Among non-users the equivalent figure is only 4 per cent.

When comparing the size of the risk group with that found in 1990, a considerable increase can be observed. This may be attributed to the increase in the number of sexual partners, in combination with consistent condom use remaining on the same level as in 1990. More general changes in youth culture, reflected in more liberal norms and an increasing use of alcohol and marijuana, may also be important background factors (compare Vogels, Brugman and Van Zessen, in press; Spanjer, 1996).

In summary, intentions to use condoms and condom use during first intercourse seem to have improved somewhat. Levels of knowledge have not changed. Even within five years, evidence was found that sexual experience tends to build up at an increasingly younger age. Among those with experience of intercourse the number of partners has increased quite strongly compared to five years ago. Protection against pregnancy has improved, but only via the pill. Condom use has ultimately remained constant, but since the number of partners has risen, the proportion that took avoidable sexual risks has risen, too.

Conclusions

This chapter described aspects of young people's sexuality in the Netherlands. Using data collected in 1990 and 1995 some clear trends are visible. The data reported here are based on (anonymous) self-reports and are as such subject to questions regarding their validity. We assume, however, that possible biasing factors will have influenced the 1990 data to a similar degree as the 1995 data. The trends described in this chapter may then be considered as reflecting trends which have occurred in reality, the more so because of the common methodology used in the 1990 and 1995 studies.

Since 1990 young people in the Netherlands have received education on sex and safe sex, as no generation before, both through the mass media and at school. We expected that these efforts would have had some effects and that these effects would be visible when comparing the 1990 and 1995 data. This, however, hardly seems to be the case. On average, level of knowledge has not improved. Intentions to use condoms have increased slightly, as has actual condom use during first intercourse. Condom use during intercourse with the most recent partner has, however, not grown. The percentage of young people who have had unprotected intercourse with someone who might have infected them with STDs, has increased.

We found an increase in number of partners, and the mean age at which one starts with the first sexual contacts has decreased. Some people might hold sex and/or AIDS education responsible for this trend. The percentage of pupils with experience of intercourse and the number of partners, however, were not related to the receipt of school-based AIDS and/or sex education. Reviews of the effectiveness of sex and/or AIDS programmes also suggest that such programmes 'do not increase sexual activity' (Kirby *et al.*, 1994; Kirby, in press). Therefore we feel it is safe to assume that AIDS education cannot be held responsible for the increase in sexual activity among young people in the Netherlands since 1990.

The data presented in this chapter make it clear that existing worries that the consistent flow of messages stressing the dangers of sex could have affected the open and free attitudes among Dutch young people towards sex were not vindicated. On the contrary, attitudes seem to have grown more liberal and there is no indication that young people are now refraining from sex in order to avoid possible health risks. On the other hand, for those expecting wholesale positive developments, as a result of all educational efforts, the results of our studies are somewhat disappointing.

This does not mean that all preventive efforts have proven fruitless.

Between 1990 and 1995 we did find an increase in condom use during first intercourse and we did find the same level of condom use during intercourse with the most recent partner, when the increased use of the contraceptive pill would have led us to expect a lower rate of condom use.

Yet, one cannot but conclude that despite all efforts, the group of young people who are at risk of HIV and other STDs has grown larger than five years ago. This is worrying because it has also become clear that old and hitherto largely hidden sexually transmitted diseases such as chlamydia infect large numbers of young Dutch people, with potentially serious consequences (Severijnen, 1993; Stichting, 1995).

In our view, the increase in the number of young people at risk is not necessarily an indication that prevention has failed. To understand what is actually going on, other developments have to be taken into account. From 1900 onwards, in the Netherlands a trend towards sex occurring at an increasingly earlier age is discernible. Several factors play a role in this trend. Physical maturation occurs at an earlier age, probably due to better nutrition and living circumstances. More liberal attitudes towards sex in society at large and the more public disclosure of all aspects of sexuality in the media in general and in youth culture in particular, may be assumed to play an important role. For the future, one must expect that the trend of earlier sexual maturation and experience will continue, leading to an increase of sexual activity among young people. The 'capacity' of a population to transmit STDs increases strongly when the mean number of partners increases and when the level of protection used remains the same.

Despite this, young people in the Netherlands do not seem prepared to take the simple message of 'always use condoms' to heart. They want to differentiate between different situations, partners and relationships. Sex education and sexual health education take place in the context of these broader developments and their effectiveness is restricted by such developments. It is within this complex context that prevention workers have to perform their difficult task to promote safer sex, which, in the Dutch situation, means increasing condom use, without decreasing the use of the contraceptive pill.

Acknowledgement

This study was funded by the Dutch Society for Preventive Medicine (28–2578) under the auspices of the Programme Coordination Committee for AIDS Research (PccAo, 94–052).

References

AIDS-BESTRIJDING (1995) 'Epidemiologie Aids in Nederland', *AIDS-Bestrijding*, **21**, p. 12.

Ton Vogels, Gertjan van Zessen and Emily Brugman

BRUGMAN, E., VAN ZESSEN, G. and VOGELS, T. (1997) 'Trends in sexual (risk) behavior among Turkish / Moroccan adolescents in the Netherlands; 1990–1995', *European Journal of Public Health* **4**, pp. 418–20.

BRUGMAN, E., GOEDHART, H., VAN ZESSEN, G. and VOGELS, T. (1995) *Jeugd en Seks 95*, Utrecht: SWP.

DANZ, M.J., VOGELS, T. and GRÜNDEMANN, R. (1993) *Jeugd en Seks: Kennis, Houding en Gedrag bij Turkse en Marokkaanse Jongeren in Nederland*, Leiden: TNO–Prevention and Health.

DEGGELER, E., DUPUIS, P.J.E., KLOOSTERMAN, G.J., KOOY, G.A., NOODHOFF, D., STRAVER, C.J., WITTE, B.S. and ZELDENRUST-NOORDANUS, M. (1969) *Sex in Nederland*, Utrecht: Het Spectrum.

JONES, E.F., DARROCH FOREST, J., GOLDMAN, N., HENSHAW, S., LINCOLN, R., ROSOFF, J.I., WETSOFF, C.F. and WULF, J. (1986) *Teenage Pregnancy in Industrialized Countries*, New Haven and London: Yale University Press.

KIRBY, D. (in press) *A Review of Educational Programs Designed to Reduce Sexual Risk-taking Behaviors among School-aged Youth in the United States*, to be published by the US Congress Office of Technology Assessment and the National Technical Information Service, Washington DC.

KIRBY, D., COLLINS, J., KOLBE, L., HOWARD, M., MILLER, B., RUGG, D., SHORT, L., SONENSTEIN, F. and ZABIN, L.S. (1994) 'School-based programs to reduce sexual risk behaviors: a review of effectiveness', *Public Health Reports*, **109**, pp. 339–60.

KOOY, G.A. (1976) *Jongeren en Seksualiteit: Sociologische Analyse van een Revolutionaire Evolutie*, Deventer: Van Loghum Slaterus.

KOOY, G.A., WEEDA, C.J., SCHELVIS, N. and MOORS, H.G. (1983) *Sex in Nederland*, Utrecht: Het Spectrum.

KRETZSCHMAR, M., REINKING, D., BROUWERS, H. and VAN ZESSEN, G. (1994) 'Network models. From paradigm to mathematical tool', in E.H. KAPLAN and M.L. BRANDEAU (Eds), *Modeling the AIDS-Epidemic: Planning, Policy and Prediction*, New York: Raven Press.

LAUMANN, E.O., GAGNON, J.H., MICHAEL, R.T. and MICHAELS, S. (1994) *The Social Organization of Sexuality: Sexual Practices in the United States*, Chicago: University of Chicago Press.

MELLINK, E.C. (1989) *Seksuele Vorming en Aidsvoorlichting. Een Inventariserend Onderzoek naar de Stand van Zaken met Betrekking tot Seksuele Vorming en Aidsvoorlichting in het Voortgezet Onderwijs*, Amsterdam: SCO-Kohnstamm Instituut UvA.

MELLINK, E.C. and GIJTENBEEK, J. (1995) *AIDS-voorlichting in het Voortgezet Onderwijs; een Herhalingsonderzoek 1989–1990*, Amsterdam: SCO-Kohnstamm Instituut UvA.

RADEMAKERS, J. (1990) *Eerste Kennismaking met Anticonceptie*, Delft: Eburon.

REISS, I.L. (1960) *Premarital Sexual Standards in America, A Sociological Investigation of the Relative Social and Cultural Integration of American Sexual Standards*, Glencohse, Illinois: Free Press.

SEVERIJNEN, A.J. (1993) *Chlamydia Trachomatis als Volksgezondheidprobleem. Prevalentie, Complicaties, Kosten en Screening*, Rotterdam: Erasmus Universiteit.

SPANJER, M. (1996) 'Dutch schoolchildren's drug-taking doubles', *Lancet*, **347**, 24 February, p. 534.

STICHTING SOA-BESTRIJDING (1995) *Fact Sheet SOA* (Fact Sheet STD), Utrecht: Stichting SOA-Bestrijding.

VAN DER VLIET, R.W.F. (1990) 'Van rijp tot ervaren; de seksuele ontwikkeling van Nederlandse scholieren', in T. VOGELS and R. VAN DER VLIET, *Jeugd en Seks, Gedrag en Gezondheidsrisico's bij Scholieren*, 's-Gravenhage: Sdu.

VOGELS, T. and VAN DER VLIET, R. (1990) *Jeugd en Seks, Gedrag en Gezondheidsrisico's bij Scholieren*, 's-Gravenhage: Sdu.

VOGELS, T., BRUGMAN, E. and VAN ZESSEN, G. (in press) 'Het gebruik van alcohol, marihuana en XTC door leerlingen in het voortgezet onderwijs; 1990–1995', *Tijdschrift voor Alcohol, Drugs en andere Psychotrope Stoffen*.

VOGELS, T., DANZ, M.J. and HOPMAN-ROCK, M. (1991) 'Weten, willen en doen, veilige seks bij leerlingen in het voortgezet onderwijs', *SOA-Bulletin*, **12**, pp. 5–9.

VOGELS, T., DANZ, M.J. and VAN DER VLIET, R. (1991) *Regionale Gegevens Jeugd en Seks*, Leiden: TNO–Prevention and Health.

VAN ZESSEN, G. and JUNGER, J.C. (Eds) (1994) *Analyse van Seksuele Netwerken*, Bilthoven: RIVM.

Chapter 14

Adoption and Maintenance of Safe Sex in a National Cohort of Gay Men in the Netherlands

Ernest de Vroome, Gerjo Kok, Hans Jager, Rob Tielman and Theo Sandfort

In this chapter we will consider behaviour change processes using the 'diffusion of innovations theory' as introduced by Rogers (1962, 1983). According to this theory, an innovation is any idea, technique or behaviour perceived as 'new' by the individual. The adoption process is the mental process through which an individual passes from first hearing about an innovation to final adoption. The stages Rogers distinguishes in the adoption process are, in summary, first the knowledge stage, in which the individual is thought to learn about an innovation. The second stage is called the persuasion stage, in which a person changes his or her attitudes about the innovation. The third stage is called the decision stage, in which someone decides whether he or she will adopt the innovation. The fourth stage is called the implementation or trial stage, in which the individual tries out the new behaviour or technique in practice. The fifth and final stage is the confirmation stage, in which maintenance of the innovative behaviour is at issue. Of course, not everyone will experience each or all of these stages separately, or at the same time. Some will go through the described stages rapidly (early adopters), others will wait and adopt an innovation later (secondary adopters), and some of course will never complete the described behaviour change process, and will not adopt the innovation. As more and more individuals permanently adopt the innovation, however, the innovation is thought to gradually diffuse within the social system concerned. A diffusion curve describes the cumulative percentage over time of the individuals who have adopted an innovation. According to the diffusion of innovations theory, such a curve resembles the typical S-shaped cumulative normal distribution curve. The adoption process differs from the diffusion process in that the adoption process deals with adoption of a new idea by an individual, while the diffusion process deals with the spread of new ideas in a social system.

Safe sex became a 'new' concept and behaviour in the gay social system during the 1980s. For many individual gay men safe sex became a new topic in that era, but also, at present, safe sex may become important for an individual where it was not an issue for him or her before. In this sense safe sex may be interpreted as an innovation according to the diffusion of innovations theory.

Although many public health officials and prevention workers would hope that because of the imminent danger of AIDS every individual would stop practising unsafe sex instantaneously, this will not occur in practice. The current approach acknowledges that not everyone is in the same stage of behaviour change, and diffusion of safe sex at the population level evolves only gradually. This approach may also elucidate which factors enhance or hinder the individual behaviour change process and thereby also the diffusion process at the population level.

When it became obvious in the beginning of the 1980s that AIDS would become a serious danger for gay men, AIDS educational interventions directed at gay men in the Netherlands began. By the second half of the 1980s, AIDS had established a prominent place in gay society, and as prevention efforts were still relatively new, this was an important era in AIDS prevention among gay men. In this chapter, the focus will be precisely on those important years at the end of the 1980s, when gay men in the Netherlands were primarily prompted to abstain from anal sex altogether. Only if the aim of having no anal sex at all proved too difficult to attain, was the use of especially strong or anal condoms recommended. Only from the beginning of the 1990s onwards has condom use been presented as an equally adequate option in AIDS education directed at gay men in the Netherlands (De Zwart, Sandfort and Van Kerkhof, 1998).

As recommended by the model of planned education (Kok, 1987; Kok and Sandfort, 1991), several studies were conducted in the 1980s to analyze the epidemiology of AIDS, the characteristic behaviours associated with the problem, and the psycho-social determinants of these behaviours. By determining the characteristics of the target group and by assessing the determinants of the behaviour that causes the problem, priorities in educating specific groups as well as priorities in AIDS educational topics can be established.

As part of this kind of needs assessment or elicitation research, the study discussed in this chapter commenced in 1986. We considered it important to study behaviour change and adoption processes at the individual level, as well as to analyze the causes of adoption and non-adoption. The current study was therefore given a longitudinal design, and the same participants were followed on a yearly basis from 1986 to 1989. To prevent basing policy decisions solely on findings from large towns like Amsterdam, men were recruited from all over the country. This resulted in a national cohort study of gay men living in the Netherlands. For a more detailed account of the study presented in this chapter see De Vroome (1994).

Methods

The majority of participants were self-selected male readers of a large circulation magazine for gays and lesbians living in the Netherlands. Additionally, male opinion leaders in the gay and lesbian movement were approached and asked to participate as well. To recruit these (public) opinion leaders, men who were active in the gay movement as educators, counsellors, politicians, journalists or otherwise were approached by letter, and were asked to become a participant in the present study. All data were collected using postal questionnaires under guaranteed confidentiality. Every year the same men filled out a questionnaire about their sexual behaviour (over the last six months), and about psycho-social factors possibly related to the adoption of safe sex.

There were 364 men who faithfully participated in each of the four yearly measurements from 1986 to 1989 (inclusive). There were also 717 men who participated in at least one measurement, but who cannot be analyzed in detail here, as they missed one or more of the measurements. We looked to see whether these two groups were different regarding recruitment (as opinion leader or otherwise), demographics, and (risky) sexual behaviour. The group that remained in study was somewhat higher educated (46 per cent at least higher professional training versus 35 per cent among those who missed at least one measurement). The work status of those who remained in the study was higher. Their urbanization level was also somewhat higher (25 versus 17 per cent in towns of at least 100000 (with the four major towns excluded)). Relatively more men among the remainders had ever been married (19 versus 12 per cent); and they less frequently had no sexual partners at all (3 versus 7 per cent). Finally, the remainders had somewhat more often practised exclusively insertive anal sex than those who did not remain in study (16 versus 11 per cent). There were no differences between these groups regarding such important aspects of their sexual behaviour as their number of sexual partners and the number of sexual partners with whom unprotected anal sex was practised.

The mean age of the remaining group was 36 years in 1986, and their educational and professional levels were relatively high (46 per cent higher professional training, 56 per cent white-collar workers). Of the remaining group, 79 per cent (287/364) had not taken an HIV antibody test before 1989; 19 per cent (69/364) reported having taken an HIV antibody test and were seronegative, and 2 per cent (8/364) reported being seropositive.

Relational status was assessed at every measurement. We asked whether the participant had had sex with steady and with casual partners. In the questionnaire a steady relationship was defined as lasting for at least six months with a person who is seen at least once a week and with whom there is regular sex; all other sexual partners were considered 'casual'. Instead of presenting each of the four yearly data sets separately in this respect, we combined the data to present the relational status as it applies to the entire study period, from 1986 to 1989. So a person whose relational status was casual-only in 1986 and 1987, but steady-only in 1988 and 1989 was defined as casual *and* steady if we look at the entire period.

Having had only casual sexual partners from 1986 to 1989, was reported by 19 per cent (69/364), and 73 per cent (264/364) had had sex with casual *and* steady partners. Adopting safe sex is considered a prerequisite for both of these groups, preferably with both their casual and their steady partners, if present. Except in the 1989 measurement, however, the questionnaire used in this study made no distinction between sexual behaviour with casual and with steady partners. At that time, the notion of 'negotiated safe sex' (Kippax *et al.*, 1993) had yet to appear on the research agenda, and safe sex with a steady and with casual partners were thought to be basically similar. In this study the adoption of safe sex with casual and steady partners will therefore be examined concurrently. The groups casual-only and casual *and* steady were combined (giving 333 participants), and relationship status was further used as a predictor variable.

A small group of 8 per cent (29/364) reported having had sex with one steady partner from 1986 to 1989. Although it is not certain whether this was always the same steady partner, relatively few partners will have been involved. Even fewer men (1 per cent, 2/364) had had no sexual partners at all. Behaviour changes in these two groups do not need to be closely examined.

Safe sex is defined here as practising no anal sex, or always using a condom during anal sex, with all partners. As we also included questions about lifetime sexual behaviour, it was possible to determine whether safe and unsafe sex had been practised in someone's entire life, that is, up to the first measurement in 1986.

As the present data are longitudinal, it is possible to determine carefully for every participant and at every point in time (that is before 1986, and at the 1986, 1987, 1988 and 1989 measurements) which of the following situations applied. First, did he have safe sex at that time and from then onwards; second, did he have safe sex at that time but practised unsafe sex later; or third, did he have unsafe sex at that time.

Related to adopting safe sex, we then defined four groups. Early Adopters are those who adopted safe sex as early as in or before 1986, and practised safe sex from then onwards. Secondary Adopters also permanently adopted safe sex; but only in or after 1987. Temporarily Safe are those who practised safe sex on one or more measurements, but had unsafe sex on one or more measurements later in time. This group can be conceptualized as the group exhibiting 'relapse' into unsafe sex, but it can also less negatively be regarded as the group representing the implementation or trial stage of the adoption process (Rogers, 1962, 1983). Continued Unsafe are considered the men who had had unprotected anal sex in each of the four waves from 1986 to 1989.

To ensure that we were really studying the *adoption* of safe sex, participants who *never* had had unprotected anal sex were excluded from this classification. Among these men, refraining from anal sex is most likely not related to the risk of HIV. Adopting safe sex should also not be confounded with stopping having sex entirely. The men who at the final measurement reported having had no sexual partners at all were therefore excluded from this classification as well.

The next question concerns whether men in these four different adoption categories differ in various psycho-social characteristics, and whether it is possible to devise a typology of each of these groups. Analyzing the determinants of adoption and non-adoption provides information about the factors that may further (or hinder) the adoption process.

To examine these psycho-social characteristics, each of the four groups was compared to the other three groups taken together. Differences were initially analyzed with bivariate t-tests, and significant results (with alpha set at 5 per cent) were further analyzed using multivariate logistic regression analyses. This technique enabled us to identify the most important and unconfounded characteristics of the various adoption categories.

The psycho-social characteristics that were studied included some social-demographic features such as age and the position of the participant in the gay subculture (for example whether he could be considered an opinion leader). Next, some aspects of his gay sexual life-style were considered (for example the proportion of gay friends, the proportion of 'anonymous' sexual partners, and at which (public) meeting places new sexual partners were met). We also asked whether he had participated in AIDS educational activities, which sources of AIDS information he had used, and what his attitudes towards AIDS education were. We also measured the participants' AIDS coping styles (based on the Ways of Coping Checklist, Folkman and Lazarus, 1980; Schreurs *et al.*, 1988), and their 'AIDS health locus of control' (based on Wallston, Wallston and Devellis, 1978). Other psycho-social factors that were measured included their knowledge regarding AIDS prevention (Fisher and Fisher, 1992), their perception of the risk of various sexual techniques (Weinstein and Nicolich, 1993), and their perceived condom or product efficacy (Ross, 1990). High product efficacy in this case means that someone has faith in condoms and their protective abilities. We also looked at the emotional value the men attached to anal sex (sometimes called the reinforcement value level of high-risk practices, Kelly, St. Lawrence and Brasfield, 1991), and their subjective acceptability of safe sex and condom use (Ross, 1990). Some questions dealt with misinterpreting the safe sex rules, sometimes resulting in inadequate personal prevention strategies (De Wit *et al.*, 1994). Further measures included the perceived social norms of the men (Fishbein *et al.*, 1992), whether there were potential cues-to-action (Janz and Becker, 1984), their level of self-efficacy (Bandura, 1989), perceived behavioural control (Ajzen and Madden, 1986) or behavioural skills (Fisher and Fisher, 1992). A major element of most models concerned with behaviour change, the intention or motivation to have safe sex, was also asked for. Finally some questions about recreational drug use were posed (Ostrow, 1994).

Though these factors derive from various theories about preventive behaviour and behaviour change, they were studied simultaneously, and were roughly ordered according to their proximity to the sexual act. For instance coping with AIDS was thought to be a distal or 'off-line' cognition, while recreational drug use during sex was thought to have a more direct impact on sexual behaviour.

Results

Figure 14.1 shows a large difference between lifetime sexual behaviours, that is before 1986, and behaviours in the six months just preceding the 1986 measurement. Only a few gay men had no experience of unprotected anal sex at all, but, probably for reasons unrelated to AIDS, anal sex had not become part of the regular sexual behaviour of a substantial group of gay men. If successive waves from 1986 up to and including 1989 are compared, this serial cross-sectional approach shows there was no significant change in the percentage that had unprotected anal sex in the casual *and* steady group. In the casual-only group, however, there was a significant decrease in unprotected anal sex (multivariate repeated-measures analysis with dummy-variables).

The frequencies of 'unsafe', 'temporarily safe', and 'safe from here on' (that is adopting safe sex) at each of the measurements are depicted in Figure 14.2. Using this longitudinal approach, which takes each participant's behavioural pattern from 1986 to 1989 into account, we can see that there was a significant diffusion of safe sex, not only in the casual-only group, but in the casual and steady group too. In the present study, S-shaped diffusion curves were fitted to the empirical data using logistic regression-analysis. This procedure models the natural logarithm of the ratio between the number of persons who adopt safe sex versus the number who do not, as a function of time. The resulting diffusion curves, shown separately for the groups with casual *and* steady partners and casual partners *only*, are also depicted in Figure 14.2 and

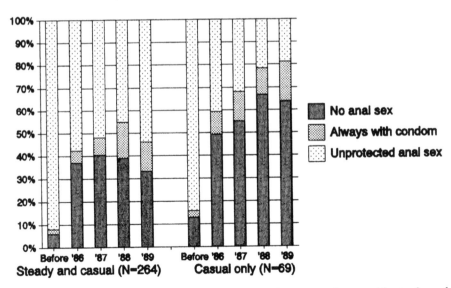

Figure 14.1 Sexual behaviour among 333 Dutch homosexual men with steady and casual partners in the years 1986–1989 (serial cross-sectional approach).

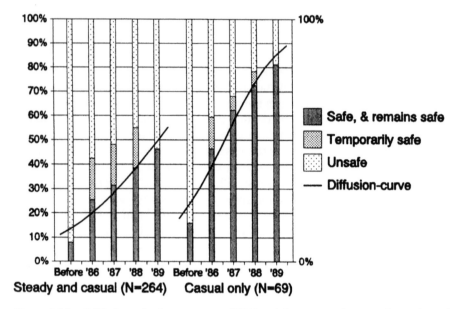

Figure 14.2 *Diffusion of safer sex among 333 Dutch homosexual men with steady and casual partners in the years 1986–1990 (longitudinal approach).*

illustrate clearly that especially among the casual-only group, safe sex rapidly diffused from 1986 to 1989.

The adoption categories that we discerned were roughly equal in size. In the studied group, 22 per cent (65/292) had adopted safe sex permanently by the time of the first measurement in 1986, and can be called Early Adopters. Another 25 per cent (72/292) had also adopted safe sex, but only in or after 1987 (Secondary Adopters). Safe at one measurement but unsafe at a later time were 28 per cent (82/292) (Temporarily Safe). Finally, unsafe at every measurement were 25 per cent (73/292) (Continued Unsafe). Forty-one participants were excluded from this classification because they had had no unprotected anal sex ever in their lives (32 men), or because they had stopped having sexual partners entirely by 1989 (9 men).

Factors that did not Differentiate between the Adopter Categories

The groups were similar regarding the environment where they met their sexual partners (for example bars, backrooms, outside cruising places). There were also no differences concerning the source from which they received their AIDS information (for example leaflets, general radio and television, or gay-specific media). There was, however, an interesting difference regarding *AIDS Info*, a widespread AIDS educational monthly newsletter: those who were unsafe at every measurement had read *AIDS Info* significantly less often than the other three groups.

Also no differences could be established regarding knowledge about HIV transmission and prevention. This was measured on a nine-item true/false scale ($\alpha = 0.62$) via statements such as: 'Anal sex carries more risk than oral sex.'

Furthermore, knowing HIV seropositive people or people with AIDS also made no distinction between the groups. The eight men who knew they were seropositive were also equally divided among the adoption categories (three seropositive men were unsafe in the six months preceding every measurement from 1986 to 1989). The factors related to being seropositive or knowing seropositive people apparently did not serve as cues-to-action as suggested by the Health Belief Model (Janz and Becker, 1984).

Early Adopters

The group of Early Adopters was somewhat older (mean = 39 years) compared to the other men in this study (mean = 35 years), and their income was somewhat higher. There were more opinion leaders among the Early Adopters (51 versus 32 per cent in the other groups), and the percentage of gay friends they had was relatively high (mean = 0.60 per cent versus mean = 49 per cent in the other groups). These characteristics of Early Adopters are in line with predictions from diffusion of innovations theory. According to Rogers (1962, 1983), Early Adopters usually have higher social status than persons who adopt an innovative idea later on or who do not adopt it at all. Early Adopters also more often had casual partners *only* (31 versus 16 per cent) rather than both casual *and* steady partners. This suggests that having a steady partner made the adoption of safe sex less likely.

Early Adopters had relatively more faith in the usefulness or effectiveness of AIDS education, compared to the other groups. A typical item of the scale which measured this construct (eight items, $\alpha = 0.64$) was: 'There should certainly be more AIDS educational meetings.' Early Adopters scored relatively high on the AIDS coping scale concerned with active problem solving (four items, $\alpha = 0.78$, for example 'I actively avoid risk during sexual intercourse'). They also had a higher 'AIDS internal health locus of control' (scale of five items, $\alpha = 0.70$, for example 'I think thoroughly about how I might avoid infection').

Early Adopters attributed more risk to having *protected* anal sex, which indicates that their perceived condom or product efficacy was *lower*. Early Adopters also attached relatively less emotional value to anal sex. Their perceived social norm regarding safe sex was somewhat higher than in the other groups. Being tested for HIV antibodies did not function as a cue-to-action for the early adoption of safe sex. Only 15 per cent of the Early Adopters had taken an HIV antibody test by 1989, compared to 28 per cent in the other groups. Early Adopters apparently assumed that by adopting safe sex early, they successfully avoided the risk of infection, making an HIV antibody test unnecessary.

Multivariate analysis revealed that the most important and unconfounded characteristics of Early Adopters were the following. First, they were somewhat older than the other groups. Second, they had relatively many gay social friends. Third, they more often had casual partners only instead of a steady partner as well. Fourth, they usually coped with AIDS in an active problem solving way. Fifth, they often had an internal AIDS health locus of control. Sixth, their perceived condom or product efficacy was relatively low. In summary, Early Adopters had a somewhat higher social-economic status, were aware of the AIDS threat, and were actively occupied with AIDS prevention. Additionally, among those who had casual partners only, early adoption appeared easier than when safe sex had to be introduced in an existing steady relationship as well.

Secondary Adopters

We will now examine the characteristics of the Secondary Adopters, defined here as the men who permanently adopted safe sex with all their sexual partners in or after 1987. First, as in the group who adopted safe sex relatively early, Secondary Adopters more often had casual partners only (31 versus 15 per cent). Furthermore, the coping style 'searching for social support' was more prevalent in the group of Secondary Adopters. An example of a typical item in this scale (seven items, $\alpha = 0.79$) is 'I ask other men how they deal with AIDS.' Similar to Early Adopters, Secondary Adopters also scored relatively high on the AIDS coping scale 'active problem solving'. Finally, Secondary Adopters typically had the strongest intention or motivation to make their behaviour entirely free of the risk of AIDS. Multivariate analysis yielded the same results although the factor 'searching for social support' did not reach significance. Secondary Adopters therefore resemble Early Adopters in some respects, but have a less prominent place in the gay subculture. Intention or motivation is apparently more important for the adoption of safe sex later on in the epidemic, than it is for early adoption.

Temporarily Safe

The group that had safe sex during the six months preceding one or more of the measurements, but later had unsafe sex again, was relatively young (mean = 34 versus 37 years in the other groups). In contrast to the Early or Secondary Adopters, many more men among the Temporarily Safe had had both casual and steady partners. This indicates once more that a steady partner is a barrier for the permanent adoption of safe sex with all partners. The men categorized as Temporarily Safe relatively often acknowledged that a steady partner may pose a risk for HIV transmission. This risk-acknowledgement may be the reason why they tried to adopt safe sex, and may simultaneously be the reason why adoption was not permanent. Acknowledging that one has taken a risk with a specific steady partner in the past, may induce the desire to only have safe sex in the future. This may also prove difficult, however, if the idea is strong that 'one cannot wipe out the risks of the past anyway'. It also appears that the Temporarily Safe do not often approach AIDS with an 'active problem solving' coping style, and this may be another reason for their not yet being successful in permanently adopting safe sex. Finally, the perceived social norm to practise safe sex is also relatively low among the Temporarily Safe, which may also contribute to their relative unsuccessfulness in permanently adopting safe sex.

Based on a multivariate analysis the main typology of the group, Temporarily Safe can be summarized as follows. First, they acknowledge that HIV transmission may also occur through a steady partner, but, second, they are less actively involved in coping with AIDS. Finally, they more often also have a steady partner apart from casual partners, which makes the adoption of safe sex with all partners apparently more difficult.

Continued Unsafe

Regarding social-demographic statistics, it appeared that the percentage of men who had been married among the Continued Unsafe was relatively high. They also more often had both (male) casual and steady partners, and in 1986 they had in fact more sexual partners in total than any other group (mean = 11 versus 7 among the other men). The more partners one has, the more difficult it apparently is to introduce safe sex among all one's partners, or to end (unsafe) relationships entirely.

Another characteristic of the Continued Unsafe was a lower score on the scale measuring whether homosexuality is an integral part of one's identity (five items, $\alpha = 0.66$, for example 'My being gay is essential to me').

In comparison to the Early Adopters particularly, the Continued Unsafe scored low on the scale measuring 'faith in AIDS education'. So in agreement with their own behaviour, there are only a few enthusiastic protagonists of AIDS prevention among the Continued Unsafe.

Members of this group also scored lower on the AIDS coping styles 'searching for social support' and 'active problem solving', and on the scale measuring an internal AIDS health locus of control.

The Continued Unsafe furthermore perceived the risk of practising anal sex with a condom to be relatively low, which may be understood as an optimistic bias regarding the risk of contracting AIDS in general as they did not habitually use condoms themselves.

This group also scored higher than any other group on the emotional value they attached to anal sex. They also often agreed with the statement that anal sex without a condom is much more exciting, indicating low condom-acceptability and high emotional condom-dislike.

They also more often expressed the misconception that having sex with a steady partner carries no risk of HIV transmission. Next, their intention or motivation to have safe sex as well as their degree of self-efficacy were lower, and the final reason for their continued practice of unsafe sex may be associated with recreational drug use. Among the Continued Unsafe alcohol consumption was somewhat higher (mean = 21 glasses per week) than in the other groups (mean = 16); and 41 per cent had used 'poppers' at least once in the preceding six months, while in the other groups only 27 per cent reported doing so.

Multivariate analysis resulted in the following typology of the Continued Unsafe. First, relatively many have been married. Second, they relatively often have a steady partner besides casual partners. Third, their internal AIDS health locus of control is relatively low. Fourth, their perceived risk of anal sex with a condom is relatively low. Fifth, anal sex is emotionally important to them. Sixth, they often assume that a steady partner is safe regarding HIV transmission. Seventh, they have less self-efficacy regarding practising safe sex. The following picture emerges. Those who continue to practise unsafe sex seem to prefer a gay life-style that includes many gay partners, using recreational drugs, and practising unprotected anal sex. As among the Continued Unsafe, the percentage of men who have been married is relatively high, their active gay life-style may in some cases be a reaction to a previous married state and possibly the associated lack of homosexual experiences. Furthermore, as the Continued Unsafe scored relatively low on a scale measuring gay identity, their focus appears more on *homosexual behaviour* than on *gay identity*. They are apparently more concerned about continuing their sexual life-style despite the threat of AIDS, than they are concerned about AIDS prevention. In fact, they do not sympathize very much with AIDS education, and seem to underestimate the risk of HIV transmission.

Conclusions

One of the generalizations Rogers (1962, 1983) formulated was that Early Adopters usually have a higher social status than later adopters, and Early Adopters are often found among opinion leaders, who in that way may start a diffusion process. This generalization was confirmed regarding the diffusion of safe sex in the studied population. This implies that as with other diffusion processes, AIDS education should gradually pay more attention to those with a relatively lower social-economic status, and who have a less prominent place in the established gay subculture. As the latter group is also a hard-to-reach target group, prevention efforts should be increasingly intense, more small-scale, more outreach based, and in some cases should even consist of face-to-face counselling.

Very evident is that adopting safe sex with a steady partner creates additional problems. In the casual-only group, the diffusion of safe sex was most rapid. Nevertheless, among those having a steady as well as casual partners, safe sex with *all* partners would certainly be preferable (Ekstrand *et al.*, 1993). Some may also want to avoid having to adopt safe sex with their steady partner through abandoning unsafe sex with casual partners. The strategy of having no casual partners at all, however, does not seem to be realistic. If we look at the entire period of four years, only 8 per cent (29/364) had had no casual partners while being involved in a steady relationship. Related to this, it is cause for concern that those who continued to practise unsafe sex, relatively often were of the opinion that sex with a steady partner carries no risk. Education should therefore be more explicit in dealing with the risk of HIV transmission within steady relationships.

Furthermore, those who continued to have unsafe sex were occasionally found to have their doubts about AIDS education. Specifically, the group 'Continued Unsafe' should be presented with AIDS educational activities that are as credible and trustworthy as possible. To help those who already adopted safe sex in maintaining this behaviour, and for those who are already in the trial stage of adopting safe sex, a monthly newsletter like *AIDS Info* seems to be an efficient means to disseminate AIDS education. Such a newsletter should not restrict itself to giving information, but should also aim at placing or maintaining safe sex on the personal and social agenda, and increasing the intention or motivation to maintain practising safe sex. Just giving information would not suffice, as knowledge was not found to be related to adopting safe sex. Although information has a prominent place in the Information Motivation Behavioural skills model (Fisher and Fisher, 1992), receiving information is particularly important in the very early stages of behaviour change. Since the level of information is high already among gay men living in the Netherlands, this factor will not be decisive in the further adoption of safe sex. In some target groups depending on geography, age and social class, however, providing basic information naturally remains essential.

Paying attention to positive coping styles ('active problem solving' and 'seeking social support'), and to the development of an internal AIDS health locus of control, seems to support early as well as secondary adoption of safe sex. To increase this kind of coping with AIDS, thinking explicitly about the threat of AIDS should be encouraged, hopefully resulting in more explicit decision making about how to prevent HIV transmission personally.

The perceived condom or product efficacy was found to be *lower* among the *Early* Adopters of safe sex. As can also be seen in Figure 14.1, Early Adopters in the Netherlands primarily became safe as a result of abstaining from anal sex and not as a result of consistent condom use. Other studies, however, found that having less trust in the protective quality of condoms predicted decreased condom use, without resulting in abstaining from anal sex (Ross, 1990). Lower perceived product efficacy may thus result in having no anal sex any more (this study), or in having unprotected anal sex (Ross, 1990). These potentially contrasting effects of lower perceived product efficacy imply that public information about the safety (or conversely, the failure rate) of condoms should be given with care.

Those who continued to have unsafe sex attached a higher emotional value to anal sex. As this attachment was very stable from 1986 to 1989 (data not shown), it appears more appropriate to promote condom use among those who emotionally value anal sex highly, than to try to change this preference and thus promote abstaining from anal sex. More problematic was the finding that condom acceptability among the Continued Unsafe was relatively low. The importance of condom acceptability has also been stressed by Ross (1990), who found that attitudes indicative of condom acceptability were an important predictor of increased condom use. Unlike the emotional value attached to anal sex, however, condom acceptability did change (increased) in our group from 1986 to 1989 (data not shown). This means that as the diffusion of safe sex proceeds, there is potentially more to gain in increasing condom acceptability and thus promoting condom use than there is to gain in decreasing the emotional value of anal sex and thus promoting abstinence.

Social norms were specifically supportive of safe sex among the Early Adopters, although this was not confirmed in multivariate analysis. Attitudes towards condoms expressing their product efficacy and their perceived acceptability were somewhat more related to safe sex. Whether attitudes towards condoms and condom use, or subjective social norms should underpin educational activities is, however, highly dependent on the specific target group (Fishbein *et al.*, 1992; Ross and McLaws, 1992). Educational interventions should therefore always be preceded by elicitation research, to determine the relative importance of different psycho-social factors related to safe sex in the target group at issue (Fisher and Fisher, 1992).

The conceptually related factors self-efficacy (Bandura, 1989), perceived behavioural control (Ajzen and Madden, 1986), and behavioural skills (Fisher and Fisher, 1992) were found to be important in adopting safe sex. Those who continued to practise unsafe sex scored relatively low in this respect. Moreover, this confirms the theoretical notion that self-efficacy becomes especially important in later stages of the adoption and thereby the diffusion process (O'Reilly and Higgins, 1991; De Vries *et al.*, 1995). Increasing self-efficacy is an important educational goal once basic information is provided, and positive attitudes and social norms are present.

Related to this, a contrast between early and later adopters should be noted. As discussed, for those who attached less emotional value to anal sex, it was relatively easy to adopt safe sex early (often by abstaining from anal sex). For Secondary Adopters though, the adoption of safe sex (often by always using a condom) seems to be less easy, and requires a stronger intention or a higher motivational level. As the diffusion of safe sex evolves, AIDS educators should therefore be ready to expect that it will become increasingly difficult to persuade those who continue to have unsafe sex to adopt safe sex. In the later stages of the diffusion process, more attention should therefore be devoted to the difficult task of increasing the level of self-efficacy as well as the motivational level of the target audience.

There have been extensive discussions in the AIDS literature about the existence and character (causal or spurious) of the relation between recreational drug use (specifically 'poppers') and unsafe sex among gay men (Ostrow, 1994). The results found in this study indicate, however, that it appears appropriate to include in AIDS educational material a discussion of the effects recreational drugs may have when having sex, and that using these substances may inadvertently result in unsafe sex.

To conclude, this study showed that AIDS prevention involves both a behaviour change process consisting of several stages at the individual level, and a diffusion process in the gay subculture. Certain social psychological elements appear more important at some stages of change than they are at other stages. As the diffusion process is time-dependent upon the individual adoption process, the weights of certain elements in AIDS education should also vary within the diffusion process. The contents of intervention messages should be adjusted to match the stages of change characteristic of most of the group members. For example, knowledge about the risk of certain sexual techniques appears more important in the earliest stage of the change process and therefore also early in the diffusion process. Self-efficacy, on the other hand, appears to become more important at the implementation or trial stage of adoption, and should therefore also receive increasing attention as the diffusion process evolves.

References

AJZEN, I. and MADDEN, T.J. (1986) 'Prediction of goal-directed behaviour: attitudes, intentions, and perceived behavioural control', *Journal of Experimental Social Psychology*, **22**, pp. 453–74.

BANDURA, A. (1989) 'Perceived self-efficacy in the exercise of control over AIDS-infection', in V.M. MAYS, G.W. ALBEE and S.F. SCHNEIDER (Eds), *Primary Prevention of AIDS*, Newbury Park, CA: Sage Publications.

EKSTRAND, M., STALL, R., KEGELES, S., HAYS, R., DeMAYO, M. and COATES, T. (1993) 'Safer sex among gay men: what is the ultimate goal?', *AIDS*, **7**, pp. 281–2.

FISHBEIN, M., CHAN, D.K.S., O'REILLY, K., SCHNELL, D., WOOD, R., BEEKER, C. and COHN, D. (1992) 'Attitudinal and normative factors as determinants of gay men's intentions to perform AIDS-related sexual behaviours: a multisite analysis', *Journal of Applied Social Psychology*, **22**, pp. 999–1011.

FISHER, J.D. and FISHER, W.A. (1992) 'Changing AIDS-risk behaviour', *Psychological Bulletin*, **111**, pp. 455–74.

FOLKMAN, S. and LAZARUS, R.S. (1980) 'An analysis of coping in a middle-aged community sample', *Journal of Health and Social Behaviour*, **21**, pp. 219–39.

JANZ, N.K. and BECKER, M.H. (1984) 'The health belief model: a decade later', *Health Education Quarterly*, **11**, pp. 1–47.

KELLY, J.A., ST. LAWRENCE, J.S. and BRASFIELD, T.L. (1991) 'Predictors of vulnerability to AIDS risk behaviour relapse', *Journal of Consulting and Clinical Psychology*, **59**, pp. 163–6.

KIPPAX, S., CRAWFORD, J., DAVIS, M., RODDEN, P. and DOWSETT, G. (1993) 'Sustaining safer sex: a longitudinal study of a sample of homosexual men', *AIDS*, **7**, pp. 257–63.

KOK, G.J. (1987) 'Gezondheidsvoorlichting en -Opvoeding, GVO', in V. DAMOISEAUX, F.M. GERARDS, G.J. KOK and F. NIJHUIS (Eds), *Gezondheidsvoorlichting en -Opvoeding. Van Analyse tot Effecten*, Assen/Maastricht: Van Gorcum.

KOK, G.J. and SANDFORT, T.G.M. (1991) 'AIDS-preventie, voorlichting en gedragsverandering', *Nederlands Tijdschrift voor de Psychologie*, **46**, pp. 238–51.

O'REILLY, K.R. and HIGGINS, D. (1991) 'AIDS community demonstration projects for HIV prevention among hard-to-reach groups', *Public Health Reports*, **106**, pp. 714–20.

OSTROW, D.G. (1994) 'Substance abuse and HIV infection', *Psychiatric Clinics of North America*, **17**, pp. 69–89.

ROGERS, E.M. (1962) *Diffusion of Innovations*, New York: Free Press.

ROGERS, E.M. (1983) *Diffusion of Innovations*, 3rd ed, New York: Free Press.

ROSS, M.W. (1990) 'Psychological determinants of increased condom use and safer sex in homosexual men: a longitudinal study', *International Journal of STD and AIDS*, **1**, pp. 98–101.

ROSS, M.W. and McLAWS, M.L. (1992) 'Subjective norms about condoms are better predictors of use and intention to use than attitudes', *Health Education Research*, **7**, pp. 335–9.

SCHREURS, P.J.G., VAN DE WILLIGE, G., TELLEGEN, B. and BROSSCHOT, J. (1988) *De Utrechtse Copinglijst*, Lisse: Swets & Zeitlinger.

DE VRIES, H., MUDDE, A., WILLEMSEN, M. and DIJKSTRA, A. (1995) 'Differences between precontemplators, contemplators, preparators and actors on attitudes, social influences, self-efficacy: the ø-hypotheses', presentation at the First Dutch Conference on Psychology and Health, Kerkrade, the Netherlands, November.

DE VROOME, E.M.M. (1994) *AIDS-voorlichting onder Homoseksuele Mannen: Diffusie van Veilig Vrijen in Nederland (1986–1989)*, Doctoral Thesis, Amsterdam: Thesis Publishers.

WALLSTON, K.A., WALLSTON, B.S. and DEVELLIS, R. (1978) 'Development of the multidimensional health locus of control (MHLC) scales', *Health*

Education Monographs, **6**, pp. 160–9.

WEINSTEIN, N.D. and NICOLICH, M. (1993) 'Correct and incorrect interpretations of correlations between risk perceptions and risk behaviours', *Health Psychology*, **12**, pp. 235–45.

DE WIT, J.B.F., TEUNIS, N., VAN GRIENSVEN, G.J.P. and SANDFORT, TH.G.M. (1994) 'Behavioural risk reduction strategies to prevent HIV infection among homosexual men: a grounded theory approach', *AIDS Education and Prevention*, **6**, pp. 493–505.

DE ZWART, O., SANDFORT, TH.G.M. and VAN KERKHOF, M.P.N. (1998) 'The message on anal sex: double Dutch, or a sensible policy?', in TH.G.M. SANDFORT (Ed.), *Pragmatism and Consensus, HIV/AIDS Policy in the Netherlands*, London: UCL Press.

Notes on Contributors

Erik van Ameijden is an infectious diseases epidemiologist at the Municipal Health Service in Amsterdam, leading several projects (for example research on AIDS, STD and tuberculosis). He completed his PhD thesis on the evaluation of AIDS prevention measures for drug users in Amsterdam (1994). Since 1996 he is projectleader of the Amsterdam Cohort Studies among drug users.

Arnold Bakker is a social psychologist who finished his PhD on *Attitudes towards safe sex* in 1995 at the University of Groningen. He is currently employed as a postdoctoral researcher at the Psychology Department of Utrecht University where he studies work-related stress and burn-out.

Cor Blom studied sociology at Erasmus University of Rotterdam. He worked as a staff member on HIV prevention policy for gay men at the SAD-Schorer Foundation, where the focus of his work was on intervention development, applying theories and research results to practice, and intervention implementation issues. He is currently employed at the AIDS Fund (Stichting AIDS Fonds) as staff member for policy and prevention.

Frans van den Boom is Director of Research, Development and Planning at the Netherlands Red Cross. From 1987 until 1992 he coordinated AIDS research at the Netherlands Institute of Mental Health (NcGv). He was a member of the social science advisory board to the Programme Coordination Committee on AIDS Research (PccAo) and participated in the task force on care of the National Committee on AIDS Control (NCAB). Currently he is a member of the Dutch committee on AIDS policy and of the international board of 'AIDS-Impact'. In the field of AIDS he has published on scenario analysis, long-term planning, mental health problems and care, grief, euthanasia, suicide, and volunteer care.

Emily Brugman studied social psychology at the University of Amsterdam. Since 1994 she has worked at TNO – Prevention and Health in Leiden, where she participated in the 1995 study on sexuality among young people in the Netherlands. Currently she takes part in the national Child Health Monitoring System, in which varying aspects of health of children and adolescents – such as weight loss behaviour, nutritional habits, psycho-social problems and food allergies – are yearly assessed.

Bram Buunk is professor of psychology at the University of Groningen. His main research interests are social comparison processes, close relationships and health-related behaviour.

Regina van den Eijnden has written a dissertation about *False Consensus and HIV-Risk Behaviour* at the University of Groningen. She is currently working at the National Institute for Health Promotion and Illness Prevention (NIGZ), Woerden.

Anton Dijker works as a social psychologist at the Department of Health Education of Maastricht University. His research focuses on the social-psychological determinants of stigmatization of chronically ill people and people with a handicap. He also studies theoretical problems in explaining behaviour and methodological aspects of evaluation research.

Ron de Graaf works as a researcher for the Netherlands Institute of Mental Health and Addiction conducted several research projects into heterosexual and homosexual sex work at the Netherlands Institute of Social Sexological Research (NISSO) and into sexual and occupational risks of HIV infection among expatriates working in AIDS-endemic areas.

Anneke van den Hoek is a medical doctor and epidemiologist. In 1985, she initiated the cohort study among drug users in Amsterdam and remained project leader until 1995. In 1990, she received her PhD for a thesis entitled *The Epidemiology of HIV Infection among Drug Users in Amsterdam*. She is head of the Department of STD, HIV/AIDS Surveillance at the Amsterdam Municipal Health Service.

Harm Hospers studied psychology at the University of Groningen. He currently teaches psychology at the University of Maastricht. His research focuses on primary prevention of HIV infection among gay men.

Hans Jager is senior researcher at the Department for Public Health Forecasting at the National Institute of Public Health and Environment (RIVM). His current research interests are in scenario analysis applied to public health and health care (cost-effectiveness analysis of medical interventions). He coordinates the European Community's Concerted Action on Multinational AIDS Scenarios.

Marty PN van Kerkhof is researcher and publicist. His main research focused on the meaning of anal sex for gay men, published in *Viewed from Behind. Anal Sex in the AIDS Era*. He has worked at the Departments of Gay and

Lesbian Studies of both Utrecht University and the Catholic University Nijmegen. He was one of the editors of *Lust for Life*, a bimonthly magazine about HIV and gay men.

Gerjo Kok is currently Dean of the faculty of Psychology (Maastricht University). Before that he was professor for health education. Since 1992 he has occupied an endowed chair for AIDS Prevention and Health Education. His research is focused on the application of behavioural science theories to health education and promotion.

Lilian Kolker works at the Dutch Foundation for STD Control and has been coordinator of the mass media campaigns on AIDS and STDs since 1990. She is responsible for long-term policy formulation on safer sex campaigns and for the supervision and control of day-to-day campaign management.

Hans Moerkerk is International AIDS Adviser to the Ministry of Health, Welfare and Sport and AIDS Coordinator of the Ministry of Foreign Affairs (Directorate-General for International Co-operation) in the Netherlands. As Director of the Health Education Centre in Amsterdam, he was one of the initiators of the Netherlands AIDS policy in 1983. Between 1987 and 1990, he acted as Executive Secretary of the Dutch National Commission on AIDS Control (NCAB). Between May 1993 and December 1995, he was Chair of the Management Committee of the Global Programme on AIDS of the World Health Organization.

Theo Sandfort is a social psychologist, is director of the Department of Gay and Lesbian Studies (Utrecht University) and a research director at the Netherlands Institute for Social Sexological Research (NISSO, Utrecht). His research focuses on determinants of HIV-preventive behaviour in gay men as well as in the general population. He is also involved in studies monitoring behavioural changes and assessing the impact of small and large scale interventions aimed at promoting safer sex behaviour. In addition to HIV/AIDS-related issues he also studies aspects of gay and lesbian lives, including coming out processes, life styles, relationships and discrimination. He has been a member of the Prevention and Education Section of the Dutch National Committee on AIDS Control (NCAB). He has recently co-edited *Sexual Behaviour and HIV/AIDS in Europe: Comparisons of National Surveys* (UCL Press).

Paul Schnabel is professor of mental health and public health at Utrecht University. From 1987 until 1992 he was a member of the Programme Coordination Committee on AIDS Research (PccAo). In 1992 he was co-chair of the VIIth International Conference on AIDS. He has published widely on AIDS, public health, sexology, mental health, social psychiatry and psychotherapy.

Frans Siero is assistant professor of psychology at the University of Groningen. His main research interests include persuasion and multivariate statistics.

Loes Singels has a masters degree in cultural anthropology. She is coordinator of the Migrants AIDS Prevention Project at the National Institute for Health Promotion and Disease Prevention (NIGZ) in Woerden.

Rob Tielman is a sociologist and received his PhD for a study of the gay and lesbian movement in the Netherlands. He has conducted research on homosexuality, AIDS and education. He was a member of the National Committee on AIDS Control (NCAB) and the Programme Coordination Committee on AIDS Research (PccAo). He is currently a professor of Humanist Studies.

Ine Vanwesenbeeck is a clinical and social psychologist and works as an assistant professor in the Department of Women's Studies at Tilburg University and as a programme coordinator in the area of sexuality, gender and emancipation at the Netherlands Institute of Social Sexological Research (NISSO). She has conducted several research projects into sex work at NISSO and into sexual conduct of young adults at the Netherlands Institute of Mental Health (NcGv).

Janherman Veenker represented the gay and lesbian community in the National Committee on Aids Control (NCAB). Since the work of this committee was taken over by the Aids Fund (Stichting AIDS Fonds) he has been a board member of this foundation. Veenker has been active in the gay and lesbian movement since 1968. Between 1975 and 1980 he was general secretary of the NVIH COC, the major Dutch organization for gays and lesbians. He studied organizational psychology and works as a consultant for cities in the area around Amsterdam on policies regarding social security and employment.

Ton Vogels studied developmental psychology at the Catholic University Nijmegen. He is senior researcher at TNO – Prevention and Health, focusing mainly on health and health behaviour of young people aged 11 to 25. Prior to this, he was project manager of both the 1990 and 1995 study on sexuality among young people in the Netherlands. Other studies concerned school drop-out, psycho-social problems in adolescence, the use of achievement-enhancing drugs among young body-builders and the quality of life of chronically ill children.

Ernest de Vroome started his involvement in social scientific AIDS research in 1984, specializing in methodology and statistics. He has co-authored many scientific publications on the epidemiology of AIDS, psychoneuroimmunologic aspects of AIDS, and on AIDS prevention and education both among gay men and among the general population. He is employed at the Department of Gay and Lesbian Studies of Utrecht University.

Gertjan van Zessen is a psychologist and sexologist and has worked at Utrecht University, the Netherlands Institute of Social Sexological Research (NISSO, Utrecht), and the Netherlands Institute of Mental Health and Addiction. He has been involved in AIDS research since 1984. Past research includes three population studies on sexual behaviour and risks of HIV infection among adults and teenagers, and quantitative and qualitative studies of sex workers and their clients, homosexual men, and young adults with multiple heterosexual and bisexual contacts.

Onno de Zwart studied history at Erasmus University in Rotterdam and at the University of Essex (UK). As a researcher at the Department of Gay and Lesbian Studies of Utrecht University, he has researched the meanings of anal sex for gay men and evaluated the Dutch prevention policy directed at men who have sex with men. He currently works as HIV Policy Coordinator at the Rotterdam Municipal Health Service.

Index